M000308445

Thinking Through Dementia

Julian C. Hughes

Consultant in Old Age Psychiatry,
Northumbria Healthcare NHS Foundation Trust, and
Honorary Professor of Philosophy of Ageing,
Institute for Ageing and Health,
Newcastle University, UK

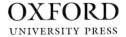

OXFORD
UNIVERSITY PRESS

OXFORD

UNIVERSITY PRESS

Great Clarendon Street, Oxford OX2 6DP

Oxford University Press is a department of the University of Oxford.
It furthers the University's objective of excellence in research, scholarship,
and education by publishing worldwide in
Oxford New York

Athens Auckland Bangkok Bogotá Buenos Aires Cape-Town
Chennai Dar-es-Salaam Delhi Florence Hong-Kong Istanbul Karachi
Kolkata Kuala-Lumpur Madrid Melbourne Mexico-City Mumbai Nairobi
Paris São-Paulo Shanghai Singapore Taipei Tokyo Toronto Warsaw

with associated companies in Berlin Ibadan

Oxford is a registered trade mark of Oxford University Press
in the UK and in certain other countries

RC
521
H84
2011

Published in the United States
by Oxford University Press Inc., New York

© Oxford University Press, 2011

The moral rights of the author have been asserted
Database right Oxford University Press (maker)

First published by Oxford University Press 2011

All rights reserved. No part of this publication may be reproduced,
stored in a retrieval system, or transmitted, in any form or by any means,
without the prior permission in writing of Oxford University Press,
or as expressly permitted by law, or under terms agreed with the appropriate
reprographics rights organization. Enquiries concerning reproduction
outside the scope of the above should be sent to the Rights Department,
Oxford University Press, at the address above

You must not circulate this book in any other binding or cover
and you must impose the same condition on any acquirer

British Library Cataloguing in Publication Data

Data available

Library of Congress Cataloging in Publication Data

Library of Congress Control Number: 2010941706

Typeset in Minion by Glyph International Bangalore, India
Printed in Great Britain
on acid-free paper by
CPI Antony Rowe, Chippenham, Wiltshire

ISBN 978–0–19–957066–9

10 9 8 7 6 5 4 3 2 1

Whilst every effort has been made to ensure that the contents of this book are as complete, accurate
and up-to-date as possible at the date of writing, Oxford University Press is not able to give any
guarantee or assurance that such is the case. Readers are urged to take appropriately qualified
medical advice in all cases. The information in this book is intended to be useful to the general
reader, but should not be used as a means of self-diagnosis or for the prescription of medication.

Preface

According to President Jed Bartlet in the television series *The West Wing*, it is almost impossible to write a good inaugural in the shadow of JFK's 1961 speech: '. . . ask not what your country can do for you . . .'. I think philosophers, and almost everyone else, should feel the same about writing Prefaces in the shadow of Sir Michael Dummett's Prefaces for the two editions of his book *Frege: Philosophy of Language* (Harvard University Press, 1973 and 1981). Dummett comes across on the page, as he does in the flesh, as a man of both towering intellect and moral integrity. He sets out in these Prefaces his views on racism and the fight against racism in the United Kingdom. Although there has surely been a significant shift in views over the last 30 years, sadly it is still a battle that has to be fought.

Dummett's Prefaces do raise, however, a rather uncomfortable thought for philosophers—and many other academics—about how worthwhile their intellectual efforts are compared with the need to attend to a variety of manifest evils in the world. My view, for what it is worth, is that clear (and detailed) thinking is absolutely essential as a way to get things right. It is hard work for the philosophers, who may at times wonder why they do it, but it is necessary for the rest of us, even if we do not realize it! Slipshod thinking quickly creeps into so many nooks and crannies of our day-to-day lives that we hardly notice. It is pervasive and we need people to point it out when it occurs.

My day-to-day life is not that of a philosopher (except in an honorary sort of way). I am a psychiatrist. My job is to look after older people with mental health problems. But in doing this I cannot help noticing that this work raises conceptual problems as well as practical ones. This book represents my reflections on those problems. In writing it, I have been surprised by some of the turns that it has taken! There are more of my other interests revealed, perhaps, than might have been strictly necessary in a book about dementia. But I have become more and more convinced, as I have reflected, that thinking through dementia leads not simply to thoughts about dementia, but to thoughts about all of our lives as we live them in the world; particularly, perhaps, as we live them in the developed world. We need to think about and understand these problems (which are about ageing and illness for instance) broadly.

Thus, I might have stepped over the philosophical mark. I might have over-reached myself philosophically. Unless it is slipshod, this does not worry me, for two reasons. First, because I am only an honorary philosopher and I can only do what I can do between ward rounds and visiting patients in their homes. If a real philosopher were to pick up my messy thoughts and present them clearly, I would be delighted. If my thinking is askew, I am happy to see it being put right. There should be a warning, however, which is that anyone who attempts this should try their hardest to make it relevant *in some way* to practice. For even though these are conceptual issues, they are also practical ones to do with how we engage with others, especially those with dementia.

Secondly, towards the end of my time writing this book (in June 2010), I was invited by *Alzheimer's Australia* to visit their country to give a two-week lecture tour in which I was to promote the work of the Nuffield Council on Bioethics, which had produced its report *Dementia: Ethical Issues* in October 2009. This was a wonderful experience, for which I remain very grateful. There was a certain amount of publicity, because I was speaking at the National Press Club and in the parliament building in Canberra to the Parliamentary Friends of Dementia. The very savvy, and immensely kind, Chief Executive Officer of *Alzheimer's Australia*, Glenn Rees, and his talented staff nudged me in the direction of saying that we needed a revolution in dementia care. This then appeared in the press release and I found myself being asked about it. So, in the talks that I gave I felt I should say it; and then I realized that I believed it! Hence, if I have over-reached myself philosophically, it is because this is too big a practical issue for me to take the cautious steps to prevent the over-reach.

We do need a revolution. We need the 700,000 people with dementia (including the 15,000 under the age of 65 years) in the United Kingdom to take to, or be let out (or wheeled out) into the streets, along with their almost 500,000 unpaid carers, (bearing in mind that these figures will double in the next 40 years, whereas they will triple in some developing countries), so that they can converge on parliament. Their families, who are also affected in numerous emotional and financial ways, would support them. They would be supported by their professional carers too. So there would easily be 2 million people on the streets of London. The people with dementia would be amongst the sickest patients that the National Health Service has to look after and some of them the most complex that social service departments have to support.

If this meant that the quality of life for people with dementia, on account of improved quality of care, were going to improve, if this meant that the amount of money spent on dementia research were going to become equitable when compared to that spent on other conditions such as cancer, if this meant that meaningful activities and person-centred care were going to become a reality in nursing and residential homes, if this meant that basic training in dementia care were going to become widespread amongst those who look after people with these conditions, if this meant that people with dementia were going to be treated with the priority and resources that are available for other conditions, if this meant that they were going to receive the quality of palliative care that some others receive, if this meant that the relatively meagre amounts of money intended to support the National Dementia Strategy were now going to be—retrospectively—ring-fenced for the good of people with dementia, then the disruption to Londoners would have been worth it!

The storyline of the book is roughly as follows. Dementia throws up a number of particular clinical, ethical, and conceptual problems, which mostly reflect complicated evaluative decisions, for instance about diagnosis and the distinction between normal and abnormal ageing (Chapter 1). These problems can be helpfully approached by adopting a broad view of what it is to be a person with dementia: the situated embodied agent view, which I introduce in Chapter 2. This view is supported by an externalist view of mental states, which locates the mind in the world, not in the head. Understanding mental states is crucial to our view of dementia: we need to have a firm grasp on what it is to be minded in order to understand the ways in which people with dementia both are and are not minded (Chapter 3). Inevitably, therefore, we shall need to understand mental states (and the implications of such understanding for dementia). But there is a critique (derived from Wittgenstein) of such theories that stresses the notion of normativity (Chapter 4). The critique involves a transcendental account of the normativity of intentional mental states. In other words, and this will be discussed in more detail in Chapter 4, the grounds for the possibility of there being ways to say that someone has remembered correctly or incorrectly must be worked out as part of our attempts to understand how the mind connects with the world. It transpires, according to the Wittgensteinian critique, that the criteria for correctness are embedded in the practices themselves as constitutive, immanent, and irreducible features. To understand what it is to remember entails understanding the criteria for veridical remembering, not as something added to the process of remembering, but as something immanent in and constitutive of the practice of remembering. This critique not only has (negative) implications for the various models that might be used to understand dementia (Chapters 5 and 6), but also suggests general thoughts about how models are used in reality in clinical practice and, in fact, suggests that we might do without models altogether (Chapter 7). Instead, we face our mutual encounters as beings-in-the-world. Our *Being-with* the Other leads to thoughts about the nature of care and solicitude. In turn, this leads to a more positive reappraisal of how we should think about people with dementia, as situated embodied agents, where dementia is regarded as dementia-in-the-world to emphasize the extent to which we and our world are one (Chapter 8). Having dementia then becomes a matter of how a person is perceived, for instance as a citizen. And the broad view that is required is then characterized as the human-person-perspective. This is the perspective which is necessary to see dementia aright. This is the perspective which should allow a unitary vision of what has to be done, where nothing is ruled out and, in a revolutionary way, everything is ruled in. In Chapter 9, using the philosophical discussion to bolster the framework suggested by the Nuffield Council on Bioethics, I hope to shed light on the particular clinical and ethical problems with which we started in Chapter 1. The final chapter summarizes the implications of dementia-in-the-world, the human-person-perspective, and the situated embodied agent view of the person. We end with the need for conversion and revolution!

The trouble with a Preface is that you have to name people. I want to attempt this, because I owe so many so much. But many of those to whom I feel gratitude I must leave out, with regret, because of space. I hope any oversights will be forgiven. I have limited myself to those whose influence I feel directly in these pages. Listing people in such a peremptory fashion is painful, but I hope excusable.

I should like to thank three lawyers and a doctor: Stephen Shea, James Lloyd, George Daly, and Dr Mark Mallet, for the formative conversations we have had from the early 1970s; the Reverend (now Professor) Brian Davies for first teaching me how to write philosophy with a little coherence and, importantly, for introducing me to the works of Wittgenstein; Dr Kieran Fletcher and Dr Michael Waters for teaching me how a good doctor ought to be with patients; Dr Jane Pearce and Dr Catherine Oppenheimer for leading me into old age psychiatry, and Professor Robin Jacoby whose influence on me has been immense; Charlie Jenkins, Tim Parry, and Jonny Cowee for showing me, through their nursing, solicitude in action; Professor John Hodges for teaching me about cognitive neuropsychology; Professor Tony Hope and Dr Clive Baldwin for huge amounts of stimulation and profitable work; my former consultant colleagues from Newcastle General Hospital, especially Dr Alan Swann and Dr Andrew Fairbairn, for giving me a job; my academic colleagues from the Institute for Ageing and Health and the Institute of Health and Society, Newcastle University, for being such a stellar bunch, but especially Professors Ian McKeith, John O'Brien, John Bond, Louise Robinson, Tom Kirkwood, Jim Edwardson, Elaine and Robert Perry, and Drs Bob Barber, Alan Thomas, Elizabeta Mukaetova-Ladinska, Lynne Corner, and Terry Aspray, along with Claire Bamford and Marie Poole, not least because of their friendship; further afield in Newcastle University, Professors Erica Haimes and Philip van der Eijk (now at the Humboldt University in Berlin), and Dr Simon Woods for stimulating other sorts of thought; all of the psychologists I have ever worked with, but currently Ian James, Angus McGregor, and Alan Howarth, for providing the other view; John Horne, Dr Marcus Redley, and Professor Tony Holland for keeping my thinking about mental capacity and human rights a little sharper; Professor Dave Jolley for being one of the greats; the Reverend Brian Allen for his kindly ear and thoughts about dementia; three professors of nursing, Charlotte Clarke, John Keady, and Wendy Moyle, for their encouragement and thoughts; the incredible Wallsend Community Psychiatry of Old Age team—Joan Lowerson, Lesley Thompson, Yvonne Bulmer, Graham Davidson, and Marion Brooks—for the amazing work they do, along with our hard-working in-patient teams; my immediate consultant colleagues at North Tyneside General Hospital, Drs Greig Ramsay, Simon Wilson, Kartini Nor, Andy Teodorczuk, for their support and, because they are also such good colleagues, Dr Joanna Cox, Dr Gbenga Afolabi, Dr Paul Paes, and Professor Richard Walker *inter alia*.

But I must thank some people more particularly. It was a thrill to come to Newcastle as a major centre for research in the fields of ageing and dementia. But soon after I arrived I had another thrill, which was to meet one of our leading moral thinkers, Dr Mary Midgley. I have then been privileged to join the meetings that Mary hosts of the Applied Philosophy Interest Section (APIS). This has been an important source of philosophical sustenance for me and I have benefited from listening to and being criticized by Mary, Michael Bavidge, William Charlton, Ian Ground, and the other members of APIS.

More than anyone else, however, I must acknowledge my most significant philosophical debts to my two PhD supervisors, Professor Bill Fulford and Professor Tim Thornton. Bill's influence on my whole career has been determinative. It is difficult to overstate this. As has been the case for many others, I know, his personal encouragement and enthusiasm have been astounding. Meanwhile, my real grip, such as it is, on Wittgenstein came from the painstaking way in which, in numerous supervision sessions, Tim guided me in how to think about the issues that concerned me. I cannot thank either of them enough. I would add here, too, thanks to Professor Michael Luntley. Apart from examining me, as these pages show, his work has been a great source of inspiration and I benefited profoundly from my conversations with him at Warwick. For similar reasons, as these pages show, I owe a great debt to Professor Eric Matthews.

Lindsay Turner, my secretary, has typed various chapters, chased up all sorts of things and generally kept the show on the road. She has my enormous thanks. Martin Baum, Charlotte Green, Abigail Stanley, and the other staff at Oxford University Press have shown their usual patience and good humour. I am grateful to them for their sensitive help.

I want to mention five further revolutionaries in particular. Readers will see that I have been very sympathetic to the work of Professor Peter Whitehouse. I am delighted to have become friendly with Peter, because the thoughts he is (constantly) having should be challenging the rest of us to think more broadly. Professor Murna Downs leads the Bradford Dementia Group and I have never been to Bradford without coming away feeling as if I have learned something valuable. She has a sensitivity of thought, combined with a robustness of approach, which is entirely refreshing. The third revolutionary is our very good friend, Dr Tom Shakespeare. I owe to Tom the title of this book: it is clever, I think, like Tom. Dr Stephen Louw has become a close friend in Newcastle. In a subtle way (for a physician) I feel Stephen has encouraged me to pursue a number of avenues of thought and work. These have always been congenial and profitable. Our work together has been a source of great pleasure and benefit to me, partly because of Stephen's humility and good humour. The final revolutionary is Professor Steve Sabat. His work has been hugely influential in this field. It has been incredibly relevant and informing for my own work. It is immensely humane. His friendship does not seem to know many bounds. For instance, he has looked at every chapter of this book. I cannot express my gratitude sufficiently; but he knows it is genuine.

Finally, I must thank my family. My parents, Ann and Peter, set me on the path safely. My siblings, Simon, Katie, Dom and Ben, and their families have supported me at different times and in different ways. To my immediate family, Olli, Emma, and Luke, I need to say very little because they know. Perhaps I should apologize: it's really taken most of their lives. But they, idiosyncratically, have been and are joys. The book is dedicated to them and to Anne, my wife, who, most idiosyncratically, has frequently poured scorn on the very possibility of this book, but has none the less ensured that it was completed, has proofread the whole manuscript, has provided me with the right environment to work and relieved me of numerous worries. She too knows. What can I say? She's a brick, but she floats.

Acknowledgements

The author would like to thank the following for permission to reproduce copyright material: Wiley-Blackwell for extracts from *Philosophical Investigations*; Cengage Learning EMEA Ltd for permission to adapt Figure 5.1 from Ellis and Young (1988); Springer for Table 7.1; and the Nuffield Council for Bioethics for use of material including Box 9.1. In addition a special thanks to Hawker publications and to John Killick for the use of *On The Move*; similar thanks to the National Gallery of Victoria in Melbourne, Australia, for permission to quote Ronnie Jackamarra Lawson from their display of aboriginal art and to Anthony Wallis on behalf of Aboriginal Artists for his advice on this matter; and finally, very sincere gratitude to Barbara Pointon for permission to use Malcolm's sketch that forms Figure 7.1. We have endeavoured to seek all appropriate permissions and apologize for any oversights, which we would seek to rectify in any future editions of the book.

Contents

Abbreviations

ADI	Alzheimer's Disease International
APP	Amyloid precursor protein
APOE	Apolipoprotein E
BPSD	Behavioural and psychological symptoms of dementia
CT	Computerized X-ray tomography
DNA	Deoxyribonucleic acid
DSM-5	Diagnostic and Statistical Manual, 5th edition
GP	General practitioner (family doctor)
HIV	Human immunodeficiency virus
ICD-10	International Classification of Diseases, 10th edition
MCI	Mild cognitive impairment
MMSE	Mini-mental state examination
MRI	Magnetic Resonance Imaging
MS	Multiple sclerosis
NHS	National Health Service
NICE	National Institute for Health and Clinical Excellence
PET	Positron emission tomography
RTM	Representational Theory of Mind (Fodor 1976)
SCIE	Social Care Institute for Excellence
SEA	Situated embodied agent (view of the person)
SPECT	Single photon emission computed tomography
UK	United Kingdom
USA	United States of America
VBM	Values-based medicine (Fulford 2004)
WHO	World Health Organization

Works by Wittgenstein

BB	*The Blue and Brown Books*
CV	*Culture and Value*
LW	*Last Writings on the Philosophy of Psychology*
OC	*On Certainty*
PG	*Philosophical Grammar*
PI	*Philosophical Investigations*
RFM	*Remarks on the Foundations of Mathematics*
RPP	*Remarks on the Philosophy of Psychology*
TLP	*Tractatus Logico-Philosophicus*
Z	*Zettel*

Part I

Introduction

Chapter 1

The clinical surround: values and versions

If in life we are surrounded by death, so too in the health
of our intellect we are surrounded by madness.
(Wittgenstein, 1980: *Culture and Value*: 44)

Introduction

A context is a surround. We are all situated or positioned in particular, but changing,
contexts; which means that we are surrounded. Inevitably, however, we are part of
our surroundings. It is perfectly true that we often feel disconnected from our
surroundings. Sometimes we are just amused, even cynical, observers; or we can feel
positively detached from what is going on around us (when it reaches a certain intensity,
this is what the psychopathologists call 'derealization'). Yet there are moments, too,
when we feel either that we reach out and embrace our world, or more profoundly that
we are part of it in an autochthonous way. The idea of being in any real sense *at one*
with nature again reflects a certain intensity of feeling captured best perhaps in works
of art; the poetry of John Keats (1795–1821) for instance:

> That I might drink, and leave the world unseen,
> And with thee fade away into the forest dim:
> Fade far away, dissolve, and quite forget
> What thou among the leaves hast never known …

> (*Ode to a Nightingale*, Keats, 1990: 286)

The idea that how we relate to our surroundings, whether via psychopathology or
poetic inspiration, is important to our understanding of dementia, is one that I shall
leave hanging, but is in the end crucial. Thinking through dementia will take us to
places we might not anticipate.

One of the aims of this chapter is to sketch the sort of problems that surround clinical practice in the field of dementia. But a lot of what I want to say in this book as a
whole is to do with surroundings. For now, more mundanely, we shall stick to the surroundings of particular clinical events, which will often be other clinical events. But
the clinical surround is itself a part of a broader field, which will usually involve ethical
concerns too.

In 1929, Wittgenstein wrote: 'You cannot lead people to what is good; you can only lead them to some place or other. The good is outside the space of facts' (CV: 3). The relationship between facts and evaluative statements in relation to the diagnosis of dementia will also dominate much of the discussion in this chapter. Wittgenstein's aphorism—'Ethics is transcendental' (TLP: §6.421)—points to an incommensurability between statements about ethics and statements about facts. Indeed, the problem of deriving a statement containing an 'ought' from a statement containing an 'is' will inevitably hover, but is not the problem with which I wish to engage (it is covered in Hudson, 1969). Rather, in talking of surrounds, an aim in this book is to highlight the ways in which the world inevitably contains facts and values and a lot more besides, a notion captured rather nicely by the title of a chapter by Mary Midgley: 'One world, but a big one' (in Midgley, 2001). This idea is antithetical to the Wittgenstein who wrote at the start of the *Tractatus* (his early work): 'The facts in logical space are the world' (TLP: §1.13), but is not inimical to his later thought, which contributes to the analysis of this book.

In any case, ethical dilemmas are a feature of the human world and they create a context, a place in the world, where there are particular circumstances linked to other circumstances involving individuals with specific and non-specific views. All of this means that decisions or events are always particular and individual, if for no other reason than that time has passed. Moreover, clinical events are always ethical in one way or another, because the surround brings in alternatives: something could have been done differently; then again, clinical decisions are ethical not just because of the *clinical* surroundings, but because they will impinge on the broader world by using up resources, by demonstrating regard for some things but not others, by infringing this or that liberty, by changing the world, perhaps by allowing someone to die.

So I shall start by sketching some typical dilemmas in dementia care. I then move on to definitions, facts, and figures; but it is important to appreciate that these are themselves surrounded: they fit in particular contexts. Some of the contexts also involve further facts. The immediate point I wish to emphasize, however, is *the link between facts and values*, the discussion of which will dominate the chapter.

Dilemmas in dementia

My aim here is to highlight the real issues that arise in the context of dementia care. They affect different people: the person with dementia, the doctor, the social worker, the nursing assistant, and the family carer. The cases that follow are real, but anonymized, and are presented only in brief to convey the day-to-day nature of ethical decision making in connection with dementia.

It can be convincingly argued that every decision in health and social care amounts at some level to an ethical decision. It is not surprising, therefore, that in dementia care, where there is the added complication that the person concerned may or may not be able to make decisions for him or herself, moral dilemmas are commonplace. In this section, I shall briefly sketch five cases that raise particular issues, which I shall discuss further in Chapter 9. The sketches are only intended to be sufficient to raise the issues as part of the process of thinking through dementia.

Mr Siders

For some while Mr Siders sensed that he was having increasing difficulty remembering people's names. He had been a teacher all his life and prided himself on his ability to learn and remember people's names very quickly. He was a bachelor, but he had a good circle of friends and each week he went to play bridge with a mixture of old colleagues and acquaintances. Initially, when Mr Siders made mistakes with people's names it was all felt to be quite humorous, but then some of his friends started to comment that they wondered whether he should seek help. Their concern was compounded by his stories of forgetfulness in one or two other spheres of his life. He had, for instance, been to the shops and then forgotten what he had gone to buy. One of the members of the bridge party had taken his wife to the local Memory Clinic. She had initially been given a diagnosis of 'mild cognitive impairment', but a year later she was told that she had Alzheimer's disease and she was put on medication. The medication had helped and his friend really thought Mr Siders should go to the Memory Clinic too. Mr Siders was far from certain that he wished to go down a road that might lead to him being told that he had Alzheimer's disease. None the less, he recognized that it made sense to get treatment early. He was far from convinced that what he had was actually a disease even though the pressure at the bridge club was now making him feel as if there might be something wrong. The moral dilemma, therefore, was this. Should he seek medical help for something that he had been regarding as humorous? Where would this lead? Given that he had always rather avoided doctors, should he now succumb to the pressure from a friend to seek medical help? If he were to attend the Memory Clinic he knew that he would be opening himself up to assessments and scrutiny that might make him feel stigmatized. What if they were to tell him that he could no longer drive? Yet, he felt completely competent to drive his car in which he had never even had a scrape. But the issue of whether or not he should be assessed had been raised and he was reminded of it every time he forgot someone's name. He reassured himself with the thought that he continued quite frequently to win at bridge!

Mrs Brownwell

Dr Smith had known Mrs Brownwell for the last 27 years. She had always been very assertive and they had sometimes clashed, but they remained on good terms. Dr Smith noted that Mrs Brownwell had been coming to see him more frequently over the last several months. The issues were generally minor. However, she had mentioned her memory on a couple of occasions, which led him to test her cognitive function in a more formal manner. He used the Mini Mental State Examination (MMSE) (Folstein, Folstein, & McHugh, 1975) on which she scored 27/30. Although this seemed like a good score, which meant that the news given to Mrs Brownwell could be reassuring, Dr Smith was nevertheless worried that this was not as good as he would have expected from someone of Mrs Brownwell's capabilities. He told her that he thought it would be worthwhile to perform some blood tests. Mrs Brownwell was on tablets for diabetes. Dr Smith was surprised to discover that the blood tests suggested the diabetic control was not as good as it might be (suggesting that she might be forgetting her tablets). Dr Smith was aware that Mrs Brownwell had a further appointment the following week, but before the appointment arrived Mrs Brownwell's daughter rang up Dr Smith and said that she wanted to know what was going on with her mother. Dr Smith could not help noticing that assertiveness seemed to be a family trait in this case. Mrs Brownwell's daughter told Dr Smith that she thought her mother was 'losing her marbles'. The family were very worried about her memory and about a decline in her personal hygiene. Dr Smith said that this was very interesting and important information, but bearing in mind Mrs Brownwell's fiercely independent nature, Dr Smith was loath to divulge confidential information. Mrs Brownwell's daughter said this was outrageous, but was pacified by Dr Smith saying that it was something he could raise with Mrs Brownwell when she next visited. In saying this, however, Dr Smith could already hear the similar outrage in Mrs Brownwell's voice at the suggestion that her doctor should be 'gossiping with all and sundry' about her health. Faced with this dilemma over the need both to respect confidentiality and to do the best for the patient, Dr Smith was in a quandary.

Dorothy Galpin

The diagnosis of a chest infection was made fairly quickly once Dorothy Galpin came into hospital. Unfortunately, her stay in hospital was prolonged because she subsequently developed diarrhoea and later a urinary tract infection. Through much of this time she was really very confused and a diagnosis of delirium was also made. Mrs Galpin was an 82-year-old widow who had lost her husband many years ago. She lived alone and she and her husband had been childless. Her closest relative was a niece who lived at the other end of the country. Once Mrs Galpin's infections were settled and attention turned to her discharge from hospital, questions arose about whether or not she would be able to manage at home. Mrs Galpin still seemed to be confused and was definitely unsafe when assessed by the occupational therapist in the kitchen on the ward. None the less a home assessment was arranged, but Mrs Galpin still seemed confused. She had problems operating her oven and she even seemed a little disorientated around her house. The medical social worker was approached to find suitable long-term care for Mrs Galpin on the grounds that she remained confused on the ward and she had not performed particularly well even when taken home. When matters were discussed with Mrs Galpin, however, she was strident in her demands to be taken home, even though she was unable to say exactly where she lived. The social worker was keen to try to support Mrs Galpin living independently in her own home, but there was considerable pressure from the medical team to move matters on more quickly; and considerable concern that Mrs Galpin would not do well at home, even with daily home care support. The dilemma for the social worker was to do with Mrs Galpin's best interests given that everyone agreed she did not have capacity herself to make decisions about her long-term care.

Mr Gupta

Mr Gupta had been in the nursing home for people with dementia for two years. He had initially been somewhat aggressive and it was for this reason that his family moved him into the home. However, he had become much more settled. He tended to walk about quietly until he became less mobile and then he simply sat and stared out of the window. He enjoyed being given books, especially if they contained pictures. He would sit thumbing through the books with some sort of interest, but with no evidence that he understood what he was looking at. He no longer spoke to anyone. His family visited at the weekends, but they never stayed long, seemingly because they found it too upsetting to see Mr Gupta in his present state. Mr Gupta had been a successful businessman. He had ensured that his children received a good education and, as a consequence, they had all done very well. Mr Gupta was obviously pleased to see them when they came into the home, although he did not communicate with them verbally, but would simply smile. One of the nurses noted that Mr Gupta, who was by now heavily dependent for all his basic needs on the care staff, was starting to cough during his meals. He would sometimes cough on solid food, but also when he was given orange squash. Initially the coughing only occurred once in a while, but it was becoming an everyday occurrence and it was clear to staff that he was developing swallowing problems. Inevitably, he contracted a chest infection, presumably because he had aspirated food or drink. After the chest infection he was weaker and the problems with swallowing and the worry about food going into his lungs became more acute. The nursing staff discussed matters with the family and with the general practitioner. No one seemed keen to pursue the possibility of artificial feeding for Mr Gupta. His family felt fairly strongly that his quality of life was not good, but some of the nursing staff felt that he was quite happy and they were uncomfortable with the thought that feeding him by mouth, as they were doing, was likely to hasten Mr Gupta's death; but they also felt uneasy about not feeding him, so artificial feeding seemed the only option. The dilemma for the nursing staff was that they had ambivalent feelings about his quality of life and, therefore, ambivalent feelings about how aggressive or otherwise treatment should be to maintain that quality of life.

Dr Montagna

Susan had always felt that it was her duty to look after her father. She had no doubts about this. Her father had always been a good man and she was more than happy to devote herself to him as his main carer. He now lived in her house and she was supported by the local general practitioner (GP) and district nurses and by carers who came into the house twice a day to help her to change her father and to wash him. She knew that she looked after him as well, if not better, than he would have been cared for in a large institution. She knew what sort of music he liked, what sort of food he enjoyed, and she was considerate in terms of planning activities to make his days more enjoyable. For instance, she would take him outside into the garden whenever it was possible. But he was becoming weaker and the family doctor, who had known them both for some time, asked her whether she would be keen to keep her father at home with her even if he were to develop a serious illness, such as an infection. She found it very hard to decide, but was keen to make plans for the future. She had previously been in touch with a community psychiatric nurse, whom she contacted. The nurse came to visit her, but in discussion they decided that it might be better for her to talk to a palliative care nurse about advance care planning. Susan had a meeting with the palliative care nurse and an interesting discussion about what might be best for her father. She continued, however, to feel quite at sea in terms of what she might do if the worst came to the worst. Another meeting was scheduled with the palliative care nurse, but before the meeting took place, the worst did happen. Dr Montagna, after a couple of days during which he did not seem his old self, in that he was generally less responsive, developed a fever. This became really apparent on a Friday evening when Susan would not be able to talk to her father's doctor again until the Monday. Instead an out-of-hours GP visited and said that Dr Montagna should be admitted to hospital. Now the dilemma was no longer theoretical: Susan had to decide whether she would allow her father to be admitted to hospital, or whether she would insist that he should stay at home with her.

Each of these cases manifests a dilemma, where the issue is that values, and judgements about values, conflict. The particular dilemmas will have to await further consideration; for now I shall focus on values in comparison with facts.

There are two types of possibility I wish to consider: first, facts may suggest evaluative concerns; secondly, facts may presuppose values.

Values from facts

The first possibility, then, is that facts suggest value judgements. There are currently estimated to be about 700,000 people in the United Kingdom (UK) with dementia (Knapp & Prince, 2007). In the world as a whole there are estimated to be 35.6 million people with dementia in 2010 (ADI, 2009: 7). The chances of developing dementia increase as we get older. Figures from the UK suggest that 1.3% of people between the ages of 65 and 69 have dementia, but this rises to 20% of those over the age of 85 (Knapp & Prince, 2007). As is well known, populations are ageing worldwide. Hence, there is predicted to be a doubling in the total number of people with dementia every 20 years. The estimates are that by 2030 there will be 65.7 million people with dementia and by 2050 the figure will have increased to 115.4 million people (ADI, 2009: 27). This rise in the total number of people with dementia will disproportionately affect those in low- and middle-income countries. Whereas in 2010 the proportion of those with dementia living in low- and middle-income countries is estimated to be 57.7%, by 2050 it is predicted to be 70.5% (*ibid.*).

These are some of the 'bare' facts. Any sort of thought about these facts, however, immediately leads to evaluative concerns. Dementia is increasing as the population ages, which immediately suggests a pull on resources. There will be issues to do with treatment and the costs associated with treatment. There is already controversy in the UK around the rationing of acetylcholinesterase inhibitors, which are currently the main drugs for treating Alzheimer's disease. In the UK, these are only available for people with moderate dementia (NICE-SCIE, 2007: section 1.6.2). This decision, which is not about the clinical efficacy of the drugs, but rather about their cost-effectiveness, clearly already reflects certain value judgements, which will include concerns about the allocation of scarce resources. As well as drug treatments, however, there are also psychosocial approaches to people with dementia. Whether someone is prone to think in terms of pharmacological or psychosocial approaches may itself tell us something about the person's interpretation of the figures. These interpretations, which are evaluative, obviously reflect different perspectives, which have a background that cannot be value-neutral.

The epidemiological facts, as well as raising concerns about resources, might also suggest the need for greater research. Once again, the type of research that is thought to be required will reflect differing background evaluations. On the one hand, there is the compelling argument that we should be seeking a cure for the various types of dementia. This might lead to a plea for an increase in the funding for basic biological research. An equally compelling case could be made, on the other hand, for more clinical research to look, for instance, at the best ways to control (what is termed) behaviour that challenges. There is great controversy concerning the best approaches to people with dementia who become agitated. Sometimes drug treatment works, but there can be side effects. For instance, antipsychotic drugs, which are known to work very well in some circumstances, are also known to increase both morbidity and mortality (Ballard & Aarsland, 2010). Other drugs may or may not be more suitable, but there are also psychosocial approaches to different behaviours in dementia that can be helpful (Stokes, 2010). Hence, in terms of the need for greater research, there may once again be quite different responses from different constituencies about exactly what is best. These different responses reflect different background surroundings. Thus, facts lead to different interpretations concerning implications, which in turn reflect different value judgements.

Values and research

Meanwhile, it is worth noting that, intentionally or not, value judgements are already at play in terms of research funding. There is already evidence that a relatively low priority is given to research on dementia compared with research on other diseases. For instance, Knapp and Prince (2007), from King's College London and the London School of Economics, in their research for the Alzheimer's Society looked at papers published since 2002 on long-term conditions and showed that, whilst 23.5% were to do with cancer and 17.6% with cardiovascular disease, only 1.4% focused on dementia. In the UK, in response to a question in the House of Commons on 16 December 2008, the British government acknowledged figures that showed that expenditure on cancer research was approximately eight times that of dementia research, whereas the prevalence of cancer was only just over twice that of dementia (House of Commons, 2008).

These figures led the Working Party of the Nuffield Council on Bioethics, which was looking at ethical issues in dementia, to conclude that more funding was required in dementia (Nuffield Council on Bioethics, 2009). The Nuffield Council report, having undertaken an extensive consultation process, further recommended that priority should be given to a broader array of research and, indeed, that there should be an increase in funding for dementia research in the following areas:

> Health services research into how people with dementia and their carers can best be supported to live well, how mainstream services can best be adapted to their needs, and how good practice can more readily be implemented; more meaningful outcome measures for

assessing the effect of particular forms of treatment or service; research into how best to improve the provision of support for ethical decision-making; all forms of research for the non-Alzheimer's dementias; and research into preventative strategies. (*ibid.*: 134)

In other words, although there needs to be an overall increase in terms of funding for research on dementia, the emphasis in this report was away from the idea of a cure purely for Alzheimer's disease. It is worth pausing over this point because it indicates the issue we are considering, namely that dementia sits in a context and the context is value-laden. There are very good reasons why a pharmaceutical company would be attracted to the idea of pursuing research on curing Alzheimer's disease—the best known of the dementias and a condition that increasingly attracts political attention. The politicization of Alzheimer's disease can be a good, if it attracts help and support for people with Alzheimer's disease and their carers, but can also be seen as potentially a bad thing if people with Alzheimer's are—if not individually, perhaps as an imper-sonal collective—seen as a threat and a problem (Robertson, 1991). Not only, there-fore, are there political agendas, at some level, which determine whether funding goes to dementia or to some other condition, but there are also political influences affec-ting where funding goes within the field of dementia. Whilst acknowledging that the economic clout of large pharmaceutical companies must have an influence within the relevant political arenas, the current point is not intended simply to snipe at large, multi-national corporations, but to highlight the pervasiveness of the influence of the *surround* at every level in connection with dementia. It is not just big businesses that focus research on cure rather than care; the same accusation is sometimes made of voluntary organizations where decisions about funding often seem to reflect the views of activist carers who are, very understandably, attracted by the idea of research that purports to uncover the basis of Alzheimer's disease and thus lead to a cure. Furthermore, at a societal level, the tendency to be seduced by the scientific possibility of curing disease, whether by genetic manipulation or by stem cell research, is potent.

Drawing attention to the potency of background concerns should raise a question about the priority of any particular background point of view. In which case, for rea-sons that will be supported by many of the arguments in this book, the views of carers of people with dementia, and not just those who have (for laudable reasons) asserted themselves to occupy positions of political influence, should be given some priority. As Widdershoven and Widdershoven-Heerding (2003) have said in another context, 'in the definition of good care, the values of both parties—the person with dementia and the surrounding care-givers—are relevant' (p. 108).

So, too, the Nuffield Council working party was keen to highlight the importance of the social context for people with dementia in connection with research in order to provide 'an evidence base to underpin better ways of supporting people with dementia and their carers' (Nuffield Council on Bioethics, 2009: 134). They went on to recom-mend that the appropriate funding bodies should,

... take active steps to encourage further research into issues such as how people live with dementia, the nature of their experience and the quality of their lives; how stigma can best be challenged; and how those working in health and social care can best be supported in providing care which genuinely respects the personhood of everyone with dementia. (*ibid.*)

This whole discussion is sparked off simply by the facts concerning the numbers of people affected by dementia and the projected increases in those figures. The facts and figures generate different types of evaluative concern depending on the particular context in which we stand or on the background from which we view the issues.

In addition to biological, social, and political backgrounds, the facts and figures can also generate evaluative concerns that are purely ethical. If, for instance, the numbers of people with dementia are going to increase and if treatments are going to improve to keep people alive for longer, then there are likely to be more ethical issues at the end of life for people with dementia. Talk of 'pure' ethical issues is, of course, misleading because, as I suggested above, ethical decision making is itself located in a context, which is social, economic, political, and so on. Resource allocation will again be an issue at the end of life, but even decisions about whether a particular person with dementia is competent to drive carries significant social importance. There is a host of issues from the use of restraint, to the use of covert medication, to the ethical demand that standards of care should help people with dementia to remain active and engaged in society—that they should not be positioned in a 'malignant' way (Sabat, 2006a)—which reflect a general ethical imperative to provide good quality care for people with dementia from the time of diagnosis until the time of death. But this ethical require-ment itself reflects and immediately engages with a broader raft of concerns that are not just ethical, but also cultural, political, economic, religious, and so forth. In short, we cannot get away from the expanding surroundings that emerge as the facts and figures are located differently from different perspectives. As we have seen, these sur-roundings are always replete with values, so the facts and figures are always subject to an evaluative interpretation.

Values in facts

It is not just that facts reflect values in the sense that values emerge from them in their interpretation. The second possibility I wish to consider is that facts themselves are value-laden: facts presuppose values. This has been recognized for some while. Gunnar Myrdal, in a collection of essays published in 1958, discusses the possibility of a purely factual analysis independent of any valuations.

> This assumption is naïve empiricism: the idea that if we observe, and continue to observe, reality without any preconceptions, the facts will somehow organize themselves into a system which is assumed to pre-exist. But without questions there are no answers. And the answers are preconceived in the formulation of the questions. The questions express our interests in the matter. The interests can never be purely scientific. They are choices, the products of our valuations. (Myrdal, 1958: 51)

He goes on to say, 'the factual analysis cannot be carried out except when guided by the value premise' (*ibid.*: 52). The same thought, that facts depend on evaluations, is true in diagnosis too. I shall discuss dementia. But the idea that diagnoses contain, depend upon, or reflect values or evaluative judgements is not new and I do not feel the need to argue the point specifically, given the standing of the existing work on values in medicine and psychiatry (Fulford, 1989; Sadler, 2004). None the less, it is worth making the point that dementia has tended to dip from view in the philosophy of psychiatry largely because it is seen as an 'organic' condition where the facts of brain pathology obscure the surrounding evaluative considerations (Hughes, Louw, & Sabat, 2006).

Some years ago, Nelson Goodman wrote *Ways of Worldmaking* in which he suggested that the same facts can be accounted for by different accounts, or what he called *versions*.

> Willingness to accept countless alternative true or right world-versions does not mean that everything goes, that tall stories are as good as short ones, that truths are no longer distinguished from falsehoods, but only that truth must be otherwise conceived than as correspondence with a ready-made world. Though we make worlds by making versions, we no more make a world by putting symbols together at random than a carpenter makes a chair by putting pieces of wood together at random. (Goodman, 1978: 94)

Different versions—we might wish to consider the different versions articulated by the different models of dementia mentioned at the end of this chapter—can be translated into each other, but what we see again is that the world of facts is surrounded by, or embedded in, a world of evaluative concerns. This means, as Goodman says (quoting Hanson, 1958), that facts are 'theory-laden'.

> Of course, we want to distinguish between versions that do and those that do not refer, and to talk about the things and worlds, if any, referred to; but these things and worlds ... are themselves fashioned by and along with the versions. ... facts are small theories, and true theories are big facts. ... We start, on any occasion, with some old version or world that we have on hand and that we are stuck with until we have the determination and skill to remake it into a new one. Some of the felt stubbornness of fact is the grip of habit: our firm foundation is indeed stolid. (Goodman, 1978: 96–7)

Facts are theory-laden, which suggests that they are value-laden too, reflecting particular versions or accounts of the world. As Myrdal said, 'the factual analysis cannot be carried out except when guided by the value premise' (*op. cit.*). Our ways of seeing dementia will also inevitably involve our world view: we shall see it in a particular surround, according to a certain version, which will include not only the perspective of our favoured model of dementia, but also our attitudes to ageing, to community, to what it is to flourish, to dependence, to suffering, to life, and to death.

Thinking through dementia involves, in part, seeing through the facts and figures to the value judgements beyond. Later I shall, first, point to value commitments in the form of models used to understand dementia and, secondly, consider the value judgements highlighted by particular dilemmas that arise in dementia care. But definitions come first.

Too much in a word

Given that 'dementia' is a term known (if not fully understood) both on the street and in the clinic, it may seem pointless to continue to emphasize its standing as a concept, as opposed to a thing (or natural kind), by the use of scare quotes. Part of the reason for doing so is that, first, many people on the Clapham omnibus would not know that dementia is not the name of a specific illness; and, secondly, the conceptual issues around the notion of 'dementia' are by no means straightforward.

No one in the field of nosology has seriously suggested that dementia is *one* thing: it describes a syndrome, a collection of symptoms and signs for which there are many causes and which manifests itself in a variety of ways. It is an umbrella term. The most common types of dementia in clinical practice are Alzheimer's dementia (about 50% of cases), followed by vascular (or multi-infarct) dementia and Lewy body dementia (each with a prevalence of about 20%); many cases are a mixture of vascular and Alzheimer's. The frontotemporal dementias are less common except in those with early onset disease (i.e. under the age of 65 years). All of this, however, is covered in standard texts and the details need not detain us (Burns, O'Brien, & Ames, 2005; Jacoby, Oppenheimer, Dening, & Thomas, 2008; Weiner & Lipton, 2009). For a beautifully succinct clinical introduction, see Jolley (2010).

The *Tenth International Classification of Diseases* (ICD-10) gives the following definition:

> Dementia is a syndrome due to disease of the brain, usually of a chronic or progressive nature in which there is disturbance of multiple higher cortical functions, including memory, thinking, orientation, comprehension, calculation, learning capacity, language and judgement. Consciousness is not clouded. Impairments of cognitive function are commonly accompanied, and occasionally preceded, by deterioration in emotional control, social behaviour, or motivation. (World Health Organization, 1992: 45)

One thing that is immediately clear in this definition is that dementia seems mainly to be conceived as a disorder of *cognitive* function (i.e. 'memory, thinking, orientation . . . . .' etc.), but this in itself represents a particular view, one which has consequences. Thus we find Stephen Post writing: 'I coined the term "hypercognitive" in 1995 to underscore a persistent bias against the deeply forgetful that is especially pronounced in modern philosophical accounts of the "person"...... Only "persons" narrowly defined, it is often argued, have moral standing' (Post, 2006: 231).

That is, if dementia is mainly a cognitive disorder and if failures in cognitive function amount to a loss of personhood, it follows that dementia must entail a loss of personhood and consequently of 'moral standing'. I shall pursue this in Chapter 2, but the important point here is that this conceptualization of dementia need not be the only alternative. Reflecting on the historical record, Berrios (1987) concluded that, 'The term "dementia" and the concept of cognitive failure came together sometime during the eighteenth century'. By the start of the next century,

> ... experimental psychology and the growth of Associationism provided laws and princi-ples, in terms of which the concept of cognitive failure could be given a quantitative defi-nition. In due course, intellectual impairment became the invariant around which the nineteenth century 'cognitive model' of dementia was formed. (Berrios, 1987)

It is interesting to note that this 'cognitive model', formed in the nineteenth century, still held sway when ICD-10 came into being towards the end of the twentieth century. But it is also interesting to note a hint that the hegemony of the 'cognitive model' is under threat. For instance, in describing dementia, a national guideline in England and Wales describes two perspectives, the medical and social, which 'are often not mutually exclusive' (NICE-SCIE, 2007: 66). The guideline describes a clinical perspective according to which, 'dementia can be described as a group of usually progressive neurodegenerative brain disorders characterized by intellectual deterioration and more or less gradual erosion of mental and later physical function' (*ibid.*).

But the guideline then continues with this important passage:

> Alternatively, from a social perspective, dementia can be viewed as one of the ways in which an individual's personal and social capacities may change for a variety of reasons, and changes in such capacities are only experienced as disabilities when environmental support (which we all depend upon to varying degrees) are not adaptable to suit them. Moreover, dementia thought of from a clinical perspective (that is, disease and disability leading to death) may also prefigure our collective social and professional approach to people with dementia as people irretrievably ill and fundamentally different from able-bodied healthy young people. This view may well underpin many of the problems faced by people with dementia and their carers when seeking help and in their experience of care in different settings' (*ibid.*).

A key intention in this book is to bring together these perspectives; or, at least, to see how they might be brought together and then to consider the clinical implications of doing so or not. But the idea is clear: the focus on cognitive impairment, if understandable, nevertheless takes us away from the broader reality of dementia. As the historical record suggests, the 'invariant core meaning' of 'dementia', according to Berrios, has included 'cognitive failure, chronic behavioural dislocation and psychosocial incompetence' (Berrios, 1987). In other words, dementia affects the whole person: not just the brain and the memory, but also a host of important aspects of daily living. If for no other reason, this suggests that our focus in thinking through dementia should be to understand the person with dementia, where—as Kitwood (1997) would have reminded us—the emphasis should be on the *person*.

So far, therefore, I have presented an international definition of 'dementia', but then I have started to show how, despite mention of emotional control, social behaviour, and motivation, the definition is inadequate. This brief discussion already indicates the extent to which dementia cannot be regarded solely from the biomedical perspective. If it cannot be pinned down in this way it is because of the surround, the context in which dementia exists. Understanding this context, however, requires a broad view, one in which dementia is seen as a condition that people live with; and thus one which quintessentially involves *persons*, where this term generates thought, *inter alia*, about psychosocial space and moral standing, as well as about pathophysiology.

It is worth noting problems associated with terminology at the simplest level. 'Dementia', from its Latin root, *demens*, suggests being out of your mind. Part of the stigma associated with dementia is connected with the fact that calling someone 'demented' is also a form of abuse. So there is a question about the political correctness of the term 'dementia'. The debate about giving people the diagnosis of dementia in an honest fashion (Bamford et al., 2004) normally involves a worry that the diagnosis might be harmful, but etymologically the worry ought to be, plain and simple, that it is *insulting*. Comparisons are made with giving the diagnosis of cancer 30 years ago, when the worry was that the news would be emotionally devastating, particularly when there was little that could be done. But telling someone they have cancer was not normally regarded as a matter of insulting them. As we have seen, the term 'dementia' is well established in international nomenclature, so to change it would seem daunting. But we no longer use 'idiot' as a diagnostic label and 'mental handicap' has been replaced by 'learning disability'. 'Dementia' would seem to be a case where political correctness makes a valid point.

Further evidence for this can be derived from the description Berrios gave, which we passed over without comment: 'cognitive failure, chronic behavioural dislocation and psychosocial incompetence' (Berrios, 1987). It is unsurprising, perhaps, that historical accounts should stress dysfunctionality—failure, dislocation, incompetence—given that these accounts are often medical. But if this way of thinking about dementia is commonplace—and it certainly is the case that 'behaviour that challenges' is often regarded as 'challenging behaviour', if not simply as 'bad behaviour'—then we can see why a diagnosis of dementia *is* insulting, because it carries with it the negative connotations of failure, dislocation, and incompetence.

Trachtenberg and Trojanowski (2008) regard the issue of terminology as a matter 'of morality and of common humanity'. Other insulting terms (e.g. mongoloid, imbecile, moron) disappeared from medical nomenclature not because of science, 'but rather primarily because of consciousness raising, educating, and lobbying by various advocacy groups. They made it abundantly evident that these types of pejorative and degrading terms were no longer acceptable. So it is now with dementia' (*ibid.*).

Conceptual problems have been identified in the literature (Thomas, 2008a): current diagnostic criteria tend to stress problems of new learning, which makes the diagnosis of Alzheimer's disease more likely, rather than executive function (i.e. the ability to plan and do things), which would encourage diagnoses of vascular dementia. Such considerations have led one acknowledged expert in the field, Vladimir Hachinski, to declare: 'The concept of dementia is obsolete' (Hachinski, 2008). He goes on to say:

> It combines categorical misclassification with etiologic imprecision. … Not only do individual sets of criteria fail to work, but none is used universally … Cognitive impairment is not a threshold, but a continuum, affecting different cognitive domains, at different rates, from different causes. All this occurs on the evolving background of aging. To achieve clarity of thought and unity of purpose, current thinking about these disorders must shift. (*ibid.*)

What, then, would be the alternative? Hachinski (2008) partly writes to encourage awareness of the fact that many 'dementias' have a vascular component, whereas currently Alzheimer's rules the diagnostic roost. Hence he commends the notion of 'vascular cognitive impairment'; beyond this he commends 'cognitive impairment, cause uncertain' as a way to keep open the possibilities for treatment. Trachtenberg and Trojanowski (2008) also favour 'cognitive impairment' or 'neurocognitive impairment', although they also advocate replacing 'dementia' with the word 'disease': 'frontotemporal disease' rather than 'frontotemporal dementia'.

Kurz and Lautenschlager (2010) feel that the 'theoretical construct' underlying the concept of 'dementia', 'continues to be valuable both for diagnosis and management, irrespective of the designation attached to it'. They go on to say, 'it directs clinicians to an underlying chronic, irreversible or progressive brain disease'. They admit that there are some limitations to the diagnostic role of the concept, because it overlooks the possibility of reversibility, does not do justice to people presenting with milder symptoms and seems biased towards the dominant paradigm of memory impairment in Alzheimer's disease. But they also see the concept as having an important role in terms of patient management. This is in large measure because it encourages attention to 'a complex pattern of impairments including cognition, behavior and functional ability, all of which are likely to worsen over time'. So the concept helps to alert us to the broader 'interpersonal concomitants' of dementia, which give it a social dimension. Nevertheless, although they see value in the concept, they feel there is a need for a change in terminology.

> The word 'dementia' is not an appropriate term for a syndrome which in current medical usage encompasses a broad spectrum of clinical severity including minor degrees of intellectual impairment. The label is particularly gloomy and distressing for patients who are still capable of managing their lives, and it causes reluctance in physicians when establishing and disclosing the diagnosis. (Kurz & Lautenschlager, 2010)

These authors do not, however, suggest an alternative to 'dementia', although they note that re-labelling has occurred in Japan, where the word for dementia, *chihoushou*, which suggests 'simple-mindedness', has been replaced by *ninchishou*, which stands for 'disease of knowledge and understanding' (*ibid.*). This is said to have had a positive effect, albeit the emphasis on the cognitive manifestations of dementia seems to remain.

Changing words

Another possibility would be to call dementia 'progressive cognitive impairment'. One objection to this is that from a relatively young age most of us have progressive cognitive impairment, although most of us do not suffer on this account. At an older age, progressive cognitive impairment is the statistical norm (Anderson, 2008). This objection could be met by adding a designating type to the overall description, e.g. 'progressive cognitive impairment—vascular type'. A difficulty with this response would be that it would logically have to entail the possibility of a diagnosis of 'progressive cognitive impairment—normal variant'. But this would be to give normal ageing a diagnostic category; that is, to make it a disease. Now, whether or not there is a biological cut-off between normal and abnormal ageing, to suggest that normal life from early middle age (if not earlier) is a disease is counter-intuitive except in the mildly humorous sense that life itself is said to be a terminal condition!

The more substantial objection, relevant to Hachinski (2008), to Trachtenberg and Trojanowski (2008), as well as to the change in Japanese terminology noted above (Kurz & Lautenschlager, 2010), is that 'progressive cognitive impairment' does not do justice to the non-cognitive aspects of dementia. It epitomizes the 'hypercognitive' tendency of society (Post, 1995). It ignores the fact that some forms of dementia present with changes in personality (e.g. frontotemporal dementia), movement disorders (e.g. Huntington's disease), or other neuropsychiatric symptoms (such as visual hallucinations in dementia with Lewy bodies), and some forms of dementia need not be progressive (e.g. those caused by vitamin deficiencies or normal pressure hydrocephalus). In addition, it does not suggest the holistic impact of dementia, as if weight loss and swallowing problems are adequately explained by the rather clean notion of 'cognitive impairment'. The cleanliness of the notion does not adequately describe the complex dysfunctions that characterize dementia in its terminal stages. These diseases are not summed up by a description that seems to bestow privilege on a mere loss of points on an intelligence test.

It appears, therefore, that the word 'dementia' is a conceptual mess. There are (at least) two ways to think about nosology, as either reflecting aetiology or as reflecting symptoms. Describing symptoms by diagnosis in a systematic, objective way is necessary when the aetiology is uncertain: bipolar affective disorder would be an example. Alternatively, a diagnosis of prostate cancer points to the pathological cause and explains why the man might have urinary symptoms, cervical lymphadenopathy (a possible sign of metastases) and back pain (a possible symptom of similar spread). Part of the difficulty in dementia is that the word implies a mixture of pathological causes and symptoms. If we are told that someone has dementia we instantly know that there will be lesions in the brain, even if we do not know their nature; and we might anticipate various symptoms, from memory problems to difficult behaviours. However, whereas 'prostate cancer' immediately tells us the nature of the problem and 'bipolar affective disorder, current episode hypomanic' (ICD-10 Code F31.0; WHO, 1992), whilst not suggesting a cause, does give us a good indication as to how the person is likely to be presenting, 'dementia' does neither. The cause could be anything from alcohol to a brain tumour and the manifestation could range from seeming normal (at least to a casual acquaintance) to being very dependent and aggressive. It really does seem as if 'dementia', the word, serves no useful (scientific or clinical) purpose and may, moreover, simply encourage stigmatizing attitudes.

In many ways this should be seen, not as a mark of failure, but as a sign of progress. We no longer have to lump together all those with 'cognitive failure, chronic behavioural dislocation and psychosocial incompetence' (Berrios, 1987) because the aetiology of the dementias is now so much better understood. This is not to say that the ultimate cause of all dementias is known, but nor is this true of most diseases (except— in a sense—those with a purely genetic cause). But the brain pathology of the dementias *is* largely known. This suggests that it should be possible to stick to categorical (aetiological) diagnoses based upon the underlying pathology. This conclusion, however, is premature. Parking this premature conclusion for a moment, the search for an alternative to 'dementia' is only a search for the umbrella term.

In the USA, at the time of writing, the *Diagnostic and Statistical Manual of Mental Disorders* (DSM) is being revised and will appear in the next few years in its fifth edition (DSM-5). The Neurocognitive Disorders Work Group has decided, partly on the basis of some of the points I have mentioned (stigma, the fact that dementia was too closely modelled on Alzheimer's disease, and so forth), to move away from the use of the term 'dementia'. Instead, they propose to talk of 'Major Neurocognitive Disorders' (see www.dsm5.org [accessed 22 March 2010]). This seems sensible in that it faces the problem. But the suggestion that this is the term that should be adopted is mostly bedevilled by the joint introduction of a new term: 'Minor Neurocognitive Disorders'. Just like Mild Cognitive Impairment (MCI), 'Minor Neurocognitive Disorders', which would include MCI, seems to be an uncertain diagnostic label, which raises all the issues to do with the boundary between normal and abnormal that I shall shortly discuss. The term 'Major' is problematic in two ways therefore: first it cries out for a 'Minor' form, whereas it can be questioned whether the minor form is a form of a disease; secondly, it sounds alarming! Of course we do not wish to give false hope, but some people may never progress beyond mild dementia and it would be stigmatizing to be told that you have a 'major' disease, albeit a mild form. Furthermore, if (as is suggested) we can have reasonable certainty that the 'minor' form is likely to progress to the 'major' form, then we give false hope in any case when we tell people they have a 'minor' form of the condition. We should do away with 'major' and 'minor' and try to be clear (pragmatically) about when a person has or has not acquired the condition. The question about a precursor condition is another question and should not influence the main question about the nomenclature for the conditions that we know to exist. My inclination is also to speak of 'dysfunction' rather than 'disorder', partly because my judgement is that 'disorder' is more stigmatizing, but also because it is possible to have dysfunction without disorder: perhaps I have some cognitive problems, but I compensate and thereby avoid 'disorder'.

So, there is a group of conditions, characterized by neurocognitive dysfunction, that are acquired (i.e. you are not born with them), that are usually chronic and progressive (but not always), which affect the brain globally, causing a variety of symptoms and signs indicative of higher cortical dysfunction, even if sub-cortical structures are also involved. But we need to be cautious. First, although medical textbooks have usually described dementia as 'global', meaning it affects more than one area of the brain, it is not actually global, it is distributed or diffuse.[1] Secondly, although it is a brain disorder, so too is a condition such as multiple (or disseminated) sclerosis (MS); people with MS can develop dementia, but we need to be able to mark the difference between these conditions. Similar points could be made about other syndromes such as schizophrenia. So the reason to commend the notion of '*neuro*cognitive' dysfunction is because this recognizes that dementias can present with symptoms other than cognitive (e.g. hallucinations, movement disorders) and can lead to a variety of physical problems (e.g. dysphagia, contractures), which are none the less connected with the nervous system more generally, whilst at the same time acknowledging that it is the cognitive symptoms that mark out these conditions.

If an umbrella (syndromal) term is required, therefore, my suggestion would be: 'acquired diffuse neurocognitive dysfunction'. It could be argued that 'chronic' is required to differentiate these conditions from acute states, such as delirium. However, since elements of delirium (e.g. a fluctuating conscious level) form part of the diagnosis of a dementia (i.e. dementia with Lewy bodies) and since fluctuating cognition can be seen in vascular dementia too (Thomas, 2008a), the clear blue water between delirium and dementia is in any case muddied. Why not include 'delirium' as a subcategory under the umbrella term? Why not add, in the description of the syndromal diagnosis, that these conditions (i.e. the dementias in contradistinction to delirium) are often (but not invariably) progressive? And the heading 'acquired diffuse neurocognitive dysfunction' need not preclude the possibility of sub-cortical conditions.

When all is said and done, this is merely a nosological term. In theory, it need not be a diagnosis that is given to patients. People might well talk in terms of the syndrome, but surely patients really want to know the nature of the particular pathology. This term, acquired diffuse neurocognitive dysfunction, would be more a way of explaining to people the nature of the problem, rather than the cause of it. The syndromal description does not commit us to a particular treatment approach. It simply allows a group of conditions, which share some common features, to be classified together, which is likely to have benefits in terms of research and public policy.

Hence, we might wish to content ourselves with the following position. The syndromal diagnosis would be 'acquired diffuse neurocognitive dysfunction'. The specific (aetiological) diagnoses would differentiate between Alzheimer's, vascular, Lewy body, frontotemporal, Creutzfeld-Jakob, Huntington's, human immunodeficiency virus (HIV), alcoholic, and so forth. If the aetiologies of these conditions become more refined or precise, the aetiological diagnosis can be adapted, but the condition would still be an acquired diffuse neurocognitive dysfunction. As suggested by Trachtenberg and Trojanowski (2008), the word 'dementia' could be replaced by 'disease' where necessary. Hence a person might have 'Lewy body disease' rather than 'dementia with Lewy bodies'—a move which in itself is likely to reduce stigma. Occasionally, where the disease manifests primarily in other ways, it might be that the syndromal diagnosis would have to be used, e.g. 'HIV acquired diffuse neurocognitive dysfunction'. Let us, for a second, accept that this solves the problems of nomenclature. To return to my main theme, it does not solve the problem of values!

Values and diagnosis

In fact, there are two big problems. The first is to do with the premature conclusion I parked above, namely that we could stick to categorical diagnoses based upon underlying pathology. The second brings into question the whole concept of disease in connection with dementia.

The difficulty with categorical diagnoses based on putative pathology is that the differences between the types of dementia at the pathological level are not clear-cut; nor indeed is there a clear distinction between normal and abnormal. Thus, in the most recent edition of a leading textbook, we read: '... the individual pathological components typical of [Alzheimer's disease] brains all occur to some extent in normal ageing ... Ischaemic brain lesions often coexist with those of [Alzheimer's disease] ... Within the spectrum of neurodegenerative diseases there is considerable overlap between Alzheimer's and Parkinson's diseases' (Nagy & Hubbard, 2008: 71–5). So, too, Holmes asserts: 'It is also increasingly clear that the spectrum of diseases that cause dementia, whilst often considered as separate disease entities clinically, have a great deal of overlap in their underlying pathogenesis' (Holmes, 2008: 104).

A large epidemiological study found that the majority of people living in the community who did not have dementia at the time of death still had Alzheimer's pathology or evidence of cerebrovascular disease in their brains (Esiri, Matthews, Brayne, &

Ince, 2001). In the textbook mentioned above, Anderson uses this to support her statement that, 'There appears to be no pathological or physiological marker that clearly distinguishes between elderly people with and without dementia' (Anderson, 2008: 33–4). She goes on to consider cognitive differences between 'normal' and 'abnormal': 'Such findings provide strong support for the continuum hypothesis in which 'normal ageing' and 'dementia' are seen as lying along a continuum of cognitive decline in old age …' (Anderson, 2008: 34).

She cautions that this should not be taken in a simplistic way to suggest that Alzheimer's is just a matter of accelerated ageing, because not all ageing leads to Alzheimer's. Nonetheless, she accepts that 'the overlap between normal ageing and Alzheimer's disease remains a problem' (*ibid.*). This is because, 'the mechanisms of biological ageing and age-related brain pathologies are hard to differentiate' (*ibid.*). There is plenty of room for conceptual confusion here. It certainly would be too simplistic to say that the evidence of a continuum meant that everything was one, as if ageing could be called a disease or all diseases could be called normal!

Part of the problem as identified by Anderson (2008) is that the difficulty in differentiating between normal ageing and pathology, 'sits alongside the view . . . that ageing is nonetheless a multifactorial phenomenon' (*ibid.*). But why should it not be the case that ageing is multifactorial and that *this explains* why it is difficult to differentiate between normal and abnormal? In a chapter intended to review the empirical work on cognition and ageing, perhaps it cannot be expected that Anderson should have worried too much about the conceptual arguments. She suggests, however, an important argument about whether it is better to undertake research into ageing itself, in order to understand the roots of age-related diseases, or whether we are best off pursuing separate research, as hitherto, into the specific diseases. But the concern running through this discussion is to do with values.

We want to be able to say two specific things: first, that this *is* a disease; secondly, that it is *this* disease and not that one. In terms of cognitive function and neuropathology, it turns out that both assertions are problematic. But the answer to the problems will not be arrived at by uncovering more facts; it has to be accepted instead that evaluative decisions have to be made. I shall pursue this point by considering the Nun Study.

The Nun Study

The Nun Study started in 1991 and has involved 678 Catholic Sisters of the Order of Notre Dame in the United States of America (USA), who were aged between 75 and 102 years when the study began (Snowdon, 2003). By 2002, the oldest surviving participant was 107 years old. In addition to background details about lifestyle, the nuns have undergone annual assessments of their physical and cognitive function. They also agreed to brain donation after death and by the end of 2003 it was expected that there would be about 400 completed neuropathological evaluations (*ibid.*). In reviewing the enormous amount of data available to the researchers, Snowdon comments, 'Given nearly the same location, type, and amount of neuropathologic lesions, participants in our study show an incredible range of clinical manifestations, from no symptoms to severe symptoms' (*ibid.*). For instance, in those with mild Alzheimer's pathology at post mortem (Braak & Braak (1991) staging one and two), 58% did not have memory impairment; and even in those with severe pathology (Braak & Braak staging five and six), 8% demonstrated no memory impairment (Snowdon, 2003).

Three things, *inter alia*, can be said about these findings. First, they *do* show a strong tendency to support the claim that the pathology is causally related to the manifestations of the disease (Riley, Snowdon, & Markesbery, 2002). As the neurofibrillary pathology spreads from the entorhinal cortex to the hippocampus and thence to the neocortex it becomes increasingly likely that the person will show evidence of dementia. Secondly, however, the Nun Study suggests that there are protective factors, to do with the social environment, nutrition in earlier life, education and intellectual stimulation, and so forth. Thirdly, it suggests that other insults to the brain, in addition to the Alzheimer's pathology (chiefly vascular damage, but potentially trauma or deficits in terms of nutrition or education) might explain why in some cases the Alzheimer's pathology becomes potent (Snowdon, 2003). It remains the case, however, that the pathology on its own is not enough to say whether or not someone has Alzheimer's disease, even if the degree, location, and type of pathology might be indicative. This does not, of course, mean that people lack the manifestations of Alzheimer's disease, which, remember, can be characterized as 'cognitive failure, chronic behavioural dislocation and psychosocial incompetence' (Berrios, 1987). It does mean, however, that a further sort of judgement is required. Is it a judgement that could be helped by knowing further facts?

The Nun Study has led to some elegant papers demonstrating how artificial neural networks can be helpful as a way to understand how pathology and other aetiologically relevant factors interact (Buscema et al., 2004; Grossi, Buscema, Snowdon, & Antuono, 2007). Artificial neural networks, which use non-linear statistical models, are based on the functioning of the brain. In this sense they are non-linear, because (just as in the brain) it is never the case that one input (or neuron) interacts neatly with just one single output (neuron). Instead, the norm is much more likely to involve multiple interactions between neurons, with positive and negative feedback, and different inputs carrying different weights depending on the strength of their previous interactions, which may decrease or increase the number of times the neurons fire, bearing in mind that the neurochemicals released when the neurons are activated can be either excitatory or inhibitory. With this degree of complexity, where indeed the surround has such a powerful influence, any change at any place will mean that the whole system may well be affected, at least to a degree. And even a small change suggests the possibility that things will subsequently be different. Artificial neural networks employ models with this level of sophistication to create a context that is more like a real brain. One of the possibilities that ensues from this complexity is that the model can demonstrate 'learning' (the scare quotes this time are used to mark my scepticism concerning whether this is learning in exactly the same sense that human beings learn, even if it approximates to it). By applying 'Back Propagation' learning rules the artificial neural network can be trained to apply different weights to particular inputs depending on the outputs. Having trained the system, it can then be used with new data to see if it achieves the outputs that are required or predicted.[2]

Buscema et al. (2004) were able to demonstrate how demographic data, cognitive and functional, or clinical variables derived from each of 117 participants during the last year of life could, using an artificial neural network, predict the presence of brain pathology. They were able to show that these variables were better at predicting the count of neurofibrillary tangles in the neocortex and hippocampus than the load of neuritic plaques, which (they suggested) strengthened the hypothesis that neurofibrillary pathology may represent the major pathological explanation of cognitive impairment in Alzheimer's disease. Grossi et al. (2007) looked at neurofibrillary tangles and neuritic plaques in the neocortex and hippocampus of 26 clinically and pathologically confirmed cases of Alzheimer's disease and 36 control subjects where, despite large differences in terms of the mean number of lesions counted in each group, there was 'a substantial overlap in the range of lesion counts'. In other words, in an individual case it probably would not have been possible to say whether or not the nun had Alzheimer's disease. They showed that artificial neural networks were able to predict which were normal and which had Alzheimer's in 100% of cases, even when they focused on the more difficult cases, where the Alzheimer's was mild. Their conclusions were, once again, that neurofibrillary tangles, especially in the cortex, were crucial in the neuropathology of Alzheimer's disease, and that, despite the complexity, artificial neural networks were able to differentiate cases from controls.

This is a remarkable achievement, although the usual caveats are required concerning the relatively small number of cases used, the uniqueness of the population, and so on. The reason for considering the Nun Study was because of the conclusion I reached above, that the pathology on its own is not enough to say whether someone has Alzheimer's disease, even if it might be indicative. These studies, contrariwise, using artificial neural networks, suggest it might be possible. The beauty of neural networks is that they mirror (at least to a degree) the ways in which we think and make judgements ourselves. And, of course, we do make decisions ourselves about whether or not people have dementia and these decisions are based on an array of data, which include demographics, clinical behaviour, cognitive tests and, ultimately, neuropathological findings.

The key thing to note, therefore, about artificial neural networks from the point of view of my discussion is that the networks must be *trained*. The essential thing is that 'the desired output (target) is defined, for each input vector, prior to the start of the learning process' (Buscema, 2004). Hence, in response to my question concerning the sort of further judgement required to distinguish normal from abnormal, the answer is that at root this judgement must be evaluative. In order to be able to say that this *is* a disease and that it is *this* disease and not that one, evaluative decisions have to be made, which might well include the idea that there is 'cognitive failure, chronic behavioural dislocation and psychosocial incompetence' (Berrios, 1987). 'Failure', 'dislocation', and 'incompetence' all suggest value judgements. Furthermore, these are judgements that have to be made in the world, that is, the social and cultural world. The remarkable thing, then, is that in this 'organic' condition, where—in contrast to other psychiatric diagnoses—there is definite neuropathology, it is not only facts that underlie the diagnosis, but facts *and* values.

Back to values

We might wish to go one step further and claim that the values come first in the sense that there must initially be the idea that there is something wrong. Fulford's (1989) analysis seems particularly apposite. The focus on disease, which is usually regarded as a physical or biological malfunctioning of the organism, is only part of the story; Fulford (1989) argues that a 'full field' perspective is required. The half of the field characterized by disease tends to focus on facts and failures of function. This is exactly as we have seen in dementia. But the other half of the field sees 'illness' rather than 'disease'. 'Illness' is a value-laden concept and, in Fulford's terms, translates as 'failure of action'. A person may have a disease, but still be able to do things; once the person is ill, he or she becomes unable to act; or, at least, the person's actions become dysfunctional by some standard.

It is easy to imagine someone with cancer who does not know that they have the disease. Perhaps they become symptomatic, that is, *ill*; or perhaps the cancer is found by chance and the person either continues to behave normally, or starts to behave dysfunctionally as a result of being given the diagnosis. All of this is quite easy to account for on Fulford's model. It makes perfect sense to say that someone has a disease like cancer but is not appearing in any way unwell or ill; and it is understandable that someone might feel unwell or ill having been given the diagnosis of cancer. In dementia, things are different.

What we have seen is that the mere presence of neurofibrillary tangles or neuritic plaques is not enough to say that someone has the disease, even if the count of tangles and plaques is very high. These lesions, which occur in dementias other than Alzheimer's disease (as well as in 'normal' brains), are called 'pathological' partly because they are not present in young brains, but mainly because of the correlation with the emergence of cognitive dysfunction and behavioural difficulties. In those cases where there is an absence of 'bad' cognitive function or behaviour and yet the lesions are present, it only makes sense to call the lesions 'pathological' as a way to highlight their absence in (what are considered to be) 'normal' brains. So, unlike the case of cancer, it is more problematic in dementia to talk of the person *having* the disease in the absence of symptoms. Since many 'normal' older brains have both tangles and plaques (Nagy & Hubbard, 2008: 69), it is difficult to say that someone *has* the disease purely on account of the 'pathology' (where the scare quotes signify that the pathology is here non-pathological, which would be an exceptionally odd thing to say about cancer cells, especially if they were extensive!). As we have seen, the temptation to think that further facts (e.g. about ischaemic damage) would save the day, if it were coupled with the ability to process like an artificial neural network, is false in the absence of the prerequisite training in the application of appropriate value judgements. There is, therefore, an evaluative problem at the level of thinking about dementia as a disease.

In addition, there is a problem thinking about it as an illness, because (above) I have talked about the person's actions becoming dysfunctional *by some standard*. Now, it makes perfect sense to ask what standard is to be used. It is equally reasonable to reply that failures of action in dementia are obvious: this person often cannot recall any new information for more than a few minutes, and this one walks in the street in the middle of the night half dressed. Well, even if these judgements about dysfunction are reasonable, which they may well be, an evaluative standard has still been applied. In the one case, you have to be able to remember new information for more than a few minutes and, in the other, you are not meant to wander half dressed in the middle of the night.

These problems are driven by values. In later developments of his work, Fulford has expounded the notion of values-based medicine (Fulford, 2004), or values-based practice (Fulford, Thornton, & Graham, 2006), which provides both a theoretical framework and a practical approach to common clinical dilemmas. The *cognoscenti* will recognize that I have already accepted the first principle of values-based medicine (VBM), namely the 'two-feet' principle, that decisions in medicine, including to do with diagnosis, depend on values as well as on facts (Fulford, 2004: 208–9). My discussion of these issues in the last few pages has also implicitly been drawing on the second principle of VBM, the 'squeaky wheel' principle. This states: 'We tend to notice values only when they are diverse or conflicting and hence are likely to be problematic' (Fulford, 2004: 209).

To return to the issue of cancer, there were no problems because we can usually take it for granted that everyone would agree: people tend to want the lump or lesion removed. Even here, however, there are sometimes marked disagreements (my use of cancer as a non-problematic example was, in fact, ironic), which then show the diversity and conflicting nature of the values at issue. When someone decides to live with their cancer and refuse treatment, or perhaps to adopt some form of 'alternative' treatment, then there are the conflicting values so keenly described by Michael Gearin-Tosh (2002) in his book about his own diagnosis of myeloma. Similarly, it might be thought that values are shared in connection with dementia, but—as in the case of cancer—in fact they are not. Perhaps they once were, but now we move into the territory of the third principle of VBM: '[s]cientific progress, in opening up choices, is increasingly bringing the full diversity of human values into play in all areas of health care (the "science-driven" principle)' (Fulford, 2004: 212).

We have already seen that great advances in our understanding of the neuropathology of Alzheimer's disease have, in a sense, increased the uncertainty. We might at one stage have said with certainty that someone had 'senile dementia', but now we have to differentiate between various types of dementia in the knowledge that, at the neuropathological level, there is considerable overlap between the dementias and between dementia and normality. Scientific advance now allows us to treat the cholinergic deficit that is regarded as a key feature of Alzheimer's disease. Depletion of the neurochemical, acetylcholine, which acts as a messenger between cells, has been known to correlate with pathology and problems with memory for many years now (Perry et al., 1978), which has led to the development of the acetylcholinesterase drugs that prolong the action of the remaining acetylcholine in the brain and improve cognitive function, at least to a degree (Wilcock, 2008). But this requires a clinical judgement as to whether the person has Alzheimer's disease, for which the drugs are licensed, or some other form of dementia, such as vascular dementia, for which they are not. A degree of complexity emerges which was not present before and which requires some evaluative decisions. For instance, a diagnosis of vascular dementia is usually confirmed by lesions revealed by brain scans, which would count against the use of the drugs. But such lesions are ubiquitous, so the clinician has to make a judgement based on a host of factors, one of which involves interpreting the brain scan (or more usually the (often briefly written) report) to decide whether it suggests the type or quantity of vascular lesions that might make a diagnosis of vascular dementia secure. But these diagnoses are rarely secure in a factual sense, because they also include this element of evaluative judgement.

Yet we might still have thought that at least the notion of 'cognitive impairment', which forms the basis of the dementia diagnosis, was itself secure and objective enough to be pinned down in an authoritative way by objective tests. Not so!

In a large, prospective, cohort study designed to investigate the prevalence of cognitive impairment using a range of published classification systems, Stephan et al. (2007) found that prevalence varied greatly, depending on the system of classification being used. Remember that these systems have been developed in response to a scientific drive to be more objective. The prevalence rates varied, when the systems were applied to the 2640 individuals in the study, from 0.1% to 42%. In addition, concordance across the systems was poor: no individual was consistently classified as impaired, and only 10.7% were always classified as not mildly cognitively impaired. 'Thus', the researchers suggested,

> ... the overall lack of convergent validity raises the questions of what exactly each set of criteria is mapping and why they are so different, especially within categories (i.e., normal or pathological). (Stephan et al., 2007)

They went on to say:

> In the rush to create new categories of disease, the clinical utility of each of these different systems may have been compromised. Criteria are generally poorly defined and difficult to apply in research and clinical settings, do not take into consideration individual trajectories, and have been criticized for removing the element of clinical judgment, which itself is unstable across or between individuals and clinicians and across time and culture. The importance of making the distinction between cognitive impairment as a result of pathological brain aging versus a clinical condition or a normal consequence of aging becomes important, especially when deciding therapeutic options. (*ibid.*)

The authors do not make the point that evaluative decisions are required, but it is clear that the scientific urge to be objective by providing clear criteria has, at least, simply led to an increase in choice, which necessitates evaluative decisions between the different systems of classification. At its worst, the study might be regarded as showing a confusing mess: depending on which system is being used, your chances of being declared cognitively impaired will range from one in a thousand to almost 50:50. More positively, we might wish to conclude from this study that it demonstrates the importance of values—the values that underpinned the development of the different systems of classification, the values that lead a clinician to choose one over another— and the need for clear conceptual thought and the right approach to these conditions, one that is cognizant of values diversity.

Summary

We shall return to the principles of VBM at various points in the course of this book. But now we need to take stock. Epidemiological facts about dementia expose the need to make value judgements about such things as treatment and research. More than that, facts are value-laden. As Hilary Putnam has suggested, the distinction between facts and values, 'is at the very least hopelessly fuzzy because factual statements themselves, and the practices of scientific inquiry upon which we rely to decide what is and what is not a fact, presuppose values' (Putnam, 1981: 128).

So we see the world according to the *versions* of reality that we tell or hold dear. Our view of the world is always from somewhere, so that what we see has a particular background or surround.

Definitions of 'dementia', therefore, that place cognitive function centre-stage, give us one view. But there are also social and personal views of dementia.[3] And there are arguments that the word itself is too stigmatizing, so that even if the construct needs to survive, the nomenclature needs to change. 'Acquired diffuse neurocognitive dysfunction' could be the syndromal diagnosis, with individual categorical diagnoses being picked out by terms that suggest pathology. At this point, however, we run up against the problem that the pathology itself does not provide clear-cut categories. There is, indeed, no clear line to be drawn between normal and abnormal; not unless, that is, we move away from the pathology back into the world in order to accommodate our background evaluative judgements. What we encounter in the world, especially as scientific understanding increases, is values diversity. Then we are left with differences: different versions, different views, different backgrounds, different contexts from which will emerge different evaluative judgements. (Remember it was Wittgenstein who once suggested he might use a line from *King Lear* as a motto for *Philosophical Investigations*: 'I'll teach you differences' (Rhees, 1981: 171).) We seem, therefore, to be in an *uncertain* world, which is strange, given that acquired diffuse neurocognitive dysfunction—at one level—is such a concrete construct.

And this takes us back to the poet Keats, who (in a letter to his brothers in December 1817) praised the idea of 'negative capability': '… that is when man is capable of being in uncertainties, Mysteries, doubts, without any irritable reaching after fact & reason …' (Keats, 1990: 370).

Poetic expression of this is famously found at the end of his *Ode on a Grecian Urn*:

'Beauty is truth, truth beauty',—that is all
Ye know on earth, and all ye need to know.

(Keats, 1990: 289)

Perhaps, then, the place we have arrived at is this: thinking through dementia will involve something that is (at least) akin to aesthetic judgement, where we shall have to accept a degree of uncertainty and doubt. The surround, we might say, suggests something more mysterious, because the questions raised will be about human life in the human world. The dilemma of acquired diffuse neurocognitive dysfunction concerns our response to the uncertainty: whether we can live with it in the way we might live with a valued aesthetic experience, or whether we need to interrogate it in the search for its underlying factual basis.

Truth, we might have thought, should be the impetus to scientific work, the value that underpins it. But against this position, which he describes as a 'strawman', Putnam asserts: '… *truth is not the bottom line*: truth itself gets its life from our criteria of rational acceptability, and these are what we must look at if we wish to discover the values which are really implicit in science' (Putnam, 1981: 130).

In Part III of this book, I shall discuss in some detail different models of dementia. In essence, the question will concern the 'criteria of rational acceptability' for each of the models. To anticipate, I shall find the models wanting, because what is required is something more mysterious (in one sense) than any model can give us. What is required, according to the Wittgensteinian analysis I shall offer in Chapter 4, is a transcendental account. Recall Wittgenstein writing in his early work: 'Ethics is transcendental' (TLP: §6.421); but we shall come to this in Chapter 2. For now we are left with the conclusion that thinking through the facts of dementia reveals a host of evaluative concerns and uncertainties. It is not apparent that further facts will clear away these uncertainties. Keats's negative capability is what is required as we contemplate the context of dementia. If the ethical dilemmas with which we started looked as if they might be susceptible to bureaucratic, procedural, or legal solutions, this is because of a failure to grasp the mystery raised by acquired diffuse neurocognitive dysfunction. It is a mystery that arises not from within the brain, but from the surroundings that situate the person *qua* person. And so it is to the concept of the person that we shall now turn.

Endnotes

[1] I am grateful to Professor Steve Sabat for discussing this point with me and for suggesting 'diffuse'.

[2] Further technical details with respect to these studies are contained in Buscema et al. (2004); further background discussion of the potential for such connectionist models can be found in Park and Young (1994).

[3] I have used scare quotes around the word 'dementia' throughout much of this chapter. This has mostly been to emphasize that the discussion has been about the term itself. But it will by now be apparent that I believe we require new terminology, e.g. acquired diffuse neurocognitive dysfunction. In the rest of the book I shall mostly avoid using scare quotes for 'dementia'; but they should be understood, because 'dementia' (as a concept) is increasingly problematic, if not vacuous.

Chapter 2

The SEA view of persons

A vast similitude interlocks all, …
All souls, all living bodies though they be ever so
different, or in different worlds, …
All nations, colors, barbarisms, civilizations, languages,
All identities that have existed or may exist on this
globe, or any globe,
All lives and deaths, all of the past, present, future,
This vast similitude spans them, and always has spann'd,
And shall forever span them and compactly hold and
enclose them.
(*On the Beach at Night Alone* from *Sea-Drift* in *Leaves of Grass*;
Walt Whitman, 1995: 196–7)

Introduction

The Romantic cry of Keats in a letter to his friend Benjamin Bailey, dated 22 November 1817, 'O for a Life of Sensations rather than of Thoughts' (Keats, 1990: 365), can easily be linked to the philosophical romanticism that is sometimes associated with Immanuel Kant's (1724–1804) criticism of reason. A disdain of reason and rationality over and against intuition and a more mystical appreciation of nature and the world may be characteristic of Romanticism generally, but the exact link between Kant's philosophy and the British Romantic poets (or Romanticism in general) needs to be treated with caution. For instance, Duffy (2005) has trenchantly argued that Shelley's treatment of the 'sublime' needs to be understood in a broader historical context (of revolution, for instance) rather than rehearsed as if it were a reflection of Kant's transcendentalism (see also Berlin [1999] for a discussion of the link between Kant and romanticism). The message, in terms of understanding the influences that motivated British Romantic poets, is that the context has to be looked at broadly.

Be all this as it may, in the United States of the nineteenth century, Walt Whitman (1819–1892) was certainly influenced by the New England Transcendentalism of Ralph W. Emerson (1803–1882). This movement saw itself standing against the 'under-standing' that typified rational approaches to practical affairs and scientific knowledge. As in the case of British Romanticism, intuition and mysticism were the preferred ways of reasoning, which allowed our oneness with nature to be seen and appreciated.

The links back to the conclusion of Chapter 1 should be obvious: the Romantic aesthetic impulse, the tendency to reject too great an emphasis on purely cognitive capabilities (instead, Keats's 'negative capability' that tolerated uncertainties and mysteries), the inclination to see our natural connectedness and, therefore, to appreciate our contextual surround. These are the inspirations that led to Walt Whitman's poems that made up *Leaves of Grass*. But these features of Romanticism and (at least one understanding of) 'transcendentalism' also anticipate some of the conclusions of the present chapter. For we turn now to the idea of the person. And the notion I shall put forward is that the person can best be characterized as a situated embodied agent, where the similitude that embraces 'All souls, all living bodies though they be ever so different, or in different worlds' (Whitman, *op. cit.*) is to the fore.

The broad situated embodied agent (SEA) view of the person (Hughes, 2001) is conceived in opposition to, or perhaps as a development of, a more limited view that can be derived from Locke and Parfit, which I shall consider first. Then, before outlining the background to and expanding on the SEA view, I shall discuss some other considerations and views about personhood. To start with, however, I shall return to Kant and transcendentalism. This is for two reasons: first, the notion of the transcendental, as used by Kant, informs the later argument of Wittgenstein that I shall subsequently consider at greater length; secondly, Kant's view is both important in its own right and relevant to arguments about the nature of selfhood in dementia.

The transcendental

Transcendentalism refers to a variety of creeds. The most obvious sense of 'transcendental' is the one that suggests realities beyond those supplied by our senses. This can then take various forms and my aim here is certainly not to attempt a thorough survey of the field. Transcendental meditation is, for example, a technique by which people can, through the use of relaxation and mantras, leave behind (in a sense) the concerns of the everyday world and get in touch (in a sense) with deeper aspects of their being—aspects that go beyond the everyday. The same inclination is evident in the Romantic poets inasmuch as they were keen to explore the reality that could be apprehended through the emotions rather than through rational thought. Thus Keats, as we have seen, wishing to:

> Fade far away, dissolve, and quite forget
> What thou among the leaves hast never known …
>
> (*Ode to a Nightingale*, Keats, 1990: 286)

A similar sentiment can be found in William Wordsworth's (1770–1850) yearning for a form of primitive encounter with the world:

> This sea that bares her bosom to the moon; …
> For this, for everything, we are out of tune; …
>
> ('*The World Is Too Much With Us* …'; see Gardner, 1972: 507)

Elsewhere Wordsworth exalts the innocent apprehension of the world by the soul, which reveals something immortal:

> Hence in a season of calm weather
> Though inland far we be,

Our souls have sight of that immortal sea
Which brought us hither, …

(*Ode: Intimations of Immortality from Recollections of Early Childhood*;
see Gardner, 1972: 512)

A more overtly philosophical sense of the transcendental is suggested by those philosophers who have posited entities that must exist (in a sense) in some sphere, which can be rationally deduced if not empirically proven. Plato (427–347 BCE), for instance, suggests that our imperfect acquaintance with beauty or truth reflects a perfect, abstract, non-material reality of Forms beyond the world of sense perception:

… the highest form of knowledge is knowledge of the form of the good.

(Plato, 1987: 229 [Book VI, Part VII: 505a])

A little later in the discussion, which occurs at the end of the famous simile of the sun, Plato has Socrates speaking as follows:

'"The good therefore may be said to be the source not only of the intelligibility of the objects of knowledge, but also of their being and reality; yet it is not itself that reality, but is beyond it, and superior to it in dignity and power."

"It really must be miraculously transcendent," remarked Glaucon to the general amusement.'

(Plato, 1987: 234 [Book VI, Part VII: 509b–c])

The idea of transcendence—of things beyond reality—does, after all, seem a markedly esoteric concern and, therefore, one likely to cause a wry smile at least. But it is one that has been pervasive and not just in philosophy. The notion of a transcendent God, for instance, is one that is widely accepted.

Kant also had things to say about non-material objects, which could not be known by the senses. He defined a noumenon—as opposed to a phenomenon (something known by the senses)—as follows:

… a thing which can never be thought as an object of the senses, but only as a thing in itself (solely through pure understanding), … (Kant, 2007: 260 [B310, A254])

The intricacies of Kant's metaphysical views about the possibility of the transcendent reality of noumena need not detain us, except to note one thing. Part of the benefit of the notion of the noumenon for Kant was that it marked the limit of what could be known through the senses. None the less, our understanding, as opposed to our 'sensible knowledge', can extend to noumena, even though we cannot say anything more about them. Kant puts it in this way:

The concept of a noumenon is also necessary to prevent sensible intuition from extending to things in themselves; that is, in order to limit the objective validity of sensible knowledge. … But, after all, we cannot understand the possibility of such noumena, and the domain beyond the sphere of appearances is (to us) empty; … (*ibid.* [B310, A254–5])

The relevance of this will become apparent in later chapters, where the similarities to Wittgenstein's thought will be more obvious. Wittgenstein would have had little truck with the idea of noumena, but he had a lot to say about the limits of our language and the way in which these limits impose a boundary to intelligibility. In Wittgenstein's earlier work this thought is clearly evident:

> *The limits of my language* mean the limits of my world. (TLP: §5.6)

In Wittgenstein's later philosophy there is a greater readiness to accept the importance of testing the boundary.

> The results of philosophy are the uncovering of one or another piece of plain nonsense and of bumps that the understanding has got by running its head up against the limits of language. (PI: § 119)

Wittgenstein, in his later work, was much more inclined to accept the idea that things can be shown—which is partly a matter of seeing our way around in language—even if they cannot be said. But there *are* things that cannot be said with sense, because of the limits of our language. The importance of this will become more evident in Chapter 4 in the discussion of quietism derived from Wittgenstein. These ideas can, then, be seen as a development of Kant's thoughts about the transcendent.

Another understanding of the notion of transcendental (as opposed to mere transcendence) was central to Kant's thinking and important to establish, because (again) I shall use the notion in Chapter 4, even though I do not intend to pursue Kant's metaphysics much further. Kant states near the start of the *Critique of Pure Reason*:

> I call all knowledge **transcendental** which deals not so much with objects as with our manner of knowing objects insofar as this manner is to be possible *a priori*. (Kant, 2007: 52 [B25, A11–12])

A transcendental argument, therefore, will be one that looks at the pre-conditions for whatever is trying to be established. Kant's broader project concerned the bringing together of experience and reason. A transcendental argument considers what is presupposed for something, some experience in the world, to be the case; given that the experience in the world is genuine, if it is the case that the presupposition is necessary for this experience to be genuine, the presupposition must be true. For instance, Kant holds that space and time are the transcendental grounds of experience itself. We have experiences, but to have them requires, as a matter of a priori truth (i.e. not as a matter that is itself based on experience or any form of empirical fact), space and time. Space and time are presupposed by experience and it would be impossible to imagine being part of a world in which this was not the case: space and time are the grounds for the possibility of experience. We shall return to this notion later. But there is a particular use of this idea that is relevant to our discussion of selfhood in dementia: Kant's idea of the transcendental unity of apperception, which needs some explanation.

The term 'apperception' refers to the perception the self has of its own experiences. These perceptions in a self seem to have a unity and this unity is transcendental in the sense that there is a single 'I' that perceives the unified view. The 'I' is presupposed in order for there to be the unity that there is: the single view that self-consciousness must and does have. As Kant states:

> It must be **possible** for the **I think** to accompany all my representations: for otherwise something would be represented within me that could not be thought at all, ... (Kant, 2007: 124 [B131–2])

Kant goes on to say that he calls this 'pure apperception',

> ... because it is that self-consciousness which, by producing the representation, **I think** (which must be capable of accompanying all other representations, and which is one and the same in all consciousness), cannot itself be accompanied by any further representations. (Kant, 2007: 125 [B132])

He goes on to explain that it is a *transcendental* unity of self-consciousness because the many representations would not be *my* representations unless they belonged to one self-consciousness.

> What I mean is that, as my representations (even though I am not conscious of them as that), they must conform to the condition under which alone they **can** stand together in one universal self-consciousness, because otherwise they would not all belong to me. (*ibid.*)

Now, the reasons for discussing Kant's ideas were, first, because his notion of the transcendental informs my later argument and, secondly, because Kant's view, as well as being important in its own right, is also relevant to arguments about the nature of selfhood in dementia. Michael Luntley argues, using a broadly Kantian conception,

> ... that the erosion of certain basic cognitive capacities central to autobiographical memory amounts to an erosion of the self. (Luntley, 2006: 105)

He goes on to say that, 'it is an empirical matter whether or not severely demented patients display the relevant erosion of cognitive capacities', but the argument shows, 'that the very idea of loss of self makes sense' (*ibid.*). Later he says,

> ... on the conception of the self I exploit, the self is that which keeps track of things. More precisely, the self is the ground for the possibility of keeping track of things. ... When the capacity for keeping track of things has been eroded there is nothing left to constitute a self. ... The point is not that under such circumstances the subject fails to keep track of their own self, for on the conception I employ, the self is not something that is ever tracked. The self is always the tracker—the ground of the possibility of keeping track of things. So the erosion at issue in the case of severe dementia is not a failure to keep track of the self, but the failure to keep track of outer things. The self is not, on this conception, an inner thing that is tracked on analogy with outer things; it is the condition for the possibility of keeping track of outer things. When that goes, the self goes too. (*ibid.*: 105–6)

Luntley also talks of the need for a 'cognitive surround' to make certain utterances meaningful. Luntley is careful to point out that, even if the self is lost, this is not necessarily a reason to change our moral attitudes to people with dementia. It also seems important to pursue the point about whether, as an empirical fact, people with dementia do lose the requisite 'cognitive surround' and the ability to keep track. We have argued elsewhere that there is some evidence to suggest that the sort of losses that would undermine selfhood do not occur until at least late in the disease. (Aquilina & Hughes, 2006)

> Is it not the case, … that selfhood—what it is that makes us the individual human creatures we are—involves capacities other than the capacity to keep track? Are we not also beings with motivations, with longings, with conation, with desires, with strivings, with humour, with emotions, with attachments, even with love? And do not these characteristics go beyond cognitive abilities and mere sentience? And may they not (empirically) persist in some form even into the very last stages of dementia in such a way as to undercut the cognitive denial of selfhood? (Hughes et al., 2006a: 32)

We went on to argue that characterizing the transcendental self as 'the ground for the possibility of keeping track of things' seems to make the self too cognitive, whereas being a human person involves so many other things. None the less, it does seem that, according to Kant's view of the transcendental unity of apperception, it is likely that at some point loss of the self becomes a *possibility* in severe dementia. However, this is *only* because Kant's view is very cognitive: the key ingredient is the 'I think'. Yet is it not at least as reasonable to regard 'I feel' as the necessary ingredient? For, it still supplies the transcendental 'I', the a priori ground for a unified view. Furthermore, the 'I' cannot be without history: the presupposed unity must be a unity across time. The arguments which start to emerge in connection with this discussion of the transcendental unity of apperception will continue to echo in the rest of the chapter and beyond: to what extent is memory crucial? Is there more to a self than a bundle of experiences and thoughts of a certain kind? Does the embedding of the person in a historical and individual, but shared, narrative provide some sort of necessary corrective to the versions that undermine the possibility of selfhood?

The Locke–Parfit view

The philosophers John Locke (1632–1704) and Derek Parfit (born 1942) are separated by three hundred years. So it has to be questioned whether it is appropriate or fair to lump them together, as if they share a single view. The tendency they both show is that they emphasize the importance of memory and consciousness. This has immediate implications for our thinking about people with dementia, which is why I think it fair to deal with their views as if they are one. In any case, Parfit talks of his view as if it were a revision of Locke (Parfit, 1984: 205–6), so it seems licit to join the two names in this way. I have to admit, however, that my treatment of their philosophies will only be in sufficient detail to make the point I wish to pit against the SEA view of the person. (For further accounts of these and other relevant views in connection with dementia see Lowe, 2006; Matthews, 2006; McMillan, 2006).

In *An Essay Concerning Human Understanding*, Locke describes the person thus:

> … a thinking intelligent being, that has reason and reflection, and can consider itself as itself, the same thinking thing, in different times and places; which it does only by that consciousness which is inseparable from thinking, and … essential to it. (Locke, 1964: 211 [II. xxvii. 9])

The person is the being with thoughts, intelligence, reason, reflection, and consciousness. My 'thinking conscious self' is bound up with my body, but—as Locke makes clear by considering what happens if a person's hand is cut off (*ibid.*: 213)—it is the conscious self that is the person: 'without consciousness there is no person' (*ibid.*: 218 [II. xxvii. 23]). Locke makes an important distinction between 'man', on the one hand, and 'person' on the other. 'Man' seems mainly (but see below) to refer to the living human body, whilst 'person' is tightly tied to consciousness (*ibid.*: 217 [II. xxvii. 20]). But 'consciousness' for Locke is 'inseparable from thinking, and … essential to it' (*vide supra*). As these quotations make clear, according to Locke, to be a person is to be a being with these psychological attributes.

The subtlety of Locke's treatment of this topic, however, must not be underestimated. Gillett points to a more holistic interpretation, according to which Locke recognizes

> … an important (internal or conceptual) connection between embodiment and the rational or metaphysical subject as the bearer of mental and moral (and even spiritual) properties. (Gillett, 2008: 14)

This interpretation is largely based on Locke's statement, just before his discussion of personal identity:

> For I presume it is not the idea of a thinking or rational being alone that makes the idea of a man in most people's sense, but of a body, so and so shaped, joined to it; and if that be the idea of a man, the same successive body not shifted all at once must, as well as the same immaterial spirit, go to the making of the same man. (Locke, 1964: 211 [II. xxvii. 8])

There are two points to make. First, if this passage refers to the same thing as the subsequent passages, then Locke is contradicting himself hugely. But, secondly, it is clear this is not the case, because here he talks of 'the idea of a man', whereas in the later passages he is talking about a mixture of 'personal identity' and 'what *person* stands for'. (The two senses of being the *same* person that might be implied by this distinction—being quantitatively the same and being qualitatively the same—also need careful handling; cf. McMillan, 2006; Radden & Fordyce, 2006) As Locke's later discussion makes plainer, he sees a real distinction and would allow the possibility of the same 'man' being a different person:

> But if it be possible for the same man to have distinct incommunicable consciousness at different times, it is past doubt the same man would at different times make different persons. (Locke, 1964: 217 [II. xxvii. 20])

Locke later talks of 'person' as a 'forensic' term, which stresses its ties to notions of agency and moral responsibility. Hence we can see that, although normally, for Locke, the 'idea of a man' involves body and spirit, at a conceptual level 'person' is tied to 'consciousness'. In terms of moral standing, it looks like 'person' wins, in which case we are thinking solely of the intelligent, rational, conscious self, not the body as such. But Gillett (2008) is surely right, in fairness, to point out the background holism of Locke.

This Lockean view of the *person*, however, stands behind the views expressed by Parfit (1984: 205–7). For instance, Locke writes: 'as far as this consciousness can be extended backwards to any past action or thought, so far reaches the identity of that person' (Locke, *op. cit.*: 212 [II. xxvii. 9]). Parfit, like Locke, feels that a person's identity is maintained by the links that join the person's former state with his or her present state. In Parfit's terminology, what is meant by personal identity is covered by 'psychological continuity', which involves 'psychological connectedness':

> *Psychological connectedness* is the holding of particular direct connections. *Psychological continuity* is the holding of overlapping chains of *strong* connectedness. (Parfit, *op. cit.*: 206)

Just as Locke suggested, my personal identity now is linked to my personal identity last week by psychological continuity between the two. Psychological continuity is maintained by memories, but also by beliefs, desires and by intentions that are later enacted (*ibid.*: 205). The consequence of these views is that personal identity is not what matters for Parfit, but psychological connectedness and/or continuity. This is called by Parfit '*Relation R*'. It is this that matters, but the psychological connectedness and/or continuity in *Relation R* must have 'the right kind of cause' (*ibid.*: 262).

Elsewhere Parfit (1987) admits to being a 'Bundle Theorist', according to whom:

> … we can't explain either the unity of consciousness at any time, or the unity of a whole life, by referring to a person. Instead we must claim that there are long series of different mental states and events—thoughts, sensations, and the like—each series is unified by various kinds of causal relation, such as the relations that hold between experiences and later memories of them.

Bundle Theorists, according to Parfit, are all those who have not believed, as 'Ego Theorists' have, that the person is some separately existing thing, 'distinct from our brains and bodies, and the various kinds of mental states and events' (*ibid.*). David Hume (1711–1776), as a successor of Locke, would be counted as a Bundle Theorist. He wrote that when he attempted to find *himself*, he found 'nothing but a bundle or collection of different perceptions' (Hume, 1962: 302 [I. iv. section vi]). Later Hume wrote:

> Had we no memory, we never should have any notion of causation, nor consequently of that chain of causes and effects, which constitute our self or person. (*ibid.*: 311)

It is clear, therefore, that for Parfit, no less than for Locke (or Hume), to be a person is just to have certain psychological states. For Parfit it is the connections between these states that amount to the person; or, rather, there is (strictly speaking) no person, there are just bundles of connected memories, intentions, thoughts, sensations, beliefs and desires, which achieve continuity. When we speak of persons we speak of no more than these continuing and connected psychological states. Inasmuch as this is a cognitive view of personhood, this is the point against which I shall pit the SEA view. An alternative, more charitable, interpretation (and note that there is some room for the possibility of sensations in Parfit's Bundle) is that the Locke–Parfit view can be expanded to the SEA view. What is required is a broader conception of 'psychological states', which I shall pursue in Part II of this book, and certainly a conception that is broader than just one type of memory.

The human person

I want now to start the process of expanding the field in which the concept of 'person' should be discussed. (We need a broader surround than simply a cognitive one.) This will not amount to a comprehensive rehearsal of every philosophical position that can be adopted concerning personhood. Instead, I shall cherry-pick to sustain the move, in the next section, to the SEA view of the person, which will in turn be supported by my later Wittgensteinian analysis.

The first important point, as the late Sir Peter Strawson (1919–2006) said, is that to see each other as persons, 'is a lot of things, but not a lot of separate and unconnected things' (Strawson, 1959: 112). The concept of a person marks these connections. We can say of the concept 'person' much the same as Wittgenstein says of 'number':

> … we extend our concept of number as in spinning a thread we twist fibre on fibre. And the strength of the thread does not reside in the fact that some one fibre runs through its whole length, but in the overlapping of many fibres. (PI: §67)

Wittgenstein accepts that boundaries can be drawn around our concepts, but this is 'for a special purpose'. He continues:

> Does it take that to make the concept usable? Not at all! (Except for that special purpose) (PI: §69).

Hence, the concept of a person is many sided, but none the less usable. Amélie Rorty notes that we want our concept of the person to fill a number of functions. Being a person, she suggests, means that we are taken seriously, with respect,

> … on grounds that can't be lost through illness, poverty, villainy, inanity, or senility. (Rorty, 1990)

She lists other functions that must be performed by the attribution of personhood: it has a legal function; it defines us as agents; and as social, interacting beings; it suggests norms which shape our lives; it reflects biology; and it encompasses a metaphysical stance towards human beings. She concludes that there cannot be a *single* concept of the person. Similarly, Adam Morton (1990) states:

> … there is nothing we can analyse and define and present as '*the* concept of a person'. Nothing whose sense will settle in advance the status of all the beings we might value for the reasons we value human persons. For these values are not any single thing.

Now, whilst the point that the concept of a person is multifarious is certainly correct, it is not clear that the concept becomes thereby problematic in the everyday setting, any more than the concepts 'number' or 'game' are problematic. As Wittgenstein suggests, concepts such as these can have a humble and everyday use (cf. PI §97 and §116). Indeed, the concept 'person' seems not to have caused Wittgenstein much worry at all. In *The Blue Book* Wittgenstein discussed the possibility of defining the identity of a person by his memories. If the memories were different on even days than they were on odd days, would that mean that there were two persons in the same body? Wittgenstein didn't really mind how the use of the word 'person' went under such circumstances. But under the ordinary circumstances we have the ordinary use.

> For the *ordinary* use of the word 'person' is what one might call a composite use suitable under the ordinary circumstances. (BB: 62)

This is true; usually we use the word without a problem. But problems can arise. Pointing out that the word can be used broadly to accommodate a variety of alternatives, that it refers widely, is a useful reminder. The problems really come when attempts are made to pin the term down by a definition to something more circumscribed. Those who are worried by the suggestion that there is some single concept of a person may well have other concerns in mind. For instance, for Morton it is the suspicion that 'person' is to be characterized in too parochial a fashion:

> The reason why we can easily give the concept of a person definiteness that it does not really have is simple. We import into it more biologically parochial characteristics of human beings than we realize. (Morton, *op. cit.*)

As Mary Midgley points out in a chapter called 'Is a dolphin a person?' the word 'person' really means a mask, which is part of a drama; and there is no direct etymological link to the concept of the 'human being' (Midgley, 1996: 109). The problem is that 'person' has been used ('for a special purpose') as a way to exclude some people (slaves and women, for instance) and some other creatures (such as dolphins) from certain sorts of concern and consideration. It has been argued, similarly, that people with severe dementia are not persons. Thus, Dan Brock (1988):

> I believe that the severely demented, while of course remaining members of the human species, approach more closely the condition of animals than normal adult humans in their psychological capacities. In some respects the severely demented are even worse off than animals such as dogs and horses who have a capacity for integrated and goal directed behavior that the severely demented substantially lack. The dementia that destroys memory in the severely demented destroys their psychological capacities to forge links across time that establish a sense of personal identity across time and hence they lack personhood.

So there are ways in which the use of this concept, as if there is a straightforward move to be made from loss of memory to loss of personal identity to loss of personhood, might be pernicious. Moreover, we can see that these thoughts are firmly based on Parfit's (1984) notion of 'psychological continuity':

> ... I believe it is not merely a judgment that the severely demented suffer a tragically diminished quality of life, though at least that much is of course true. Instead, the point is that the severely demented have been cut off from the self-conscious psychological continuity with their past and future that is the basis for the sense of personal identity through time and which is a necessary condition of personhood. ... Personhood involves criteria of psychological continuity that are not satisfied in the severely demented. (Brock, *op. cit.*)

The antidote to this way of thinking is to take a broader view of what constitutes a person, which might be considered a better tactic than simply denying its status as a concept or changing it somewhat randomly. In connection with 'person', Rorty spoke of 'respect' and Morton mentioned 'values'. Part of the usefulness of the concept is that these fibres—respect and values (we might add dignity)—run through it, add to its strength, and should not be discarded.

Pace Morton (*op. cit.*), Wilkes, for one, sees no problem with parochialism:

> Speciesism ... is not unreasonable; ... there just are no persons around who are *not* human beings, and so on solid inductive grounds we are usually justified in assuming that all

humans are persons and vice versa. That is, membership of the species *homo sapiens* is taken to be, and usually is, all we need to validate the ascription of personhood, and hence there is an a priori reason for adopting the 'person stance' to them alone. (Wilkes, 1988: 97)

There might, then, be reasons for accepting the link between 'person' and 'human being' and Wiggins (1987) suggests that these reasons are not just empirical but conceptual:

… if the references of 'person' and 'human being' were theoretically discernible but … determined the same principle of individuation,

then the word 'person' will inevitably,

… lean secretly for its support upon our understanding of 'human being' and our empirical notions of what a human being is. (Wiggins, 1987)

It is not completely clear to me how successful this argument really is in the face of those, like Morton and Midgley, who point to the possibility of there being a loose correspondence between persons and human beings. Midgley also commends the notion of 'emotional fellowship' rather than 'intellectual capacity' and she continues by commending the relevance of,

… sensibility, social and emotional complexity of the kind which is expressed by the forming of deep, subtle and lasting relationships. (Midgley, 1996:116)

In brief, we may wish, 'for a special purpose', to ascribe these possibilities to non-human beings.

Rather than pursuing this argument directly, it seems more fruitful to consider the context in which we use these concepts. We use them in particular contexts for specific, but multifarious, tasks. Smith recognizes, too, that it would be difficult to define the notion of a person independently of our understanding of human beings. Hence, he commends the notion of a 'human person' understood 'in terms of … its manner of living' (Smith, 1990).

A 'human person' is someone who stands in the Right Relation to one of us:

… someone stands in the Right Relation to count as one of us if he shares with us enough of the human world constituted by interpersonal relationships. (*ibid.*)

Examples of such relationships are:

Jack and Jill talk to each other, habitually read each other's face and gestures, go out together for meals, lend each other books, laugh together at the same silent movies, occasionally play tennis, and so on and so forth—these and many more are the sort of ties which go to make up the web of our shared human life. (*ibid.*)

So there is a way of unifying the multifarious strands of the concepts 'person' and 'human being' by considering instead the notion of the 'human person'. For Smith, this notion is one that is embedded in the shared human world. It is in this world, after all, that people wish to show respect and concern to persons along the lines set out by Kant's 'practical imperative':

Act in such a way that you treat humanity, whether in your own person or in the person of another, always at the same time as an end and never simply as a means. (Kant, 1993: 36 [429])

This does rather depend, however, on there being a shared set of values around the notion 'human person', which (if Brock's (1988) view is anything to go by) cannot be presumed. We cannot simply stipulate that we are speaking of a *human* person, because there are still questions that can be raised about what a *person* is; and, as we have seen, although mostly the term can be used unproblematically, it can be defined in ways that do cause problems. We are back to Fulford's (2004) second principle of values-based medicine (the 'squeaky wheel' principle): we tend to notice values when they are diverse.

Perhaps all we can say is that in this context, this way of living, there is something captured by the Kantian moral sense of person, which is to do with sensibility and certain types of relationship as Midgley (*op. cit.*) suggests. This thought supports Strawson's claim that the concept of 'person' is primitive (Strawson, *op. cit.*: 101). Wiggins characterizes this claim thus:

> ... if you did not have the idea of a person from the start, then you could never build up to it from any combination of ideas like those of experience, material body, and causality. (Wiggins, *op. cit.*)

Explanations act as elucidations of the concept; there is no sense in which a definition of 'person' will suffice. The claim of primitiveness has the status, says Wiggins, of an elucidation,

> —or a reminder, helpful only to those who already know what a person is, of *what* it is that they already know. (*ibid.*)

The elucidation, according to Strawson, is that,

> ... the concept of a person is the concept of a type of entity such that both predicates ascribing states of consciousness [P-predicates] and predicates ascribing corporeal characteristics [M-predicates], a physical situation &c. are equally applicable to a single individual of that single type. (Strawson, *op. cit.*: 101–2)

Strawson argues there is a type of P-predicate,—'going for a walk', 'coiling a rope' etc.—that mostly involves a characteristic bodily movement rather than a particular sensation or experience. So, in these cases, bodily movements will dominate the ascription of such P-predicates to others. (*ibid.*: 111)

With this in mind, Wiggins suggests that, although we cannot build *up* from the notion of persons as objects of biological inquiry to the notion of persons as subjects of consciousness, yet we may be able to build *down* from persons as subjects of consciousness to persons as biological objects. Just as P-predicates can involve bodily movement and gesture, so the concept of the person inevitably seems to involve, or rely on, the concept of the human being. Wiggins finally argues that the actual *extensions* of the two concepts, 'human being' and 'person', will coincide, whether or not we wish to say that the concepts themselves coincide (Wiggins, *op. cit.*). This allows, in other words, the truth of Midgley's (1996: 109) point, that these just are different concepts, but suggests that all the occurrences of what we mean by a human being will turn out to be a person. It is still possible, however, that we shall wish to designate some things as persons that are not human beings, as in law (when e.g. corporate bodies might be regarded as 'legal persons' [Midgley, *ibid.*]), but this is decidedly an example of what Wittgenstein called a 'special purpose' (PI: §69).

This discussion of the concept of person leads to four points.

- First, the analysis of 'person' requires attention to the embedding context or surround, because the concept plays a role and functions as it does on account of this context; I shall later show how the Wittgensteinian analysis of intentional mental states supports this broader view.

- Secondly, personhood—as usually understood and used—is situated, or embedded, in the *human* world. Whilst there are undoubtedly good reasons for cautioning against the use of a restrictive notion of 'person', it is still the case that there are empirical and conceptual ties between being a person and being a human being. The ties can be broken and stretched, but the concept of the person typically reflects a human perspective and involves the concept of the human being.

- Thirdly, ascriptions of P-predicates can involve the ascription of bodily movements and behaviours. Persons are beings to whom states of consciousness *and* corporeal characteristics can be ascribed. That is, being a human person, embedded in the context of the world, involves physical embodiment. It also entails (at least potentially) the agentive ability to participate in the practices that help to constitute what it is to be a human person.

- But appreciating this point requires, fourthly, an appreciation of the multifarious nature of personhood.

According to Wiggins:

> … there is no clear limit to what concerns and capacities and perception[s] and feelings … we shall have to credit our fellows with if we are to make sense of them. (Wiggins, *op. cit.*)

In other words, the possibilities for persons cannot be circumscribed. This is true at both an empirical and at a conceptual level. Empirically, we are constantly amazed by the interests, abilities, and concerns of human beings *qua* persons. This amazement often (perhaps typically) has an aesthetic quality: creativity in art, in science, in sport, in adversity, is often what hooks our amazed attention. There seem to be no limits to the possibility for amazement: 'Now I've seen everything!' actually means 'Now I've seen one more thing I didn't ever expect to see!' Conceptually, once 'person' is seen in its full surround it becomes obvious that the uniqueness of every context—derived from history and experience, as well as from biology, psychology, and the social environment—entails that the possibilities for persons seem infinite. Of course, this is not to say that living human beings *qua* persons can do anything. We are bounded (by birth and death for example), which contributes to our standing as individuals with a personal identity (Lesser, 2006), because (among other things) the boundedness helps to establish the nature of the narrative drama that makes up a life. But there are two particular points. First, the considerations that limit the possibilities for an individual life do not thereby limit the possibilities for other lives, so the concept need not be circumscribed on this account. Secondly, the drama that involves *personae*, albeit there is a beginning and an end, nevertheless contains uncircumscribed possibilities: we genuinely do not know what is going to happen and (almost) nothing would surprise us, whilst at the same time what happens is a surprise.

> To treat a person like a thing (like a billboard), what I have to be ready to do is to suspend all the impulses on which that uncircumscribed possibility precisely depended. (Wiggins, *op. cit.*)

And it is for this reason that treating a person like an object is so objectionable. As Kant recognized, we have to treat humanity, 'always … as an end and never simply as a means' (*vide supra*).

Having set out a philosophical background I shall now proceed to describe the SEA view of the person. This amounts to what Wiggins (*op. cit.*) described above as an elucidation or a reminder. I am characterizing personhood by way of elucidation, not defining it. It is not a definition because it is open-ended. In keeping with the discussion above, the SEA view of the person is not circumscribed.

The situated embodied agent view

In its most general form, the SEA view suggests that psychological phenomena are properly understood only in a contextually embedded manner: they cannot be characterized independently of the situated context. This marks a major distinction between this view and the Locke–Parfit view. According to the Locke–Parfit view, a person is constituted *solely* by psychological phenomena. So this view is reductive of the notion of the person. Given the SEA view of the person, it is not possible to characterize psychological phenomena independently of an embedding context. So psychological phenomena are given a broad construal and the notion of the person is not reduced, but enlarged.

To anticipate, we are partly situated as human beings by our bodies, which place us in an historical context of time and place. So, in contradistinction to Locke, the concept of the (human) person *constitutively* involves what Anscombe called the 'living human body'. At least on account of its being droll, it is worth giving the full quotation:

> … when I use the word 'person' here, I use it in the sense in which it occurs in 'offences against the person'. At this point people will betray how deeply they are infected by dualism, they will say: 'You are using "person" in the sense of "body"'—and what they mean by 'body' is something that is still there when someone is dead. But that is to misunderstand 'offences against the person'. None such can be committed against a corpse. 'The person' is a living human body. (Anscombe, 1975: 60–1)

We have already rehearsed the possibility that 'person' might refer to other entities for 'a special purpose', but the context of the human person is clearly implied here and in this context the embodied nature of persons does refer to the human body. But non-human persons will, according to this characterization, also need to be embodied in some form or other. The Trinitarian God, for instance, is still embodied in the (incarnate) person of Jesus; and other manifestations of God (as Father or as Holy Spirit) require bodily forms from a burning bush (*The Bible* Exodus 3:4) to a dove (*The Bible* John 1:32).

In addition, the situated context involves human agency, because we act and interact with our surroundings in a way that can be interpreted humanly. According to

Toulmin (1980), having 'goals, purposes, and interests of their own', makes human beings 'agents', and gives them a certain moral status. This agency is manifest in bodily action and used in historical and cultural human contexts.

Gillett points to this sort of conception of the person too:

> The understanding of mental predicates is tied to our experience of identifiable and re-identifiable persons. ... To know that I am a person is to know that I fit, in a reciprocating way, into those forms of life where interpersonal discourse occurs. (Gillett 1992: 38–9)

For Gillett it is true both that our conception of persons is closely tied to psychological phenomena and that to be a person is to be situated in a certain form of life. Gillett later derives some support for his view from clinical practice:

> A pertinent empirical fact is that a person with dementia retains a sense of self and the ability to make simple verbal and conceptual judgements longer than other cognitive abilities and well after spatio-temporal orientation is lost. ... self-identification and self-awareness go hand in hand with making judgements. (*ibid.*: 45)

He argues that making judgements conceptually entails 'I' thoughts. It seems right to notice that even those diagnosed as having severe dementia, in showing mastery of some concepts, can thereby be reaffirming a sense of self. Gillett goes on to say:

> ... the 'I' who is a subject of conceptual thought is not only the 'subject of these conscious states', but also an objectively identifiable and engaged member of a set of conceptual practices, or, as Strawson puts it, 'a person among others'. (Gillett, *ibid.*: 39; reference to Strawson, 1959: 103)

Now this sort of conception of the person is in contrast to the Locke–Parfit view, which takes no account of other persons, or the context in which a person is embedded. I shall later argue that intentional psychological states have to be understood constitutively as potentially involving others on account of their normative nature. As I shall suggest, our mental states at least require the potential involvement of other people and the world. But if it is correct to argue that psychological states can be understood constitutively as culturally and historically embedded, then the situated view of the person is supported. If persons are regarded as agents, personhood cannot simply be conceived as consciousness, for consciousness must be embodied in order to act. As Strawson (*op. cit.*) suggested, it is both P-predicates and M-predicates: states of consciousness involve corporeal realization.

I shall now consider the elements of the SEA view in more detail.

Situatedness

The notion of a situated self stresses context and the external factors that go to make up a person. Luntley suggests, 'We become situated selves when we acknowledge the existence of principles of substantive rationality' (Luntley, 1995: 188). This notion of 'substantive rationality' is to be cashed out in terms of our 'sensibilities', by which Luntley implies,

> ... our capacities not just for feeling, but for knowing what must be done and how to deliberate about it. ... sensibilities that provide perspectives on human goods, purposes and our sense of what makes life worth living. (*ibid.*: 195).

Luntley allies his thoughts to those of Taylor, who considers that a crucial fact about a self or person is that we are not selves in the way that we are organisms,

> ... we are only selves insofar as we move in a certain space of questions, as we seek and find an orientation to the good. (Taylor, 1989: 34)

Taylor asserts that a basic condition of making sense of ourselves is, 'that we grasp our lives in a *narrative*' (*ibid.*: 47). He uses this conception to counter the Locke–Parfit view of the person. For Taylor, human persons as selves,

> ... exist only in a certain space of questions, through certain constitutive concerns. ... And what is in question is, generally and characteristically, the shape of my life *as a whole*. (*ibid.*: 50)

Taylor rejects the Parfitian notion that there are successive selves. Rather, 'there is something like an a priori unity of a human life through its whole extent' (*ibid.*: 51). He accepts that this is not quite true, because we can imagine cultures in which a conceptual split could (in theory) be made between the younger and older person, but there is no such cultural understanding in our world: 'It runs against the structural features of a self as a being who exists in a space of concerns' (*ibid.*). So, again, persons are situated in a 'space of concerns', but also in a narrative. Understanding a person must now involve an understanding of the narrative in which they are embedded.

MacIntyre also suggests that the notion of the unity of the self 'resides in the unity of a narrative which links birth to life to death as narrative beginning to middle to end' (MacIntyre, 1985: 205). He suggests that,

> ... the histories of individual agents not only are, but have to be, situated, just because without the setting and its changes through time the history of the individual agent and his changes through time will be unintelligible (*ibid.*: 206–7)

MacIntyre then emphasizes,

> ... that what the agent is able to say intelligibly as an actor is deeply affected by the fact that we are never more (and sometimes less) than the co-authors of our own narratives. (*ibid.*: 213)

He, too, criticizes the Locke–Parfit view of personal identity. According to MacIntyre, both empiricists and analytical philosophers have failed to see that,

> ... a background has been omitted, the lack of which makes the problems [of the connections between psychological states and events and strict personal identity] insoluble. That background is provided by the concept of a story and of that kind of unity of character which a story requires. (*ibid.*: 217)

One danger in the way that Taylor sometimes puts things is that he seems to allow that a conception of past or future is constitutive of the self. For example,

> In order to have a sense of who we are, we have to have a notion of how we have become, and of where we are going. (Taylor, 1989: 47)

This suggests, however, that the self requires psychological continuity, in which case the Parfitian argument takes hold. But this is clearly not Taylor's intention and, elsewhere, he has made it clear that the exercise of the sort of capacities to which he refers must be a possibility in principle, if not in fact:

> A person is a being who has a sense of self, has a notion of the future and the past, can hold values, make choices; in short, can adopt life-plans. At least, a person must be the kind of being who is in principle capable of all this, however damaged these capacities may be in practice. (Taylor, 1985: 97)

The importance Taylor has attached to the notions of 'embodied agency and social embedding' (Taylor, 1995: 169) means that the concept of a person is tied to external contextual factors, which become themselves constitutive of our conception of the person.

One final reflection on the notion of persons as situated beings is that it is an idea contained in the characterization, by Martin Heidegger (1889–1976), of the human existent (*Dasein*) as 'Being-in-the-world'. Not only is it a necessary feature of *Dasein*, but also this embeddedness means that *Dasein* is, '. . . bound up in its existence with the Being of those entities which it encounters within its own world' (Mulhall, 1990: 110). As Heidegger puts it:

> There is no such thing as the 'side-by-sideness' of an entity called '*Dasein*' with another entity called 'world'. (Heidegger, 1962: 81)

Our acquaintance with other humans is also a matter of 'Being-with' and this raises the possibility that our encounters in the world require what the late Hans-Georg Gadamer (1900–2002) referred to as 'pre-understanding' (Gadamer, 1960). There is a transcendental argument here: certain prerequisites are presumed in our encounters in the world. Specifically human encounters involve significance or meaning as part of what it is for things to be understood. This parallels the Wittgensteinian thought (which will emerge in Part II) that understanding meaning is a matter of grasping a practice in a form of life (cf. PI §§ 238–42).

Embodiment

There is a straightforward sense in which I know what it is to be a body. To be a body means that I am susceptible to causal (including pathological) processes, including those that lead to acquired diffuse neurocognitive dysfunction. But, in addition, to be a body means that I occupy a space and, as a matter of fact, I share that space with others: hence Heidegger's notion of 'Being-with' (*Mitsein*) (Heidegger, 1962: 149–63). Moreover, through my body I impinge on others, physically and verbally. So, how I communicate is a matter of my embodiment. The space occupied by our bodily selves and others is also a space in which values and concerns become known. This sense of 'public space' depends on having a language by which we can communicate our concerns. It is 'a common vantage point' (Taylor, 1985: 259). In other words, our bodily involvement (our situatedness) in the space of language amounts to an involvement with shared concerns and values.

Taylor discusses the notion of embodiment as an important antidote to 'monological consciousness' (Taylor, 1995: 168–73). According to this monological view,

> We are in contact with an 'outside' world, including other agents, the objects we and they deal with, our own and others' bodies, but this contact is through the representations we

have 'within'. ... But what 'I' am, as a being capable of having such representations, the inner space itself, is definable independently of body or other. (*ibid.*: 169)

This sort of consciousness leaves out 'the body and the other' (*ibid.*). Against this, asserts Taylor, philosophers such as Heidegger, Merleau-Ponty, and Wittgenstein, have seen the person (as an agent),

> ... not primarily as the locus of representations, but as engaged in practices, as a being who acts in and on a world. (*ibid.*: 170)

Not only does this description capture the sense of persons as being situated agents, but it also leads Taylor to emphasize the importance of embodiment. Thus,

> Our body is not just the executant of the goals we frame, nor just the locus of causal factors shaping our representations. Our understanding is itself embodied. That is, our bodily know-how, and the way we act and move, can encode components of our understanding of self and world. ... My sense of myself, of the footing I am on with others, is in large part also embodied. (*ibid.*: 170–1)

The importance of the body is also emphasized by Slors, who contends that:

> ... the body can play the part that is usually ascribed to the immaterial ego; it can provide a deeper psycho-biographical unity... (Slors, 1998)

Slors makes use of the notion of narrative to give a fuller account of psychological connectedness than that given by Parfit, because—according to the narrative view—connectedness must also take into account the content of psychological states *by virtue of which* successive states have meaning:

> Narrative connectedness between particular psychological contents, then, is a relation between contents such that one or more contents are a necessary prerequisite for another content's full meaning and the intelligibility of its occurrence. (*ibid.*)

According to this view, whereas our psychological lives may be 'gappy' (lacking in the ideal fluidity and coherence and occasionally disrupted by loss of consciousness), there is a 'basic narrative ... represented by our consecutive perceptual contents. (*ibid.*). And,

> ... successive perceptions acquire narrative coherence in virtue of the fact that we know them to be caused by one body's movements through a stable (not static) physical world with whose character and proceedings we are acquainted. (*ibid.*)

So we must be situated in the world, of which we have an understanding (or a pre-understanding), in order to make sense of our perceptions, which are, however, the bodily perceptions of a situated being. Hence,

> ... we cannot but think of our past experiences and thoughts as being had by a person-stage whose objective whereabouts were represented by perceptual contents that are narratively related to our present ones. (*ibid.*)

Slors links the embodiment of persons to their situatedness through the notion of narrative. In so doing he shows that the Locke–Parfit view needs to be expanded to take into account the reality of mental content, which acquires meaning (via narrative connectedness) within the context of the world in which the person, *qua* body, perceives and moves. It is not just *psychological* continuity. According to philosophers such as Slors and Taylor, the body cannot just be thought of as standing over against psychological states (P-predicates separate from M-predicates). It is inextricably involved in such states (P-predicates and M-predicates are ascribed together).

Let us return to Heidegger's idea of 'Being-with', or community, which is taken as a basic facet of human existence. Macquarrie put it this way:

> Just as there is no existence apart from a world, so there is no existence apart from other existents. But the other existent is not seen as an object within the world but as a *co-Dasein*. Thus we are related to the other existent not in terms of the 'concern' (handling, producing and the like) by which we relate to things, but in terms of a personal concern or 'solicitude' that characterizes relations between selves. (Macquarrie, 1968: 18)

Typically, on this view, we do not relate to other human beings in the same way that we relate to other *objects* in the world, that is instrumentally.

> Even 'concern' with food and clothing, and the nursing of the sick body, are forms of solicitude. But we understand the expression 'solicitude' in a way that corresponds to our use of 'concern' ... For example, 'welfare work', ... is grounded in Dasein's state of being as Being-with. (Heidegger, 1962: 158)

Earlier, Heidegger had made a distinction between the way in which we are close to the ground on which we walk, which is in contrast to the way in which instantly we are closer to another person, or human existent, further down the street (*ibid.*: 141). Of course, as he suggests in the later passage, we can *not matter* for one another, we can *pass each other by* and be *indifferent*, but these are (what he calls) 'deficient modes of solicitude' (*ibid.*: 158). As he says, from the point of view of Being,

> ... ontologically there is an essential distinction between the 'indifferent' way in which Things at random occur together and the way in which entities who are with one another do not 'matter' to one another. (*ibid.*)

Perhaps I just pass someone in the street and then cannot even recall having done so; but still, from Heidegger's viewpoint, what has just happened is not like when I walk past the postbox and can't remember it. As he says:

> Dasein's spatiality is not to be defined by citing the position at which some corporeal Thing is present-at-hand. (*ibid.*: 142)

Remember that, in Heidegger's terminology, being 'present-at-hand' describes the relationship I might have to things or objects that are just there and are of no real concern to me. But this, I think, brings us neatly back to the topic of embodiment. Just prior to this last sentence Heidegger wrote:

> If Dasein, in its concern, brings something close by, this does not signify that it fixes something at a spatial position with a minimal distance from some point of the body. ... Bringing-close is not oriented towards the I-Thing encumbered with a body, but towards concernful Being-in-the-world—that is, towards whatever is proximally encountered in such Being. (*ibid.*)

What I want to draw from this is: something about the essential importance of 'concern' and 'solicitude', used none the less in their technical sense in Heidegger (to which I shall return in Chapters 7 and 8); something about how, on this view, the nature of our Being, *as human beings*, gives us a different standing towards the world and towards each other, summarized perhaps by Martin Buber's (1878–1965) talk of *I-Thou* (Buber, 2004); and, therefore, something about the human body, which is almost seen as an encumbrance, and yet is the unavoidable, quintessential means by which we encounter and be *in-the-world*.

The world has a *significance*, to return to Charles Taylor's idea, for us *as* human beings because of *the nature of our being*, which is in large measure determined by our bodies, which just *are* our way of being-in-the-world. Taylor talked of 'bodily know-how' encoding 'components of our understanding of self and world' (Taylor, 1995: 170). Similarly, it is interesting to find Maurice Merleau-Ponty (1908–1961) writing:

> The body is our general medium for having a world. (Merleau-Ponty, 1962: 169)

What we see in Merleau-Ponty is a detailed examination of a physiological phenomenon—the bodily experience of perception—which nevertheless reveals the true nature of that physical phenomenon as being situated historically, culturally, psychologically, as well as physically. The body participates in the world and makes it *our* world. Hence, Merleau-Ponty states:

> In so far as I have a body through which I act in the world, space and time are not, for me, a collection of adjacent points nor are they a limitless number of relations synthesized by my consciousness, and into which it draws my body. I am not in space and time, nor do I conceive space and time; I belong to them, my body combines with them and includes them. (*ibid.*: 162)

Merleau-Ponty is often summed up by talk of the 'body-subject', an expression he seems not to have used himself, but intended to convey the idea that our subjectivity is embodied and our bodies are minded, as it were. This is the antithesis of Cartesian dualism. But, interestingly, Merleau-Ponty makes reference to René Descartes (1596–1650) and his letter to Princess Elizabeth of Bohemia (1618–1680), dated 28 June 1643. In this, Descartes is discussing for Princess Elizabeth the relationship of soul and body. It is quite instructive to look at what Descartes actually said. He is taxed to explain 'the notion of the union between body and soul'. In essence, having pointed out how the intellect can distinguish the body and the soul as distinct, he then says that we can conceive of them as *one* thing only when we suspend intellectual thought and resume normal, everyday life. This seems to anticipate 'ordinary language' philosophy: Wittgenstein for instance saying that it is only when we philosophize that certain things seem odd to us so that the treatment is to stop philosophizing; and it also could be regarded as anticipating those existentialists, like Merleau-Ponty and Heidegger, who emphasize the importance of our worldly encounters, of our being-in-the-world. Thus as Descartes states:

> ... those who never do philosophise and make use only of their senses have no doubt that the soul moves the body and the body acts on the soul; indeed, they consider the two as a single thing, i.e. they conceive of their union; for to conceive of the union between two things is to conceive of them as a single thing. Metaphysical reflections, which exercise the

pure intellect, are what make us familiar with the notion of soul; the study of mathematics ... accustoms us to form very distinct notions of body; finally, it is just by means of ordinary life and conversation, by abstaining from meditating and from studying things that exercise the imagination, that one learns to conceive the union of soul and body. (Descartes, 1954: 279–80)

This notion of the union between body and soul resonates with Merleau-Ponty's notion of the 'body-subject'. But the whole idea seems nevertheless profoundly anti-Cartesian: as if the body has some sort of primacy in terms of our way of being-in-the-world. Eric Matthews, in his book *The Philosophy of Merleau-Ponty*, put it this way:

> ... as soon as we recognize that the subject of experience is a 'body-subject', whose being is essentially *in* the world experienced, then the objects of our perception cease to be simply objects that causally affect our sense organs and constitute instead the 'field' in which we move about and act and to which we respond. The 'meanings' that we find in the world are no longer ... the simple result of causal processes ... Instead, they become part of a reciprocal relationship in which the human body becomes the expression of a certain way of being-in-the-world. (Matthews, 2002: 59)

The idea of the 'body-subject' allows that part of what I am is determined in a real sense by my genes. Who I am as a person appears through my body, even if my personality is also shaped by my situatedness in a particular socio-cultural environment and so forth. But equally, my body points in various ways because it is not just a body, it's a 'body-subject', with a subjective view and engagement with the world.

There is an interesting way in which our bodies instantly convey our subjective states. There is no gap between the bodily manifestation and our awareness of the bodily state that is betokened. Wittgenstein talked about cases in which we could be fooled, for example where we might not know whether someone was in pain, but his point is I think that cases of doubt are unusual. Normally, we can be in *no doubt* that someone is in pain. And the reason for this is not because they necessarily do something that rules out the possibility that they are pretending, it is because the rest of the proceedings help to give the meaning or show the *significance* of the bodily gesture, groan or movement. Similarly, the notion of the 'body-subject' helps to get rid of the idea that the inner is always hidden (as Wittgenstein once ironically put it). Instead, the subjective feeling of 'hope', for instance, is what it is on account of its *significance*, which in turn comes from the surroundings:

> The surroundings give it its importance. And the word 'hope' refers to a phenomenon of human life. (A smiling mouth *smiles* only in a human face.) (PI: §583)

Of course a person might keep their hopefulness hidden; but the first part of this quote makes the point that the subjective phenomenon has the significance it does only in its particular surroundings, without which it is not a manifestation of hope. If you are hopeful, there are certain other things that must follow *in the world*; whether or not they do *actually* follow is another question, but the meaning of 'hope' is as it is in the human world because of all that goes with it as a notion, because of all that we say and do in connection with our use of the word. And the second part of the quote, 'A smiling mouth *smiles* only in a human face', refers us clearly back to the human body.

The significance of a smile is what it is because it is a smile in a human face; which takes us to the famous Wittgensteinian comment:

> The human body is the best picture of the human soul. (PI: 178)

Drawing on Merleau-Ponty, in a paper entitled 'Ethnographic reflections on selfhood, embodiment and Alzheimer's disease', Pia Kontos suggests:

> The notion of embodied selfhood that is advocated refers to the complex inter-relationship between primordial and social characteristics of the body, all of which reside below the threshold of cognition, are grounded in the pre-reflective level of experience, and are manifest primarily in corporeal ways. (Kontos, 2004)

The point is that the significance of the body is 'primordial' or pre-reflective. This is why Merleau-Ponty cites Descartes's letter with approval. This idea reflects the earlier work of Edmund Husserl (1859–1938), whom Merleau-Ponty studied, and the central importance of the notion of the *Lebenswelt* or 'life-world'. Eric Matthews describes it thus:

> The life-world is the 'pre-given' or 'everyday' world that is the basis for all our theoretical constructions in the sciences and philosophy. ... It is the world in which we actually *live*, in which we must live before we can begin to theorize or try to explain it. (Matthews, 2002: 28)

Once again, parallels can be drawn between this idea and Gadamer's (1960) later notion of 'pre-understanding': that which is basic to our lives but which makes understanding possible.

Perhaps the point is made more strongly by considering the case of language itself. There are links to be made with the rule-following argument in Wittgenstein (which I shall discuss in Chapter 4), where it is shown that underlying the normativity of the language of intentional mental states lie practices, which are simply givens. To have language we simply have to have a certain form of life (*Lebensform*), or perhaps life-worlds, which ensure that our articulations have meaning, but which cannot themselves be justified: they have to be accepted. Kontos (2004) describes Merleau-Ponty's view in this way:

> ... words do not do their work by arousing representations associated with them. Language has inner content but the meaning of words is not entirely contained in the words themselves; rather, their meaning emerges from and is influenced by the contextual discourse. During interactions, words assume a gestural significance ...

The key point is that words require a background against which they have meaning and, in human life, this is provided by human bodies and society. Kontos spent some months observing in a home for people with dementia. Her work clearly shows the many and various ways in which individuals maintained their selfhood by way of their bodily movements. At an extreme, where language was lost, communication was mainly by gestures, which accompanied inarticulate noises and made them meaningful. In this sense there was 'gestural significance', an example of the body pointing, in this case to meaning. But the people being observed also showed evidence of 'bodily know-how', with various complex skills preserved.

Agency

But 'gestural significance' is also a sign of agency. An agent acts 'in and on a world' (Taylor, 1995: 170). Moreover, it is the human world and, therefore, it follows that the agent is both situated and embodied. Discussing the move from a linguistic turn to a practical turn in philosophy, Luntley suggests that this shift,

> … makes visible a concept of practice and practical know-how that is not merely descriptive of socially constituted ways of doing things. … it also offers a fresh way of understanding the practical and seeing how the practical is not rooted in the social, but in the way the individual relates in thought to the world. (Luntley, 1999: 344–5)

For, according to Luntley, the subject of thought is an agent, engaged with the world. Wilkes (1988) makes the point that Aristotle's account similarly stresses that the human being is active. Aristotle's human is an agent whose highest good is to live and do well. Thus,

> We become the people that we are by choosing, deciding, acting; we have the responsibility for shaping ourselves, our characters, and our lives. (Wilkes, 1988: 213)

Human beings are considered as active agents in the world, not as passive observers. An agent acts from a point of view and with a purpose. In the next chapter I shall discuss intentionality, which (in its technical philosophical sense) is said to be a distinguishing feature of states of mind, namely that they demonstrate 'aboutness'. When I think, I think *about* something, for instance. Intentionality is also sometimes described as 'ofness': my memories are intentional (in this technical sense) because they are memories *of* something. Now, there is a temptation to think that 'states of mind' are in the head—they are inner—but as we shall see, this is not the case. Intentionality helps to make the link between the inner and the outer. And the reason for raising this here is because human agency demonstrates intentionality, which

> … consists not in its capacity for surveying and rearranging its inner symbols, but in its capacity for acting in and manipulating the world. (Luntley, 1999: 319)

Our standing as creatures with the sort of mental life that we have entails that we act on and in the world in a particular way, with a particular sort of agency. Furthermore, actions will usually have causal effects and involve others, whether directly or indirectly. Agency involves context too.

It is these considerations that Taylor has in mind when he discusses agency. According to Taylor, Heidegger and Wittgenstein had to overcome the 'disengaged', 'view from nowhere' approach to the human being. They had to recover,

> … an understanding of the agent as engaged, as embedded in a culture, a form of life, a 'world' of involvements, ultimately to understand the agent as embodied. (Taylor, 1995: 61–2)

By 'engagement', Taylor implies that 'the world of the agent is shaped by one's form of life, or history, or bodily existence' (*ibid.*: 62). Later he suggests that the arguments against disengaged agency tend to emphasize the notion of a background or pre-understanding which make the actions of the agent intelligible, but which remain largely unarticulated (*ibid.*: 70). Thus, the notion of agency itself involves a sense both of the embeddedness and embodiment of human persons.

The idea that as human persons we are agents needs, on the face of it, neither much explication nor defence. We are people in the world who do things. The human world is as it is because of our agency. We might wish to add, as I have suggested above, that this form of agency carries the uniquely human characteristic of being informed or supported by our mental capabilities, which show intentionality and which also involve the complexities of language. We are not agents in the world like dogs and cats, because of our abilities for conscious self-reflection, and so on. Hence, given that this much about agency seems obvious, little more might need to be said. But I shall make two more comments.

First, the notion of agency is often linked to that of autonomy. We might, then, be inclined to define ourselves (quintessentially) as autonomous agents. This does, however, raise problems in the context of dementia, where people are often not able to act as autonomous agents. In a way this takes us straight back to the discussion in Chapter 1 about society's hypercognitivism (Post, 1995, 2006). To stress autonomy in this context is to stress rational decision making, which requires particular cognitive abilities.

The importance of autonomy as a defining principle in ethics goes back to Kant. As a matter of historical academic interest, however, Kant did not say what people might think he said. He talks of autonomy as being 'the sole principle of morals', but he is speaking of autonomy in a particular sense.

> Autonomy of the will is the property that the will has of being a law to itself (independently of any property of the objects of volition). The principle of autonomy is this: Always choose in such a way that in the same volition the maxims of the choice are at the same time present as universal law. (Kant, 1993: 44 [440])

This is some way from our contemporary notion of autonomy, which tends to emphasize self-determination in the sense that whatever I will I should be able to choose. In Kant's terminology this is not 'autonomy' of the will, but 'heteronomy' of the will. 'Heteronomy' suggests looking outside yourself for a guiding maxim—doing something because something else perceived as good will result, which would include maintaining one's reputation (*ibid.*: 45 [441])—but the point about 'autonomy' is not just that you look 'internally'. Rather, it is that when you do look inside yourself for the rational maxims that should guide specifically moral decisions, you should find (according to Kant's lights) the categorical imperative. We have already seen one formulation of the categorical imperative, which is fleshed out in connection with persons thus:

> ... rational beings are called persons inasmuch as their nature already marks them out as ends in themselves, i.e., as something which is not to be used merely as means and hence there is imposed thereby a limit on all arbitrary use of such beings, which are thus objects of respect. (*ibid.*: 36 [428])

The academic point, therefore, is that autonomy of the will was, for Kant, not a case of people being free to choose *simpliciter*, it was a matter of choosing in accordance with right reason as set out by the categorical imperative. But this is not *merely* an academic point, because it links to a theme that has run through this discussion of being a person. Numerous thinkers have pointed out the extent to which we are persons in a context of relationships. Our surroundings, naturally and conceptually, are social and relational. Hence, if agency raises the issue of autonomy, even if we do not buy into Kant's vision of the world, we should see this as *relational* autonomy. I shall say more about this later. For now we might simply note that autonomy—if it is relational—is limited by the surround. We cannot just do anything we want as agents; it would be more realistic to abide by the Biblical injunction ('the Golden Rule'), which is sometimes given as a further formulation of the categorical imperative: 'Do as you would be done by'. In this way, our agency is situated in a moral field where the 'emotional fellowship' of which Mary Midgley spoke is important (Midgley, 1996:116).

My second comment follows on from this. In discussing the different components of the SEA view, we should not forget they are synergistic. We are not just talking about agency, but about situated agency; it is embodied agency too. The importance of this is that it would be easy to presuppose that, in severe dementia, agency was inevitably lost. I shall have more to say about this later. But it is as well to remember the possibility that even in severe dementia there can be meaningful acts that suggest agency, in which case it is human agency because of the embedding context (Aquilina & Hughes, 2006). Recall Kontos (2004):

> ... meaning emerges from and is influenced by the contextual discourse. During interactions, words assume a gestural significance.

Thus, situated agency may take on various forms, but is none the less agency, even if under certain circumstances greater efforts at meaning-making are required (Widdershoven & Berghmans, 2006). If we are to show persons respect, however, to treat them as ends in themselves, if we are to exercise our Being-with in a fully authentic way, we shall need to recognize agency even in the person with dementia.

Summary

This chapter has been concerned with shedding light on the nature of personhood. The elucidation of what it is to be a person has required an extensive (but not exhaustive) survey. Starting with the views of Locke and Parfit, I have broadened the perspective by characterizing the person as a situated embodied agent. The SEA view depends on multifarious background lights, but the effect is essentially simple: the person is seen against an uncircumscribable surround.

Concluding remarks

In general, because of the overwhelming tendency to conceive persons in a narrow light, as self-conscious, rational, cognitive beings, with little attention to our emotional, social, volitional, historical, cultural aspects, and so on, talk of personhood in connection with moral status is usually fairly facile (Newson, 2007).[1] The agenda is mostly reductionist and problematic in that, as we have seen, the tendency is to argue that certain sorts of human beings are not persons. But this is because the literature is more keen to define what a person is (narrowly) rather than to encourage a broader elucidation of the possibilities for persons. Once such an elucidation is attempted and the non-circumscribable nature of personhood is grasped, so that the ground for the possibility of my perspective on the world is seen to be not just a transcendental ego, but an embodied and situated ego, then the view of the person becomes infinitely richer. The connection with moral status is also thereby made more secure and given more depth. The SEA view of the person provides a background context in which we can (later) discuss again issues around diagnosis, quality of life, best interests, and end-of-life decisions.

And, after all, the broader view of the self is nothing new.

> One's-self I sing, a simple separate person,
> Yet utter the word Democratic, the word En-Masse.
> Of physiology from top to toe I sing,
> Not physiognomy alone nor brain alone is worthy for the Muse, I say the Form complete
> is worthier far,
> The Female equally with the Male I sing.
> Of Life immense in passion, pulse, and power,
> Cheerful, for freest action form'd under the laws divine,
> The Modern Man I sing.
>
> (*One's-Self I Sing* from *Inscriptions* in *Leaves of Grass*; Walt Whitman, 1995: 3)

Endnotes

[1] I am not suggesting that Newson's discussion is facile! It is perfectly proper and competent. But the literature she reviews remains at one level and does not engage with the sort of (more metaphysical) issues I am touching on.

Part II

Mental states and normativity

Chapter 3

The mind and the world

Meanwhile the Mind from pleasure less
Withdraws into its happiness:
The mind, that Ocean where each kind
Does straight its own resemblance find;
Yet it creates, transcending these,
Far other worlds, and other seas;
Annihilating all that's made
To a green thought in a green shade.
(Andrew Marvell [1621–1678], from *The Garden*;
Gardner, 1972: 336)

Introduction

Once again, in Marvell's poem, we encounter the inclination to transcendence, to go beyond the mere pleasures of made objects in the world. Once again, it is the contemplation of the world of nature that moves the poet. But here it is specifically the mind that will bring about the transcendent experience. There is an element of metaphysical conceit in the idea that the mind is like the ocean: we might accept that the mind can be deep, but might not expect the mind to roll out and cover much of the world. It suggests, in a way that is also typical of the metaphysical poets, a strong philosophical stance, namely that just as (it was believed) the creatures of the sea mirror the creatures on the land, so too the content of the mind must have a 'resemblance'. But, the argument continues, the mind can do more than this: it also creates 'Far other worlds, and other seas'. So we have a picture of the mind having resemblances (presumably of the world) and the mind constructing other realities (transcendental worlds). The mind as an ocean conjures up a picture of its vastness, of something that cannot be pinned down, which is uncircumscribable perhaps.

All of which helps to make a connection with what has gone before and with what is to come. For the mind is critically important to our consideration of dementia, which after all means to be out of one's mind. Thinking through dementia, therefore, entails thinking about the mind. Moreover, my preferred way to think of acquired diffuse neurocognitive dysfunction is to think in the context of personhood, so the mental life of persons, how we construe mental content, will be critical, therefore, to our conception of the person. I want my thinking about the mind to support my thinking about the person; and I want my thinking about the person to inform and enhance my thinking about dementia.

In this chapter, I shall present some ways in which philosophers have understood the mind. I shall do this briefly, in part because the issues are too far-reaching and have been discussed in more detail by more competent philosophers.[1] But there is another reason for my being brief in terms of covering the issues in the philosophy of mind. The question I am really interested in is: what are the implications of these philosophical approaches for our understanding of acquired diffuse neurocognitive dysfunction? I shall outline classical dualism and three physicalist accounts of the mind (those of the Churchlands, Jerry Fodor, and Donald Davidson). I shall go on to describe the view of the mind that emerges in discursive psychology or social constructionism. Then I shall discuss the nature of intentional psychological states, before concluding with a discussion of the notion of the externality of mind. In each case I shall ask how the theory presented might be understood as relevant to acquired diffuse neurocognitive dysfunction. To make this question real, I shall reflect on the case of Miss Breen.

Miss Breen

She is 82 years old and has lived in her Elderly Mentally Infirm (EMI) nursing home for three years. She has a diagnosis of Alzheimer's disease. When she arrived she could speak with reasonable fluency, but now her language is disjointed, with only short snatches of sense. When I visit she is always walking around aimlessly. She is rather expressionless, but smiles when she is addressed by name. If you speak with her, she'll sit down and she tends to hold and stroke my hand in a way that seems to indicate an urgency or anxiety. In response to direct questions about how she feels, she always says that she is well, but she does this in a way that suggests a well-learned social response. At other times she smiles at me but also looks worried and says things like 'I can't' and 'What is it?'. Her constant walking has been having a bad effect on her pre-existing arthritis and sometimes she seems to be in pain. She is not at all keen to take her medication. She waves to me when I leave, but does not obviously recognize me when I visit a few months later.

Mind and world: the dualist background

The letter that Descartes sent to Princess Elizabeth on 28 June 1643, which I cited in Chapter 2, is highly significant because it shows the depth of the problem that faced Descartes. Dualism, as will be well known, is the theory that the mind and the body are entirely separate. Of course, the separation between what is immaterial (i.e. the mind or the soul) and material (i.e. those things that have extension in space, in other words shape, and other physical attributes such as weight and temperature) is also a distinction between the mind and the world. Descartes arrived at the distinction by his method of doubt. In brief, his argument was that he could doubt everything except the 'I' that doubts. He says, for instance, that if I convince myself that nothing exists then I must have existed otherwise there would have been nothing to do the convincing. He concludes, '… that this proposition "I am", "I exist," whenever I utter it or conceive it in my mind is necessarily true' (Descartes, 1954: 67). He goes on to say:

> … 'I am' precisely taken refers only to a conscious being; that is a mind, a soul (*animus*), an intellect, a reason … I am a real being, and really exist; but what sort of being? As I said, a conscious being (*cogitans*) (*ibid.*: 69)

This led to the more famous formulation, 'I think, therefore I am' (*Cogito ergo sum*).

Now, there is a huge literature concerning Descartes and the *cogito* argument (e.g. Kenny, 1968). I shall only focus on two concerns about Descartes' dualism. First, there is the status of the argument itself. Secondly, there was the question that particularly vexed Princess Elizabeth, namely how something immaterial (such as the mind) could have an effect on something material (such as the body).

The problem with the status of the argument is that it can be questioned whether, indeed, it was meant as an argument. The alternative is that it should be regarded as a sort of 'intuition'. Kenny divides 'intuition' into introspection or a type of performance in which there is, 'recognition of the self-confirmatory character of an utterance such as "I think"' (Kenny, *op. cit.*: 41). In broad terms, the problem for Descartes's argument—if it is meant as a proof—is that, having raised the possibility of doubt, the premise, 'I think', can be doubted in a more radical way than Descartes intended. Descartes attempts to head off this radical doubt by appeal to the notion of God. There are various reasons why this move fails; but chiefly, if it is possible for me to be mistaken about everything, it would be possible for me to be mistaken about God. Hence, the radical scepticism that Descartes has unleashed holds sway. Remember, by the way, that Descartes was hoping to establish by this argument a foundation for all scientific knowledge but, in which case, the rigour of the proof, regarded purely as an argument, would require to be more firmly established. In any case, Descartes suggests in various places that he never meant his argument to be a logical proof, as if it were some sort of syllogism. For instance, in the reply to a second set of objections to his *Meditations on First Philosophy*, Descartes says:

> For when we observe that we are conscious beings (*res cogitantes*), this is a sort of primary notion, which is not the conclusion of any syllogism; … This is clear from the fact that if he were deducing it syllogistically, he would first have to know the major premise: *whatever experiences is or exists:* whereas really it is rather that this principle is learnt through his observing in his own case the impossibility of having experience without existing. (Descartes, *op. cit.*: 299).

So, if it were not syllogistic reasoning, then the argument would appear to be a matter of intuition. This seems to be confirmed in a famous letter of March or April 1648 to the Marquis of Newcastle. Descartes wrote:

> … I admit that <our intuitions—*connoissances directes*> are slightly obscured by being mixed up with the body; but still, the knowledge they give us is primary, unacquired (*gratuite*) and certain; and we touch upon the mind with more confidence than we give to the evidence of our eyes. You will surely admit that you are less assured of the presence of the object you see than of the truth of the proposition: *I experience* (je pense) *therefore I am?* Now, this knowledge is no product of your reasoning, no less in that your masters have taught you; it is something that your mind sees, feels, handles; and although your imagination, which insistently mixes itself up with your thoughts (*pensées*), reduces the clearness of this knowledge, it is, nevertheless, a proof of our soul's capacity for receiving from God an intuitive kind of knowledge' (Descartes, *op. cit.*: 300–1)

In summing up the debate concerning whether the *cogito* is an intuition or an inference, Kenny (1968) is easygoing. It can be regarded as an inference in that there is a conclusion that follows from a premise. In addition,

> Those who think of the *cogito* as an appeal to introspection are right in that the indubitability of the premise '*cogito*' results from its truth only because thought is by definition

something of which the thinker is immediately conscious. Those who claim that the *cogito* is performative have this much truth, that the particular event that makes the premise '*cogito*' true may be a mental performance; but it need not be, and a headache will do just as well. (Kenny, 1968: 55)

So, there are debates to be had about the status of the *cogito* as an argument, about whether it is valid and whether it really proves what Descartes intended it to prove. The second point I wish to highlight was the one raised by Princess Elizabeth when she asked how something that was immaterial could have an effect on a body. Later in the letter of 28 June 1643 to Princess Elizabeth, Descartes said the following:

I supposed that your Highness still had very much in mind the arguments proving the distinction of soul and body; and I did not wish to ask you to allay them aside, in order to represent to yourself that notion of their union which everybody always has in himself without doing philosophy—viz. that there is one single person who has at once body and consciousness, so that this consciousness can move the body and be aware of the events that happen to it. Accordingly, I used in my previous letter the simile of gravity and other qualities which we imagine to be united to bodies as consciousness is united to ours. I did not worry over the fact that this simile is lame, … for I thought your Highness was already fully convinced that the soul is a substance distinct from the body. (Descartes, *op. cit.*: 281)

Kenny summarizes this letter by pointing out that Descartes only had two things to say:

… first, that the action of soul on body was rather like that which the scholastics mistakenly attributed to gravity; second, that the union of soul and body was perceived better by sense than by intellect, and therefore it was best not to philosophize too much about it. (Kenny, *op. cit.*: 224)

The truth is that Descartes could not really answer the point that Princess Elizabeth was putting to him. Or, at best, Descartes's answer was the one of which Merleau-Ponty approved, namely that:

… it is just by means of ordinary life and conversation … that one learns to conceive the union of soul and body. (Descartes, *op. cit.*: 280)

Nevertheless, Descartes persisted in stating that there was a separation between the substance of the mind and the substance of the body.

Descartes, therefore, remained a dualist, but he could also be called an *interactionist*. In *The Passions of the Soul* Descartes gave his fullest account of the relationship between the soul and the body and said,

Although the soul is joined to the whole body, there is yet in that a certain part in which it exercises its function more particularly than in all the others. (cited in Kenny, *op. cit.*: 224)

The point at which the mind or soul interacts with the brain is, according to Descartes, the pineal gland on the grounds that it is in the centre of the brain and is single and not divided into a left and a right. Recourse to the pineal gland, however, does not really free Descartes from the hook. For, as Kenny says,

If interaction between thought and matter is inconceivable, then interaction between soul and gland presents no less a problem than interaction between soul and body. (*ibid.*: 225)

Before we write off this interactionism as risible, we should note that in our own time no less a figure than the eminent Nobel Prize winner, Sir John Eccles (1903–1997), in collaboration with the equally eminent philosopher Sir Karl Popper (1902–1994), has also put forward a theory of dualist interactionism (Popper & Eccles, 1977). In two highly detailed papers, Eccles (1986, 1990) argued, first that non-material mental events can act on the brain at the level of the presynaptic vesicles. The synapse is the gap between one nerve and another; and the vesicles are the bubble-like packets which contain the neurotransmitter chemicals. An electrical impulse down the nerve causes the release of the neurotransmitters. Eccles argued that the release of a single vesicle in response to a presynaptic impulse would occur in a probabilistic manner, which he felt would be modified by a mental influence working analogously to the probabilistic fields of quantum mechanics. That is, the communication between nerves in the brain, which occurs at the synapses, has to be seen as probabilistic in the sense that the release of the contents of a single synaptic vesicle does not happen regularly, but probabilistically. Just as at the level of quantum mechanics it is not possible to say exactly which events will occur, so too at the level of the synaptic vesicle. In the second paper, Eccles (1990) takes on the materialist belief that mental events exist 'in an enigmatic sort of identity with neural events'. Concerning this, Eccles states:

> This strange postulate of identity is never explained, but it is believed that it will be resolved when we have a more complete scientific understanding of the brain, perhaps in hundreds of years; hence this belief is ironically termed promissory materialism. (Eccles, 1990)

Eccles recognizes that his theory is accused of contravening the first law of thermo-dynamics, namely that energy can be transformed but can neither be created nor destroyed. In his later paper, Eccles points to the groupings of the dendrites (which are the branched projections from a neurone) into a neural unit, which he calls a dendron. Eccles then puts forward a 'new hypothesis', which is that any mental event or experience is:

> … a composite of elemental or unitary mental events, which we may call psychons. It is further proposed that each of these psychons is reciprocally linked in some unique manner to its dendron. (Eccles, 1990)

The suggestion is that each dendron is linked with a psychon to give its own characteristic unitary experience. Eccles accepts that the psychon is an hypothesis, as is the matching of dendrons to psychons. However, he argues that, because the structures involved in synaptic transmission are small enough to operate analogously to quantum probability fields, the energy required to cause the exocytosis of a vesicle (i.e. the process by which the vesicle opens out from the end of the nerve to release its neurotransmitter), 'could be paid back at the same time and place by the escaping transmitter molecules from a high to a low concentration' (*ibid.*). Eccles explains:

> In quantum physics at microsites energy can be borrowed provided it is paid back at once. So the transaction of exocytosis need involve no violation of the conservation laws of physics. (*ibid.*)

Eccles contends that the quantum explanation and the dendron–psychon hypothesis help to explain both attention and intention. In other words, he feels that he can explain, at least hypothetically, both how the world acts on the mind and how the mind acts on the world. Now, the immediate reaction to all this might be to suggest that, although the neurophysiology has improved, the philosophical argument has been taken no further by Eccles since the time of Descartes. One thing, however, that Eccles can argue is that we know that intentions (i.e. mental events) do indeed have a physical outcome: I intended to put on my glasses and I have just done so. Eccles would question how this is possible. He is, at least, making an attempt to combine a scientific and philosophical account. What remains puzzling, however, is the nature of the psychon and consequently the way in which it can have any influence on something as material as the body, even at a quantum level. In other words, Princess Elizabeth would still be asking her same question. None the less, Eccles surely has some right on his side when he implies that the identity theorists, those who think that the mind and the body are one substance, seem simply to be ignoring the conceptual issue raised by mental events.

In ending this discussion of dualism, therefore, it seems apposite to restate the challenge that Hywel Lewis (1910–1992) set, in his book *The Elusive Self*, for those who questioned dualism:

> … do they seriously deny that there is an ingredient in our behaviour, and in that of other creatures, which it is not plausible to reduce to purely physiological terms? Do we not feel pain, do we not perceive coloured entities, whatever their status, do we not hear sounds? And however full the explanation may be at the physical and physiological levels of all that occurs in this way, there is also, over and above all that, something vital for the proper understanding of such situations. This is where the dualist takes his stance. (Lewis, 1982: 5)

Even if the arguments for dualism are not particularly convincing, the dualist does at least serve the function of emphasizing just how strange, how mystical one might say, the mind is. In ordinary life, as Descartes accepted, we take it and its union with the body for granted. But now I shall consider, albeit tentatively, what dualism might mean for Miss Breen.

Dr Descartes and Miss Breen

In all likelihood Descartes would meet Miss Breen as he would anyone else. In the everydayness of such an encounter, especially when he was not particularly thinking about the separation of mind and body, Descartes would treat Miss Breen in the normal way. As he says, in our day-to-day encounters body and soul seem to be one. It would seem perfectly legitimate, however, for us to press Descartes about what he really thinks of Miss Breen when he considers her more seriously. There may be one way in which his dualism is helpful; but there are several ways in which it is problematic and perhaps even positively unhelpful.

The potentially helpful thing is that Descartes may see Miss Breen in the light of the mystery that surrounds the nature of the soul. Given his belief in God and his belief that God maintains a benign supporting presence to ensure that the self is not mistaken about itself, Descartes would be likely to show considerable reverence to

Miss Breen inasmuch as, despite her cognitive difficulties, he would tend to recognize her essential spiritual nature.

There are, however, a number of problems. I suppose, for instance, that Descartes might regard Miss Breen's mind as being in some sense 'locked in'. He might regard the problem as being something to do with her deteriorating body, but given that he thinks the soul is entirely separate, there is no reason for him to think that the soul also disintegrates. Indeed, his religious beliefs would tend to make him think in terms of the soul being immortal. So he would have to explain what was happening to Miss Breen's soul despite all the outer appearances. He would, further, have to say whether, given that there is some evidence of distress, Miss Breen was suffering in terms of her soul or her body. It is, then, not completely clear how her body suffers, unless it is united to a soul. But why should the soul itself suffer merely on account of the deteriorating body? The thought that there might be a suffering soul within the deteriorating body is, of course, not an unnatural one: it is one which occurs to many people faced with dementia. The question for Descartes is how he thinks we might be able to affect the soul in any potentially beneficial way.

He could simply rely on the spirit or soul in the hope that his spirit, as the healing physician, might touch Miss Breen's spirit in a therapeutic way. Now, there is a sense in which this could be regarded as quite helpful in that it could be seen as encouraging a psychotherapeutic way of 'being with', in which the person's spirit is in some way reassured or touched by the presence of the other spiritual being. This is not outlandish and many of us could attest to the fact that 'being with' someone (rather than 'doing to') can be helpful and positively beneficial. But there is a way of interpreting this that could seem not just mysterious, but primitive and objectionable. If inside Miss Breen (as it were) we think there is a fully fledged, fully functioning soul, and if Descartes is himself essentially a soul, we might ask why they cannot communicate directly by some form of telepathy, soul to soul? This seems very primitive, as if the way to deal with Miss Breen might be to indulge in a séance. But it could even be used (objectionably) to suggest that dementia is not such a bad thing, if it is believed that the immaterial soul persists untouched by the disease. Why, then, can we not communicate with Miss Breen by something akin to telepathy? Is our failure to do so a failure in terms of our standing as essentially spiritual beings?

All of this seems to suggest that we do actually need the body. We need the body to touch the soul. The body seems to be required as the *locus* of interaction. Speech, for instance, which requires a body, would seem on the face of it to be our way of influencing the soul. This raises again, however, the issue of interaction between body and soul, which seems to remain as mysterious as the hypothetical entities that Eccles called psychons.

Furthermore, despite the importance that Miss Breen seems to attach to physical contact with me, dualism undermines the importance of such bodily communication. Remember that, for Descartes, the answer to the question 'What am I?' must be 'I am a thinking thing' (*sum res cogitans*). If I am essentially spirit, then the body seems less important. In which case, why do I place so much importance on Miss Breen's physical actions? Do they not provide us, as Wittgenstein might have said, with the best picture of the state of her soul (cf. Wittgenstein, 1968: §178)? Would it not be better, as Merleau-Ponty might have suggested, to regard Miss Breen as a 'body-subject'? These options are not open to Descartes. In short, the dualist approach to Miss Breen is much more problematic than it is helpful. Even the fairly simple therapeutic option of considering medication to calm her anxiety is problematic except insofar as there exists a justifiable account of mind–brain interaction. I think Dr Descartes would have to regard his patient with so much puzzlement, if he were to take his dualism seriously, that he would simply not be able to offer her treatment. He might pray for her, but it could be questioned why he should do this given the possibility that her spirit is not suffering. How do we know her spirit is suffering unless we presume the unity of the body and soul not just when we are idling, but in our everyday dealings, through and through, with Miss Breen? Dualism seems to offer a large dose of therapeutic nihilism.

Causal and constitutive

The problem that faces a dualistic account of Miss Breen is that it will be thin in terms of its explanation of her condition. Descartes might be able to speak of the bodily causes of Miss Breen's deterioration, but (unless interactionism can be given strong enough support) it will be impossible to explain how physical causes affect the immaterial mind. There is an alternative account, which is the constitutive one. It seems appropriate to discuss these two types of account before moving on. After all, if we wish to understand dementia, we should understand its causes. Perhaps Miss Breen's problems can be explained by physical, psychological, or social causes. For instance, there are the physical, pathological, lesions in the brain. Alternatively, we might give a psychological explanation, in terms of the failure of one or other cognitive function, as to why she can no longer do certain things. Finally, it might be that certain social environments or responses to her tend to make Miss Breen's behaviour worse in one way or another. Notwithstanding these sorts of explanation, there is still something that we cannot understand about someone like Miss Breen. This is to do with the personal meaning of her condition, or the subjective experience of it. Understanding the meaning of cognitive deficits in acquired diffuse neurocognitive dysfunction will require something other than *causal* explanations. A *constitutive* account, on the other hand, involves saying what it actually *is* to remember or to forget. A constitutive account will flesh out the phenomena of dementia. In so doing, a constitutive account allows a broader view, because it brings into play meaning and surround. Meanwhile, such an account does not preclude the possibility of a causal account, because understanding what constitutes memory failure does not exclude a discussion of causes. What it *does* preclude is both a *narrow* discussion of causes and a discussion that *only* looks at causes and not at the phenomenon itself as something of meaning and significance in a person's life.

The distinction I am drawing between causal and constitutive accounts parallels the distinction found in Karl Jaspers (1883–1969) between *Erklären* (the explanation of natural sciences) and *Verstehen* (the understanding of human sciences) (cf. Jaspers, 1923: 27). According to this distinction *explanation* (typical of the sciences) helps us to see causal connections, whereas *understanding* (which relies on empathy) helps us to perceive meaning. Not everyone agrees that there is a distinction to be made here.

For instance, Bolton and Hill (1996) wish to argue that causal explanations are meaningful and the distinction between explanation and understanding is undermined by the commitment of cognitive psychology to meaningful states (cf. Bolton & Hill, 1996: 32–4). I shall discuss their views further in Chapter 5, but whether or not the distinction is philosophically robust, there is certainly a difference between the understanding a friend might have of Miss Breen and that of a neuroscientist. We need causal, scientific explanations, but if we are to understand dementia thoroughly, we also need a constitutive account to explain what it actually is to experience these psychological phenomena. Such an account will bring in context and meaning. As we shall see, if dualism has problems with causal accounts, extreme materialism (or physicalism) has problems with constitutive accounts. One way to castigate physicalism is to suggest that it can *only* provide a causal account of the mind. We shall have to see whether this is true of all physicalist accounts, but the suggestion is that the causal account *is* the constitutive account. This amounts to (what is called) a type–type identity theory of the mind and brain. According to this theory, remembering something is a type of mental event and it is identical with a certain type of brain event. The strict identity implied by such a theory means that *anything* involved in remembering can be accounted for in terms of brain states. I shall pursue this by considering the work of Armstrong (1968) and the Churchlands (e.g. 1984).

Extreme materialism

According to Armstrong's 'central state theory', mental states are to be identified with purely physical states of the central nervous system. As he says:

> If the mind is thought of as 'that which has mental states', then we can say that ... the mind is simply the central nervous system. (Armstrong, 1968: 73)

This is a reaction, not only to dualism, but also to behaviourism, which emphasizes outer behaviour but denies inner psychology. Armstrong's physicalism accepts that inner mental states exist—he says: 'they are physical states of the brain' (*ibid.*: 75)—and it gets rid of the problem of explaining how the mind and brain interact, since they are one and the same thing. Mental causation exists because it is, in a real sense, physical causation. Everything that is mental, therefore, is on this view contingently identical with states of the central nervous system. Armstrong makes it plain that he considers there are two steps in his analysis. The first, the 'causal analysis', is a logical analysis of mental concepts. The second step identifies mental states with physico-chemical states of the brain, which he describes as, 'a contingent or scientific identification' (*ibid.*: 90–1). He accepts that there could, logically, be something other than the brain doing what the brain is in fact doing. Armstrong argues that,

> ... mental states are states of the person defined solely in terms of causal relations, of a more or less complex sort, to the objects or situations that bring the mental states about and the physical behaviour that constitutes their 'expression'. (*ibid.*: 356)

The account is most certainly causal. Mental states (which turn out on empirical [contingent] grounds to be brain states) are caused by objects or situations and, in turn, cause behaviour. So, the mental state of recognizing Churchill's face is brought about by seeing a picture of Churchill, and this mental state leads me to say: 'the finest British wartime Prime Minister'. And that mental state, as it happens, which stands in these causal relations, is a state of my brain caused to be in this state by the picture and, in turn, causing a vocal response. Moreover, not only is the account causal, but it is constitutive too, inasmuch as it suggests that to have a mental state of this type is simply to have a brain state of this type. There is nothing else to a mental state. This leads me on nicely to the eliminative materialism of the Churchlands, although it should not be presumed that Armstrong would have approved of eliminativism. He once described a similar theory as 'desperate indeed' (Armstrong, *ibid*.: 78).

In a book notionally to do with Alzheimer's disease, the Churchlands considered the objection to eliminative materialism that,

> … what constitutes a human consciousness is not just the intrinsic character of the creature itself, but also the rich matrix of relations it bears to other humans, practices, and institutions of its embedding culture. A reductionistic account … cannot hope to capture more than a small part of what is explanatorily important. (Churchland & Churchland, 1992: 26)

Neuroscientists, they respond, should embrace the objection:

> … any adequate neuro-computational account of human consciousness must take into account the manner in which a brain comes to represent, not just the gross features of the physical world, but also the character of the other cognitive creatures with which it interacts, and the details of the social, moral, and political world in which they all live … we confront no problem in principle here. Only a major challenge. (*ibid*.: 26–7)

According to eliminativists every aspect of human life will finally be accounted for in neuro-computational terms and, furthermore, the folksy modes of description will be eliminated in favour of neuroscientific terms. In other words, when we speak of beliefs, intentions, desires, memories, and so on, we are using out-of-date terminology. These words, according to the Churchlands, reflect theories that should now fall into disuse. These 'folk' psychological theories must be replaced by more modern neuroscientific accounts. The implication is that the folk theories will literally be eliminated. So, instead of talking about my beliefs, I shall instead have to refer to the activities in the brain that occur when I have a belief.

One immediate consequence of eliminativism, is that, strictly speaking, I cannot say I *believe* in it! The notion of a belief in eliminativism goes out of the window. But, rather than pursue the pros and cons of that particular philosophical argument, I shall for now return to Miss Breen, although all of the theories being put forward in this chapter will be returned to later following the Wittgensteinian analysis of intentional mental states in Chapter 4.

Miss Breen and the materialists

I am sure that even extreme materialists such as the eliminativists, like the Churchlands, would still be perfectly pleasant if they were to meet Miss Breen. But how would they (seriously) think of her and how might this (at some level) show itself? They could not think of her sadness, or of the likelihood that she was either sad or anxious.

The eliminativists would have to dismiss such notions and instead simply make statements about, for instance, certain serotonergic pathways in the brain that might causally account for symptoms of low mood and anxiety. (Serotonin, or 5-hydroxy-tryptamine, is one of the neurochemicals which acts as a neurotransmitter and relays messages across synapses from one nerve cell to another). So, in their attitude towards Miss Breen they would have to reduce the constitutive account of her potential suffering to a causal account. The thing that goes out of the window is the notion of suffering as we understand it. The meaning of 'suffering' would have to be dismissed as mere folk psychology. In its place, according to eliminativism, we should have to say something about the lack of serotonergic activity in some part of the brain or other. Meanwhile, of course, there would still be our own sense of sadness or worry in meeting Miss Breen. These feelings, too, would have to be discounted as a mere remnant of some form of sentimental folk psychology, because we would know that it only represented some particular goings-on in our brains. Any attempt or inclination to make such feelings *significant* would have to be dismissed similarly as folk psychology nonsense.

Hence, even if we could keep up the appearance of kindness towards Miss Breen—which we would not, by the way, be able to label as 'kindness'—the possibility of true empathic understanding must necessarily be ruled out as far as Miss Breen (or any other feeling creatures) might be concerned. Empathic understanding, remember, requires that we can put ourselves into the shoes of the other person and attempt to experience what they are experiencing. But if all that their subjective experience amounts to is some sort of deficiency in terms of neurotransmitters, then attempts at empathy are simply attempts to experience the same deficiency, which is not, however, what is referred to by the notion of 'subjective experience'. Eliminating 'sadness' or 'kindness' from the vocabulary would not in itself eliminate the subjective experience of sadness or kindness, but for that subjective experience to be the experience that it is, it cannot simply be conceived as a particular flip-flop in some specific part of the brain. To have the true nature of sadness or kindness, we need to move from the causal to the constitutive. The folk experience is the experience; and the experience is the thing. A merely causal account misses the thing altogether. It is precisely to give it no experiential reality at all. And lacking access to such contentful, experiential reality means that empathy is impossible.

Thus, the meeting between Miss Breen and the Churchlands would presumably be interesting for the Churchlands, but unlikely to provide Miss Breen with much solace unless there were to be some unexpected benefit in being regarded as a bundle of neurophysiological and neuropathological processes, albeit processes without feeling or meaningful content.

Not all materialists, however, are eliminativists. None the less, as I shall show in Chapter 6 when I return to this theme, unless materialists recognize the problem, namely that they are in danger of only giving a one-sided (causal) account rather than a causal and constitutive account of mental phenomena, materialists might as well be eliminativists. But not all of them are, which is lucky because there is a sense in which we are all materialists, or physicalists, now. It would be really quite difficult to maintain that there was no causal link between mental states and brain states. Functional neuroimaging, for instance, can show very precisely which bits of the brain are activated during particular mental tasks (Haynes & Rees, 2006). The challenge is to give an account of the mind and brain that makes conceptual sense. Eliminating the mind would seem to be nonsense: simply a way of avoiding the difficulty. It would involve, moreover, a complete denial of Miss Breen's suffering; a denial which seems not only conceptually implausible, but also ethically wrong.

The Fodorian Paradigm

In this section I shall discuss another physicalist approach to the mind, but one based very firmly on an analogy with computers. Jerry Fodor provides a functionalist approach to the mind, which (as we shall see in Chapter 5), seems at first blush to provide an extremely good philosophical paradigm for cognitive neuropsychology. He calls his paradigm the Representational Theory of Mind (RTM).

Fodor's RTM is a species of functionalism. There are differences between Fodor's functionalism and other breeds. According to functionalism, mental states with content are connected in a causal fashion. Fodor treats such states as linguistic-type entities that can be combined to form a language in a systematic way. He calls this a 'Language of Thought' (Fodor, 1976). This language is a system of representations that explains our behaviour. Functionalism itself does not require such a language; it only requires that one mental state should cause another. It has been well recognized that functionalism provides a useful model for cognitive science generally. Fodor himself calls functionalism the 'ontological doctrine' of cognitive science:

> For, if Functionalism is true, then there is plausibly a level of explanation between common-sense belief/desire psychology … and neurological … explanation … (Fodor, 1985)

This looks very promising, therefore, as a way to provide a physicalist, causal explanation, making use of our understanding of how computers work, along with commonsense, folk psychology accounts of our beliefs and desires. Fodor's RTM requires a belief in respresentationalism. Fodor describes this as follows:

> Mental states, insofar as psychology can account for them, must be the consequences of mental processes. Mental processes … are processes in which internal representations are transformed. (Fodor, 1976: 200)

As we shall see, this is fully in the spirit of cognitive neuropsychology in which a representation acting as an input, for instance hearing a word, is processed into another representation that can lead to an output, such as a word being spoken or spelt out. Fodor characterizes the RTM as follows:

> At the heart of the RTM is the postulation of a language of thought: an infinite set of 'mental representations' which function both as the immediate objects of propositional attitudes and as the domains of mental processes. (Fodor, 1987: 16)

Fodor fleshes out his account of the RTM by making two claims. The first claim is about propositional attitudes:

> For any organism O, and any attitude A, toward the proposition P, there is a ('computational'/'functional') relation R, and a mental representation MP, such that MP means that P, and O has A iff [i.e. if and only if] O bears R to MP. … to believe that such

and such is to have a mental symbol that means that such and such tokened in your head in a certain way; it's to have such a token 'in your belief box'... (*ibid.*: 16–17)

The second claim concerns the nature of mental processes, which are regarded as 'causal sequences of tokenings of mental representations' (*ibid.*: 17). Both claims bring out the importance of mental representations to RTM.

Elsewhere, Fodor has put forward two arguments in favour of RTM. The first starts by noting there are infinite thoughts and asks how a theory of mind accounts for this 'productivity'. The answer is, by appealing to what constitutes a propositional attitude, namely a symbol. 'What kind of symbol do you have to token to token an attitude? A mental representation, of course. Hence RTM' (Fodor, 1985). This argument makes use of the first claim made above. Thus, RTM accounts for the fact that we can go on making up new sentences and having new thoughts. All that is required is the ability to compose new thoughts from the vehicles of content, namely the representations, which, once possessed, can be combined in an infinite number of ways. The 'productivity' of thought poses no problem for Fodor's account and, moreover, fits neatly with the cognitive neuropsychology model, which we shall discuss in Chapter 5: the stored representations of words can be accessed and then used in a huge variety of ways.

Similarly, the second argument relates to the second claim. It requires that 'mental processes are causal sequences of mental states' (*ibid.*). Fodor argues: 'you connect the causal properties of a symbol with its semantic properties via its syntax' (*ibid.*). The syntax of a symbol is, roughly, its shape. The shape determines its causal role. It then becomes possible to conceive of machines (computers or brains) that operate to change symbols by changing their shapes. Such transformations will only occur if the symbols bear certain semantic relations to one another. Fodor continues:

> But, patently, there are going to have to be mental representations if this proposal is going to work. In computer design, causal role is brought into phase with content by exploiting parallelisms between the syntax of a symbol and its semantics. But that idea won't do the theory of *mind* any good unless there are *mental* symbols; mental particulars possessed of semantic *and syntactic* properties. There must be mental symbols because ... only symbols have syntax, and our best available theory of mental processes ... needs the picture of the mind as a syntax-driven machine. (*ibid.*)

Fodor makes it clear that thoughts, or mental content, must be explicitly represented for RTM to be true. Postponing further discussion of Fodor's views to later chapters, what would all of this mean in clinical terms for Miss Breen?

Jerry Fodor meets Miss Breen

This encounter would be much more empathic than the encounter between the Churchlands and Miss Breen. For one thing, Fodor believes in 'belief boxes'. He may or may not recognize the possibility that Miss Breen still has a 'belief box', but he would certainly allow the possibility that she has other boxes that might explain her worry or even her sadness. Fodor can certainly explain on his view why Miss Breen is unable to do certain things. If the pathways to her 'speech box' are interrupted, or if the representations in her 'language box' have degraded, then she will not be able to express herself adequately in spoken language. If Fodor's theory of mind, which is based on his theory of language, makes sense, he will be able to give a good account of the problems that Miss Breen faces. As we shall see, however, there are problems precisely with Fodor's resrepresentationalism. This will have consequences for whether or not Fodor can give a convincing account of content and what it is that constitutes mental states. For Fodor this must all boil down to having the right sort of representation, or mental symbol, one with the right syntax (or shape) to allow it to have semantic (i.e. meaningful) properties. Hence, if Fodor's theory works, he could give a perfectly adequate account of Miss Breen's state.

But still, would Fodor be able to show the sort of empathic understanding that was beyond the Churchlands? In one sense this would be possible. Fodor's observations of Miss Breen would cause certain sorts of representation to be formed in his mind and it is perfectly possible to talk in terms of these representations then leading to particular outputs showing concern and care. So, on the whole, the encounter would be much more therapeutic. In another sense, however, there is a theoretical problem. This stems from the computer analogy. We might be able to imagine two computers set up so that the output from one computer leads to (what seems like) an appropriate output in response from the other computer. For instance, one computer could make incoherent noises that seemed to represent fear and anxiety. In response to this, the other computer could generate the following words: 'Don't worry, I'm here'. But what sort of encounter would this have been? Not one, I think, which shows true empathic understanding. Even if the second computer were set up with a hand that could be extended to place itself on the hand of the first computer, we would still not have reached the level of empathic understanding that perhaps Miss Breen is entitled to expect. The difficulty this scenario highlights for Fodor points to the heart of the problem with representationalism. Representations can work in a simple functional way, as in a computer, but in a human context or surround (e.g. Miss Breen's) they need something else, some sort of manifest *significance*, which is what it is for them to be meaningful.

Lacking really meaningful empathy, however, would not stop Fodor from performing a useful function in terms of performing cognitive tests on Miss Breen. As we have suggested, functionalism forms a useful philosophical paradigm for cognitive neuropsychology. So Fodor could perform a perfectly useful task in meeting Miss Breen in much the same way that our computer could interrogate its fellow computer, judging its outputs in a great variety of ways in order to build up a picture of those elements of the computer or brain that are dysfunctional. Given the level of Miss Breen's problems, however, it is not clear how beneficial this would be for her and I am not even sure that Fodor himself would relish being cast in this role. I shall quickly add that the cognitive neuropsychologists I know and have known do not solely function in this way. But this is because they do not solely function as computers, even if some of what they do could be done (and is done) by computers. No, the real Jerry Fodor, like the real cognitive neuropsychologists I have known, would also, I am sure, function humanly, with *significance*, which means out of the box.

Anomalous monism to the rescue?

Donald Davidson (1917–2003) accepts that 'all events [including mental events] are physical' (Davidson, 1980: 214). He holds this view in an attempt to account for the causal role that mental events have in the physical world. He states:

> Psychological events and intentional actions are causally related to physical events. (*ibid.*: 231)

Whilst his monistic stance rejects dualism (and is, therefore, to this extent, in line with other forms of materialism), he regards mental events as 'anomalous' in that they 'resist capture in the nomological net of physical theory' (*ibid.*: 207); in other words, they do not abide by the sort of rules and laws that are associated with scientific theories covering physical phenomena. Davidson's 'anomalous monism' is anomalous, 'because it insists that events do not fall under strict laws when described in psychological terms' (*ibid.*: 231). More bluntly, there are no precise psychophysical laws.[2] His arguments for this are predicated on his views about mental autonomy and holism (*ibid.*: 217). Thus,

> Mental events as a class cannot be explained by physical science; particular mental events can when we know particular identities. But the explanations of mental events in which we are typically interested relate them to other mental events and conditions. We explain a man's free actions, for example, by appeal to his desires, habits, knowledge and perceptions. (*ibid.*: 225)

That is, whilst for other reasons Davidson accepts that mental events are physical events, he also recognizes the radical difference that exists between the language of the physical sciences and the language of the mental. There are differences between mental and physical predicates which stem from their different degrees of law-likeness. Not only will physical predicates never give rise in a law-like manner to terms that can capture the full meaning of mental predicates, but there is also a radical difference between the closed system of a physical science and the generalizations of mental predicates (*ibid.*: 211). Because of their differing roles, the physical and the mental cannot be tightly bound together, as would be required by strict psychophysical laws. This allows the freedom that is entailed by the notion of rationality.

> When we attribute a belief, a desire, a goal, an intention or a meaning to an agent, we necessarily operate within a system of concepts in part determined by the structure of beliefs and desires of the agent himself. Short of changing the subject, we cannot escape this feature of the psychological; but this feature has no counterpart in the world of physics. (*ibid.*: 230)

So we see Davidson being unequivocal about his physicalism, but also unequivocal about the realm of the mental. The physical world will work in a law-like manner, but when we bring desires and beliefs into the picture, things become less law-like. This is not to deny the physical pre-conditions for such mental states, it is simply to note that these mental states themselves enmesh with other mental states, with other concerns and beliefs. Davidson is recognizing, that is, that what is constitutive here (the way mental states enmesh with each other) is more important, at least as regards the mental realm, than what is causal. Unfortunately, however, Davidson must *both* locate mental states within a realm of rational and normative connections *and* maintain links to physical and causal events in the brain in order for the theory to remain monist. Trying to maintain an anti-dualist position whilst marking out separate realms for physical and mental predicates is difficult. For, on the one hand, there is the commitment to the link between the mental and the physical; whilst, on the other hand, there can be no psychophysical laws. Nevertheless (and this is the difficulty), for any description of a mental state there is, according to anomalous monism, a particular physical state that must, in some way, specify the normative relations of the mental state to other states without which it would not be the mental state that it is. This is not possible, however, if there are no psychophysical laws.

One response to this is to say that it has missed the point, which is that Davidson proposes a *token* identity theory.[3] The links between mental states and physical states of the brain, according to Davidson, are not type–type links, where one type of mental state maps on to a type of physical state. Rather the token theory allows that there will be a variety of ways in which a particular mental or physical state can be realized (or tokened). None the less, there are grounds for arguing that the token theory just cannot get round the need to establish some sort of closer conceptual links between the physical and the mental once the dichotomy has been allowed to appear. Meanwhile, the mental state will also be particular (recognizing Winston Churchill, say), which will mean that this mental state will have particular (normative) relations to other mental states (remembering the cavalry charge at Omdurman). But, as Thornton has observed,

> ... this places constraints on its physical properties which will have to be such that its causal role fits its rational role such that it is causally related to other token states that realise those other mental abilities and states. The normative relations constitutive of content impose general constraints on the physical level. (Thornton, 1998: 200–1)

In other words, mental content, since it is also surrounded by normative relations (i.e. rule-like connections) that actually constitute those states, seems to require more harmony between the physical and the mental than the notion of 'anomalous monism' suggests. These sorts of problems have led one commentator to suggest that Davidson should be characterized as a dualist:

> ... in spite of his anomalous monism, dualism in the form of a commitment to the mental as an autonomous domain is a nonnegotiable premise of Davidson's overall position in 'Mental Events'. (Kim, 1985: 385)

Davidson has attempted to avoid this dualism by linking the non-relational mental states to non-relational physical descriptions. He has also tried to allow room for human rationality (and anomalousness) by making another link between non-relational mental states and relational mental descriptions. The problem is that the *mental state* of recognizing Churchill's face is itself relational, not just the *description* of recognizing Churchill.

So, although Davidson makes a distinction between the homonomic (strict) laws of physics and the heteronomic laws governing mental predicates (which are relational and subject to human rationality and the content of customs and practices), this is at odds with his insistence that mental events are physical events. Something has to succumb: either mental events are physical (and susceptible to causal explanations as free-standing, non-relational items) or mental events are anomalous (and subject to understanding within the relational context of human rationality). Hence, although the intentions behind Davidson's theory of anomalous monism seem right, in that he wishes to maintain a sort of freedom in the mental realm, whilst allowing that, in the physical realm, things must behave in a law-like fashion, none the less maintaining the balance between these inclinations is theoretically challenging.

The anomalous monism of Miss Breen

Davidson would undoubtedly treat Miss Breen as an agent operating within a world structured by beliefs and desires. He would almost certainly understand the content of Miss Breen's anxiety as reflecting the historical development of her condition in which she has been more or less aware of the deterioration in terms of her mental capabilities. Davidson would also be at home in terms of the causal explanation of her presentation. The difficulty in Davidson's encounter with Miss Breen, however, would be for Davidson himself since he would have to decide whether he was inclined to think about Miss Breen's mental life as being a physical life and subject in some sort of tight way to causal explanations, or whether he would wish to think of her mental life as more anomalous, as more understandable in terms of human relationships and rationality. Would Davidson wish to look inside the head at the physical goings on, or would he wish to look at Miss Breen as someone in a context, surrounded by a psychosocial environment that might be good or bad in terms of its effects? The two sides of this divide cannot, on Davidson's account, be brought together by psychophysical laws: this is necessary to maintain the anomalous state. As we have seen, however, this is problematic in that it seems to incline us towards dualism, where the psychological side and the physical side are distinct. But Davidson cannot say this, if he also wishes to continue to maintain that mental events are physical events. So, the encounter between Davidson and Miss Breen would perhaps be therapeutic for Miss Breen, but immensely intellectually upsetting for Davidson.

The social construction of mind

Social constructionism emanates from a variety of sources. Elements of social constructionist thought are pre-figured in the works of George Herbert Mead (1863–1931), who argued that the self arises through the process of social experience and activity (Mead, 1934), and Lev Semyonovich Vygotsky (1896–1934), who held that speech develops 'from the social to the individual' (Vygotsky, 1934: 20). More recently, Rom Harré stated thus:

> The central thesis of social constructionism is the claim that most psychological phenomena are created in and have their primal being in social encounters. (Harré, 1993: 95)

Indeed, Harré has split contemporary psychology between, on the one hand, those following Freud, Piaget, and Dennett, who have embraced the individualism of the cognitivists who think of human action as stemming from individual mental proc-esses, and, on the other hand, those in the camp of Wittgenstein, Vygotsky, and Mead, sharing,

> ... the collectivism of the social constructivists, who conceive of human action as the joint intentional actions of minded creatures whose minds are structured and stocked from a social and interpersonal reality. (Harré, 1983: 8)

Harré has associated himself with the general spirit of social constructionism:

> I share with many the idea that people and what they do are artefacts, products of social processes. (Harré, 1993: 2–3)

Elsewhere, Harré has identified the thesis that he thinks is shared by all versions of social constructionism:

> ... all psychological phenomena *and the beings in which they are realized* are produced discursively. (Harré, 1992)

According to Gergen, one of the assumptions of social constructionism is that,

> The terms in which the world is understood are social artefacts, products of historically situated interchanges among people. (Gergen, 1985)

Gergen explicitly recognizes related themes in the work of Wittgenstein:

> Wittgenstein brought into poignant clarity the extent to which the use of mental predi-cates is convention-bound ... many classic problems both in psychology and philosophy appear to be products of linguistic entanglement. (*ibid.*)

The social constructionist movement begins in earnest 'when one challenges the concept of knowledge as mental representation' and replaces it with the view that 'knowledge is not something people possess somewhere in their heads, but rather, something people do together' (*ibid.*) mostly by means of language. The ontological basis of mind or self, according to social constructionism, is not in the head but is 'within the sphere of social discourse' (*ibid.*). Again, this analysis is supported by a Wittgensteinian spin:

> ... one ceases to view mental predicates as possessing a syntactic relationship with a world of mental events; rather, ... such terms are cashed out in terms of the social practices in which they function. (*ibid.*)

According to Harré, it is in discourse, ordinary conversations, that the construction of selves and of psychological phenomena occurs.

> I take the array of persons as a primary human reality. I take the conversations in which those persons are engaged as completing the primary structure, bringing into being social and psychological reality. Conversation is to be thought of as creating a social world just as causality generates a physical one. (Harré, 1993: 64–5)

Harré's inclination to stress the intersubjective nature of persons constitutes a direct assault on what he sees as the old paradigm of psychology:

> We must really stop thinking of psychology as the science of what happens in and around individual people. We must turn to the most tantalizing and difficult aspect of human action, namely conversing, to find the empirical basis of our studies. (Harré, 1989a)

Elsewhere, Davies and Harré (1990) argue that, 'the constitutive force of each discursive practice lies in its provision of subject positions'. Now, the notion of positioning within a discourse, which acknowledges the importance of understanding the relationship between participants in a conversation, is itself relevant to any consideration of discourse between a person with dementia and his or her carers. This point is summarized by Harré and Gillett thus:

> Positioning highlights the importance of 'making something of a situation' as one participates in it and according to one's perceptions of it. This idea in turn underpins the concept of subjectivity, which expresses the way things appear to be or are signified by the speech and action of a person seen in relation to a discursive context. This is the closest our present approach comes to an account of the Cartesian 'inner'. (Harré & Gillett, 1994: 35)

Hence, mental phenomena are made, or constructed, from continuing human practices. Our understanding of a mental state, therefore, will be contingent upon social interactions and, in particular, on human conversation and discourse.

Discourse with Miss Breen

There are grounds for arguing, in my view, that Miss Breen will do best with the social constructionists. This may be a prejudice on my part, one which I hope to justify, but it stems in part from the inclination of social constructionists to stay out of Miss Breen's head. They are not particularly concerned by what might be going on there. And, of course, neither is Miss Breen. Inasmuch as we can say what she is concerned by, it would seem reasonable to suggest that she is concerned by what is happening to her here and now. Here and now, in this conversation, there may be things occurring that help to give her some sense of being valued, or there may be things occurring that help to make her feel more like an object: an object of intellectual curiosity, an object for testing, an object that feels it may be being used *solely* as a means to something else, rather than as a Kantian end in itself. The discourse that is occurring may not be coherent. It may involve touch and gesture, but the social constructionist will be trying to understand the meaning of these things, rather than looking towards the causal explanations that lie behind them. Miss Breen can be 'positioned' by the discourse as someone who is confused, or as someone who is valued. Her subjectivity, her mental life, will emerge, according to the social constructionists, in the context of these discursive encounters. It does not have to be postulated as existing elsewhere. It certainly does not have to be seen as sitting somewhere inside her head. In short, my prejudice is to think that the social constructionists will provide the greatest therapeutic benefit for Miss Breen.

I shall discuss the theory behind discursive psychology with a more critical eye in Chapter 5. But some will feel that the social constructionists have been let off somewhat lightly from at least one perspective. The perspective is that of the physicalist. This point does seem to have at least some justification. For despite the great value in approaching Miss Breen as a social being, whose mental life is also exhibited and affected by the social surround, she is also physical, has a physical brain, and may indeed benefit from the physical understanding that, for instance, it could be beneficial to her (and to her mental life) to alter some of the physical goings-on in her brain. Perhaps, after all, she needs more serotonin!

Intentionality and externalism

Still, social constructionism seems to hold out the most hope for Miss Breen, at least as things stand, in terms of an encounter that might in some way provide a degree of empathic understanding and psychotherapeutic benefit. As we have seen, it also offers a picture of the mind as something that is outside the head, or more public than the inner physiology of materialism and the inner representations of functionalism. In this section, I shall introduce in a little more depth two notions that also support the idea that the mind is not solely confined to the inner, whether that be the inner soul of dualism, the inner boxes of representationalism, or inner neurophysiology. The first notion is that of intentionality; and the second is that of the externality of mind. Both notions will figure significantly in much that follows, either overtly, or in the background. We have already had some suggestion of the second notion, both in Harré's talk of conversation 'creating a social world' (Harré, 1983: 65) and in Marvel's poem (*vide supra*), in which the Mind creates, 'Far other Worlds, and other Seas'. So I shall start with intentionality.

Intentionality is a technical philosophical term used to describe a certain property of some mental states. It is the property of 'aboutness'. What this means is that there are certain mental or psychological states that are, in their nature, *about* or *of* something. If I say that I am *hoping* the snow does not upset my travel arrangements, my mental state is *about* the snow and so forth. To *remember* something is to have a mental state that is *about* the thing remembered. Similar things can be said about most of the concepts used to define the cognitive deficits associated with dementia. My judgements and speech are about something. Nor do I simply comprehend, calculate or learn, but I comprehend, calculate, and learn something. Other phenomena too— reading, writing, copying, attending, and concentrating (*inter alia*)—can all be construed in intentional terms.

Not all mental states, however, show the property of intentionality. Pain is said not to be about something, it just is *pain*. Now, there is some controversy here, because it can be argued that the interesting thing about *intentional* mental states is also interesting about *non-intentional* mental states, namely that they both set up conceptual links with the world in a way that exhibits normativity (cf. McDowell, 1991). I shall have more to say about normativity in the next chapter. I do not need, however, to become caught up in this controversy. It is enough for me that intentional mental states are as they are; namely that they make a link with the world because, conceptually, they must be *about* or *of* something. The normative nature of the link is something to which I shall come. It is worth noting, however, that the word 'intentionality' should not be confused with *having an intention*. My *intention* to do something *does* show the property of intentionality but only in the same way as my *hope* does.

I also wanted to introduce the notion of the externality of mind. But, in some ways, the idea is already to be found in the discussion of social constructionism. It is the idea that, 'the mind just ain't in the head' (McCulloch, 2003: 12). It is also in the world. According to Thornton,

> Externalism … claims that mental (and linguistic) content depends upon, or is constituted by, states of the non-mental world. (Thornton, 1998: 123)

The notion of the world being *constitutive* of the mind is central. It is important because it implies the world is inherent to the nature of mental states: without some item in the world (X), the thought would not be the thought that it is (a thought of X):

> … the world enters constitutively into the individuation of states of mind. (McGinn, 1989: 9)

This is to make the same point that we have made about intentionality: to have a mental state, for instance to be thinking of something, requires that there are things in the world. For a thought to be a thought of a garden, for it to have meaning or content, the requirement is that there should be a garden. Without this, it would be a thought without content or meaning. As Luntley puts it, mental content,

> … is not characterizable independently of that (the environment) which it represents. (Luntley, 1999: 9)

The external world (a garden) is constitutive of the mental state (thinking of or remembering a garden). The world penetrates the mind, in a sense, and the mind embraces the world.

If the mind is not in the head, then, in a very real sense we can share our thoughts:

> … the walls of the mind seem … built to be breached by other substances; the mind is only too willing to share its domicile with other substances (it keeps the front door always open). (McGinn, *op. cit.*: 22)

Thus, different minds embrace the same objects, which is a prerequisite for the sharing of meanings, that is, communication. Thus we can know what someone else is thinking. It is the external world, in which people act and interact, that allows meanings to be conveyed. As McCulloch says:

> Doings and sayings are the primary bearers of content. (McCulloch, *op.cit.*: 105)

Commenting on this elsewhere, I have said:

> But, of course, 'doings and sayings' are out there in the world. Much of our mental life, therefore, goes on in external space, in which our minds must engage with objects and with each other. (Hughes, 2006a)

This takes us back to think about Miss Breen. If the mind is shareable in public space, there is the possibility of a meeting of minds even when acquired diffuse neuro-cognitive dysfunction is marked, not through rational, cognitive processes, but by the act of *being with* the person. As we have commented elsewhere:

> … externalism's push outwards, whereby content becomes necessarily shared, or at least shareable, makes sense of the attitude towards people with dementia according to which, however muddled their language, it might still be possible to hear their meaning through genuine attempts to engage with them phenomenologically. (Hughes et al., 2006a: 18)

Indeed, especially as dementia worsens, it becomes necessary to work harder in order to interpret the person's meaning. But the person with dementia retains the ability to convey meaning (Sabat & Harré, 1994), even if what is required from us is a greater effort at meaning-making (Widdershoven & Berghmans, 2006). The emphasis is on communication. And, indeed, there is evidence that attention to communication can help to restore the possibility of meaningful (if sometimes incoherent) exchange even in severe cases of acquired diffuse neurocognitive dysfunction (Allan & Killick, 2010). But more of this later.

Conclusion

The point of this chapter was to give a brief view of some theories of the mind. Dualism is perhaps the best known, but holds the least sway these days. Interactionism does not convincingly get around the problems of dualism. Extreme materialism, involving the elimination of everything mental, seems egregious. But other forms of physicalism, whether involving representationalism or anomalous monism, are also problematic. As we have seen, the issue is often to do with the inadequacy of the constitutive, over against the causal, accounts provided by these approaches to the mind. Physicalism, after all, seems to provide an adequate account of the causal structures that underpin mental events. Social constructionism is radically different and has the benefit of bringing *others* into the equation. The externality of mind links with a social constructionist approach and accounts for at least some of the constitutive features of the mind that are not readily accommodated by physicalism or materialism: the way in which much of our mental life seems essentially shared; it is certainly not all in our heads.

In turn, this helps to highlight the importance and remarkable nature of intentionality, concerning which Michael Luntley has written:

> *Aboutness* does not look natural. It might be ubiquitous, for us at least, but the aboutness of our thought and talk is not, unlike the colour of our hair, a straightforward natural fact. (Luntley, 2003a: 1)

How it is that our 'thought and talk' latches on to the world—whether indeed it is right to give the world precedence, rather than regard it as one of the 'Far other Worlds, and other Seas' that the mind (through thought and discourse) creates—is a major philosophical issue. In particular, philosophers have been concerned with the normative nature of intentionality, how it is that our 'thought and talk' about the world can be correct or incorrect. It is this to which I shall now turn.

But we should not forget Miss Breen. The importance of our conception of the mind is because it will have implications for our conception of the person. Part of the reason for sketching some of the theories of the mind was to demonstrate their inadequacies as far as Miss Breen is concerned. An egregious account of the mind leads to an egregious approach to Miss Breen. An inadequate or deficient or incomplete account is just as bad. We need to find an account of the mind that allows Miss Breen to be approached meaningfully, where the significance of her ways of engaging with her surroundings can be understood.

My argument is an attempt to bring together the philosophical and the clinical. If there were a way to understand mental phenomena which would allow us to move towards a better understanding of Miss Breen's otherwise incoherent engagements with the world, this would be of tremendous help in terms of our clinical encounters with her in her current context. But understanding mental phenomena in the human context is to understand *at some level* what it is to be a human person. What we have seen so far is how difficult it is to give an account of our intentionality—of how the mind makes contact with the world—partly because we cannot even give a straightforward account of how the mind links with the body. My answer will be to point eventually to the importance of our concept of the person as the *locus* of our intentionality. It is through the person that contact is made between the mind and the world. But we need a fully fledged account of the person (including Miss Breen), one which encompasses the mind and its being about something else. The mind can, perhaps, as Marvell suggests (*vide supra*), transcend the world and annihilate all that's made; but 'a green thought in a green shade' is still a thought *of* something. Even this transcendent thought is parasitic on the world; and the question to which we turn concerns how our 'thought and talk' quite generally is to be understood and judged as far as its rightness and wrongness goes.

Endnotes

[1] There are numerous introductory guides to the philosophy of mind, but the books I have most recently used for general purposes are Kenny (1989) and Lowe (2000). I would also recommend Matthews (2005), which gives a very clear account of the topics raised in this chapter. For more focused attention on the problems that arise to do with the mind in connection with the philosophy of psychiatry, I have tended to be parochial by depending on the works of my mentors: Thornton (1998), Luntley (1999), Fulford et al. (2006), and Thornton (2007). I would commend these works for the greater depth of their philosophical discussion.

[2] I am grateful to Professor Steve Sabat for pointing out to me that there is at least one area where a law-like relationship is said to hold between psychological and physical realms. Gustav Fechner (1801–1887) was the founder of psychophysics. Through a series of experiments using different sensory systems and drawing on the experimental findings of E.H. Weber (1795–1878), Fechner arrived at a relationship between the psychological intensity of a sensory experience and the physical intensity of the outside stimuli that lead to those experiences. That relationship, called Fechner's Law, was:

$$S = k \log I$$

where S is the subjective (psychological) magnitude of a sensation, I is the physical intensity of the stimulus, and k is a constant. Although Fechner's Law does not hold true at extreme values of physical intensities, it is valid for a wide range of physical intensities of diverse sensory stimuli. This does appear to contradict the rather bold statement that there are *no* precise psychophysical laws; but readers will have to judge whether it contradicts Davidson's broader point that mental and physical predicates are (as it were) qualitatively different and, therefore, cannot be related in a law-like way.

[3] A 'token' is a particular; a 'type' is an abstract entity, a concept. There is a type, which is a belief—in the abstract—that Anne is making lunch (you can now think conceptually about the belief that Anne is making lunch); and there is the particular manifestation of that belief type, the token, which is my belief (right now) that Anne *is* making lunch.

Chapter 4

Normativity in the world

It is impossible for me to say one word in my book about all that music has meant in my life. How then can I hope to be understood?

(Wittgenstein to Drury, 1949; Rhees, 1981:173)

Introduction

The transcendentalism implicit in Wordsworth's Ode: *Intimations of Immortality from Recollections of Early Childhood*, which we noted in Chapter 2, was one of the features that probably appealed to Gerald Finzi (1901–1956) when he decided to set the poem to music. Both because of the standing of the poem itself and because of its themes, it was a long and difficult task. According to Finzi's wife, Joy, '*Intimations* was certainly with us all our married days …' (Banfield, 1997: 370). There were mixed reviews after its first performance in 1950, but subsequently the piece (as with much else in Finzi's work) has become clearly established in the repertoire of twentieth century English music.

One way to set up the topic of this chapter is to ask a specific question about this music: whence does the sense of its Englishness come? When someone says, 'This is so English!', how is this justified? Or what are the criteria for such a statement being correct or incorrect? Of course, a similar question could be asked of the Frenchness of Claude Debussy (1862–1918) or of the American character of Aaron Copland (1900–1990). For whichever nationality we might wish to enquire, the answer is probably the same. In an Editorial (1965) in *Music and Letters*, reviewing a book on Edwardian England, the author wisely states: 'The question of "Englishness" in music cannot be pinned down to a single element.' The Editorial goes on to comment on the 'Englishness' of Frederick Delius (1862–1934) and Edward Elgar (1857–1934). In both cases, as with Finzi, it is remarkably easy to discover influences on and to see elements in their music that are decidedly not 'English'. But, in which case, how are *these* judgements—about the elements that *lack* 'Englishness'—to be justified as correct or incorrect? I am not going to answer this aesthetic question. I simply note its force. There is something really compelling about the conviction that Elgar—despite his links with music of the European continent—is quintessentially English. What I also note, however, is that, despite the potency of this Englishness, it cannot be explained in a convincing way, apart from gesturing to something that cannot be pinned down. Concerning Elgar, Kennedy says:

No technical analysis can discover for certain just how he took something from the air of the Malvern Hills, from the banks of the Teme and Severn, from the cloisters of Worcester

Cathedral, and turned it into music which speaks immediately and directly of these things to his fellow-countrymen. Walk in Worcestershire and the music of Elgar is in the air around you, fantastic as this may seem to the prosaically minded. Genius has the right to retain its mysteries and its magic. (Kennedy, 1970: 16–17)

The question is: what allows us, with right, to call this music English, that American, this humorous, and that sad? Where do the standards of correctness or incorrectness come from? My aim is not to become enmeshed in the philosophy of music, but the connection with our theme, which concerns thought and language, is one that Wittgenstein clearly felt.

Understanding a sentence is much more akin to understanding a theme in music than one may think. What I mean is that understanding a sentence lies nearer than one thinks to what is ordinarily called understanding a musical theme. Why is just *this* the pattern of variation in loudness and tempo? One would like to say 'Because I know what it's all about.' But what is it all about? I should not be able to say. In order to 'explain' I could only compare it with something else which has the same rhythm (I mean the same pattern). (PI §527)

Wittgenstein goes on to say that there are sentences where the words could be replaced by other words without any loss of sense; but there are other cases where the words could not be replaced, 'Any more than one musical theme can be replaced by another' (PI §531). Wittgenstein then asks how, in this sort of case, one can 'transmit one's comprehension'; and he replies:

Ask yourself: How does one *lead* anyone to comprehension of a poem or of a theme? The answer to this tells us how meaning is explained here. (PI §533)

I shall return to this point towards the end of the chapter. But, to recapitulate, I have discussed in Chapter 1 how dementia throws up a number of particular clinical, ethical, and conceptual problems. These can be helpfully approached by adopting the broad view of what it is to be a person described in Chapter 2: the situated embodied agent view. This view gains support from a broad view of mental states and, as I sketched in the last chapter, understanding mental states is crucial to our view of acquired diffuse neurocognitive dysfunction. Inevitably, therefore, I need to deal with ways in which mental states might be understood (and the implications of such understanding for acquired diffuse neurocognitive dysfunction), which I do by concentrating on Wittgenstein's discussion of rule-following.

The eventual aim is to understand dementia and my argument is based on the thought that intentional psychological states must be understood as a first step. The insight from Wittgenstein concerns how these states are normative; he does this by discussing rules. Whilst it is possible to take a thoroughly sceptical approach to the normativity demonstrated by rules, this route is blocked if rules are considered as practices insofar as practices are conceptualized as embedded in the world.

In more detail, the argument starts by establishing that intentional psychological states are normative and that normativity is a matter of rule-following. But what actually constitutes rule-following? Wittgenstein dismisses various suggestions. It is not a matter of metaphysical tracks leading us. Neither is it a matter of causal processes, nor of internal mental processes. Each of these possibilities can be thought of as supporting a different view of intentional psychological states and, therefore, different ways of understanding dementia. Another possibility, famously advocated by Kripke, is that a thoroughly sceptical view of rule-following can be adopted. Kripke interprets Wittgenstein as saying that no account can be given to justify our insistence on the reality of rules. Such scepticism is erroneous, but its challenge has philosophical force. The challenge is met by emphasizing the role of practices and customs. I shall consider the 'community view' and 'constructivism' as two possible accounts of what this emphasis on practices amounts to. However, I shall level arguments against both accounts. Instead, I shall commend the notion that these practices must be understood as embedded in the human world. The account I shall give is a transcendental one, in that it depends on looking at the pre-conditions of intentional mental states, but the embeddedness of the practices stresses the immanence of normativity, in that normativity lies within our practice of language use. It also suggests the externalism of mind already encountered in Chapter 3. I shall end by discussing the notion of quietism. This chapter will establish that the normativity of intentional psychological states is a matter of worldly embedded practices. This account can then be used as a critique of various models of dementia, which I shall deal with in the coming chapters.

Psychological states, rules, and normativity

In this section I shall set out two of the premises that motivate the rest of the discussion. The first needs some explanation; the second is more like an analytical truth. They are:

- intentional psychological states are normative;
- normativity can be thought of as rule-following.

Psychological states and normativity

As a preliminary to the discussion of rules, Wittgenstein points out that the experience of understanding is something that can occur 'in a flash', but this seems contrary to the notion of meaning as use, which implies a process over time (PI §138). He amplifies this by asking, 'can the whole *use* of the word come before my mind, when I understand it …?' (PI §139). This central question concerns the problem of intentionality as it relates to understanding. The problem is that understanding is *about* something and it seems, therefore, as if the something should 'come before my mind' when I have understood. If in the present I say, 'Now I understand', I am committed to certain things in the future. So how does the thing before my mind *now* constrain the future? Given that 'the meaning of a word is its use in the language'(PI §43), Wittgenstein's question is: how can all the future uses come before my mind when I understand the meaning of a word or phrase? But when it is said that I have understood, say, the meaning of the word 'chair', it is implied that I shall call a chair 'a chair' and not 'a table', not just today, but tomorrow and for the foreseeable future. This *just is what it is* to understand the word 'chair'. In which case, it might seem, 'in a *queer way*' (PI §195), that I must have the potential uses of 'chair' already in mind, otherwise it would not be the case that I understand its meaning. All of this follows from the intentional nature of the concept of 'understanding', but also from the supposition that understanding involves something coming 'before my mind'.

For the sake of clarity, I should observe that there is a trivial sense in which all concept-use is normative. It is trivially true that the concept 'chair' refers to some things and not others. Similarly, a word such as 'understand' must retain its meaning. But intentional psychological states, such as 'my understanding that p', seem to involve a further commitment. For when I say, 'I understand the Cyrillic alphabet', the mental state of understanding at once determines something in the world, namely what must be the case when I am presented with a text written in the Cyrillic alphabet. What is true of understanding is also true of intending and remembering. The unique aspect of intentional psychological states is the way in which they make contact with and constrain the actual instances that justify my saying I understand, intend, or mean something, even when these instantiations are not yet in existence. The normativity thus demonstrated is absent, however, in a starkly contrasting way when I consider the *physical* state of being a chair. There is nothing more to being a chair than being a chair! But an *intentional psychological* state constitutively and normatively involves something else being the case. The question is how our 'thought and talk' represent reality (Luntley, 2003a: 1): what are the standards of correctness or incorrectness that allow us to say that someone has or has not understood a phrase (in language or in music) correctly? The first step is to be gripped by the issue. How our thoughts latch onto, or connect with, reality is as big a mystery as the Englishness of Elgar's music or the American nature of Copland's *Appalachian Spring*.

Often what is constrained will be in the future. But the temporal relationship is not crucial, although it is striking. Rather, the point is that being in a mental state normatively constrains the world. All intentional psychological states, that is, raise the question that motivates Wittgenstein's discussion of rule-following: how can it be that something that happens 'in a flash' (the meaning of a word occurring to me, i.e. a mental state) fits something extended over time (namely, my actual use of the word, i.e. something that features in the world) (PI §§ 138–9)?

There is the potential for confusion since the normativity that governs the usage of *any* word is ultimately a matter of meaning; and meaning something involves an intentional psychological state. So, when I say 'That's a chair', the meaning of the phrase is constrained intentionally because it is a way of connecting a mental state (viz. meaning 'chair') to a state of the world. But there is also the simple act of *seeing*, which is clearly a mental state, but *not* an intentional one, in that it does not have the feature of *aboutness*. My thought is about something—it cannot be a thought that is not about something—but the actual act of seeing is not about anything; it is just what it is: the mental experience of redness or something similar.

There is more to be said about *non*-intentional states than I can cover here. But, for instance, McDowell (1991) has made a specific connection between *non*-intentional states and normativity. He argues that the relevant non-intentional concepts cannot be understood simply from the subject's point of view. The concepts set up normative links between both the mental states and the 'publicly accessible circumstances' (McDowell, *op. cit.*: 160) in which the normal expression of the concepts takes place.

If I say, 'I see a red patch', the mental state in itself does not constrain the world. If anything, on this view, matters are the reverse: redness in the world constrains my mental state. In intentional mental states, the mental states constrain the world. None the less, when I state, 'I see a red patch', in McDowell's view normative links are established between the relevant mental state and the public circumstances—the surround one might say—in which it makes sense to claim that the statement is correct.

When Wittgenstein starts to consider understanding, the notion of normativity quickly comes into view. My understanding of the meaning of 'chair' determines (for me) how I should use the word 'chair' and this is determined for as long as I am able to use this language. Wittgenstein notices that, rather than this sort of fact being shocking, it is expected and accepted in our everyday use of language. In normal cases, 'the use of a word is clearly prescribed' (PI §142), and people generally, 'apply *this* picture like *this*' (PI §141). We expect, as we do when we weigh things, constancy and predictability (PI §142). Normativity is, at least, expected in *normal* cases. But if normality did not hold,

> ... if rule became exception and exception rule ... this would make our normal language-games lose their point. (*ibid.*)

Wittgenstein immediately sets about considering a language-game in which signs are used in accordance with a rule in response to orders.

It is worth noting that there is an issue regarding the connection between normativity and the normal. Later in the chapter I shall discuss whether normativity, through its connection to practice, might either be a matter of the normal practice of the community, or a reflection of the normal unfolding of human propensities and conventions. In my view, normativity is not simply a matter of (e.g.) normal dispositions, although there is a connection between what we normally do and normativity. Whilst the normal and abnormal use of words is the stuff of normativity, in that it is concerned with correct and incorrect usage, this refers to the normativity that governs all words, rather than the normativity of intentional mental content, where the issue is how thoughts link to the world. There are important things to note about what comes naturally to us, as in Eldridge (1986) stating: '. . . our selves are partially determined by the practices we find natural'. But this is almost a truism rather than the sort of account of normativity I am pursuing. The view I shall endorse, however, is a transcendental argument that looks at the preconditions for normal usage and the normativity of intentional psychological phenomena has to be understood in this light.

What needs to be kept in mind is that the normativity relevant to intentional psychological states is constitutive. It is not something that is optional: I cannot allow that my pupil has understood how to 'add 2' when he or she continues the series by saying '1004' after '1000'. The meaning of 'add 2' is powerfully constraining. It is *powerfully* constraining because it is constitutive of 'add 2' that only by adding 2 have I acted in accord with the meaning of 'add 2'. Luntley put the point thus:

> The normativity of content means that understanding the meaning of an expression requires that you grasp certain patterns of use. These are patterns of use that you have to grasp if you understand the concept. ... Understanding the concept places certain obligations upon the speaker to use the concept in a patterned manner. (Luntley, 1999: 16)

Recall Wittgenstein talking of music and how to explain, for example, what a theme might mean (and note the added emphasis): 'In order to "explain" I could only compare it with something else which has the same rhythm (I mean the same *pattern*)' (PI §527).

Intentional psychological states involve normativity as a constitutive feature. This particular mental state (e.g. understanding, intending, or remembering) that I now experience involves the norms that govern whether or not the mental state can be assessed as correct or incorrect, even if those norms will be realized in the future.

The rule-governed nature of normativity

The claim that intentional psychological states are constitutively normative depends partly upon the analogy with rules. It clearly is constitutive of rules that they should constrain, that they should lay down norms. The point that Wittgenstein employs is that we can similarly think of psychological phenomena. In the example of completing an arithmetical series, indeed, the two things coincide: understanding how to complete the series (a psychological phenomenon) is the ability to apply the arithmetical rule. In Wittgenstein's discussion of reading, it is the way in which the written words ineluctably (or normatively) guide the reader that is crucially puzzling. Wittgenstein describes this in various ways: it is the experience,

> ... of being influenced, of causal connexion, of being guided ... I as it were feel the movement of the lever which connects seeing the letters with speaking. (PI §170)

Or, I might describe it by saying that,

> ... the written word *intimates* the sound to me.—Or again, ... letter and sound form a *unity*—as it were an alloy. (PI §171)

Wittgenstein adds:

> In the same way e.g. the faces of famous men and the sound of their names are fused together. This name strikes me as the only right one for this face. (*ibid.*)

The normative relation between the face and the name, or (in the case of reading) between the word and its sound, can be discussed in terms of rules. (Failure to recognize familiar faces can be a symptom in acquired diffuse neurocognitive dysfunction, to which I shall return in Chapter 5. Understanding what constitutes face-recognition, therefore, is important for our constitutive understanding of dementia). Wittgenstein's so-called rule-following considerations are all about the normativity of intentional psychological states, such as understanding and reading, and the way in which these can be construed in terms of rule-following. Moreover, normativity is a feature of intentional psychological phenomena that is generalizable:

> A wish seems already to know what will or would satisfy it; a proposition, a thought, what makes it true—even when that thing is not there at all! Whence this *determining* of what is not yet there? This despotic demand? (PI § 437)

In this section, I have established the basis of the argument that follows. Intentional psychological states are normative. This is a constitutive feature: they constrain how the world will be. What is special about intentional psychological concepts is that they involve, constitutively, a link being made between a particular mental state and something constrained in the world to satisfy the mental state. This constraining works in the way that rules work. One way to understand normativity, therefore, is to understand the nature of rule-following.

Negative conclusions

Even if a proper appreciation of Wittgenstein's remarks is to see them in their positive light, the rule-following discussion seems largely concerned with the negative task of undermining a number of possible explanations of the normativity of understanding. How it is that something we 'grasp in a flash' can constrain the future might be explained by underlying (i) metaphysical, (ii) mental or (iii) causal processes, but the rule-following discussion shows that such explanations are deficient. In the rest of this section I shall briefly consider the negative arguments used by Wittgenstein to show what does *not* constitute rule-following. On the way, I shall advertise some possible implications of the discarded theories for our understanding of dementia.[1]

(i) Rules and Platonism

Platonism makes normativity a metaphysical notion. I briefly mentioned the transcendental nature of Plato's forms in Chapter 2. Platonism postulates fixed rails of correct usage. The rails are laid out in advance and somehow guide the intentions implicit in my use of concepts. Luntley describes matters thus:

> The Platonist account of the source of grammar holds that what constrains our use of a sign is the existence of abstract patterns of use to which our use must conform. (Luntley, 2003a: 9)

The idea that there is some ideal (a fixed track) to which concepts conform has, at least, some intuitive appeal in mathematics. Wittgenstein considers the idea (only to reject it) in his discussion of rule-following in connection with the giving of the order to 'add 2' (cf. PI §§185–7). The suggestion is that, having given this order, it is somehow predetermined that when the pupil reaches 1000, the next number will be 1002, and not 1004, even if this possibility has not actually occurred to the teacher. Wittgenstein's description of the Platonist's thought is as follows:

> ... your idea was that that act of meaning the order had in its own way already traversed all those steps: that when you meant it your mind as it were flew ahead and took all the steps before you physically arrived at this or that one.
>
> Thus you were inclined to use such expressions as: 'the steps are *really* already taken, even before I take them in writing or orally or in thought'. And it seemed as if they were in some *unique* way predetermined, anticipated—as only the act of meaning can anticipate reality. (PI §188)

Before indicating what is wrong with this view, it is illuminating to consider the implications for our understanding of dementia. Say that following a rule is a matter of adhering to metaphysical tracks, then intentional psychological phenomena would have to be accounted for constitutively in such terms. Therefore, when I calculate something I am (in some sense) steered as I make the calculation towards the solution. I might take a wrong turning, because I have not latched on to the rails sufficiently. But there is a metaphysical sense in which, once I have the track in view, I can be sure that my calculation is correct. Because others will have access to the same metaphysical rails, they will agree. What makes a calculation correct is not the agreement, but the Platonic ideal to which we all conform. In which case the person with acquired diffuse neurocognitive dysfunction, who used to be able to calculate but can no longer, must be—in some sense—derailed. He or she has lost track, which is what, therefore, the loss of mind of dementia amounts to.

Although the thought that normativity is present as some sort of 'superlative fact' (PI §192) is tempting as a way of accounting for its force, it is problematic. The main problem is that, even if there were a Platonist realm containing the standards to which we had to conform to follow a series or use a word with meaning, there would be within that realm another standard according to which, having reached 1000, the pupil ought to say '1004' rather than '1002'. The question then becomes how will we know which standard to choose? That is, the Platonic realm, which is supposed to supply normativity, requires some normatively constrained means of choosing within it. It just is not possible to track a metaphysical standard without already having some notion of what is and is not correct, but this is the account of normativity that the metaphysical standard is intended to supply (Thornton, 1998: 42).

Pears takes an approach that emphasizes that speaking a language is a practice:

> Wittgenstein's objection to [Platonism] is that it removes the basis of the distinction between obeying and disobeying a linguistic rule. Speaking a language is a practice and it is an essential feat of any practice that its followers cannot slavishly conform to any fixed paradigm, even a metaphysical one. What they actually do necessarily makes some contribution to determining what counts as what they ought to do. (Pears, 1988: 363; and cf. 460–501)

Luntley is more damning:

> … the Platonist purports to have an account of the source of grammar that really amounts to no more than a positing of the existence of grammar! Furthermore, the existence of grammar is posited not in actual ordinary sign use, but in an abstract Platonic realm that then, somehow or other, interacts with ordinary sign use. (Luntley, 2003a: 10)

Rather than pursue Wittgenstein's thoughts about Platonism further, I simply wish to note that, despite any intuitive appeal at first blush (cf. PI §§ 218–21), Platonism cannot provide a coherent account of normativity. So intentional psychological states are not a matter of a metaphysical attachment and, however appealing as figurative speech, dementia is not some sort of metaphysical derailment.

(ii) Rules and mental processes

What, then, of the possibility that rule-following is a matter of an internal mental process? A comparison can be made between following a rule and understanding a series. Wittgenstein points out various ways in which a pupil might go wrong when asked to write down a series of numbers. He suggests (ironically) the impossibility of stating for certain when the series has been mastered (PI §145). Understanding how to go on in a series may lead to an exclamation, 'Now I can go on!' (PI §151), as if the understanding appeared in a flash, but it is not the case that just *one* thing may have happened in this flash. It may be that a formula has occurred to the person, or it may be that the pupil simply realized that he knew the series (say he had seen it before, but did not recall it until this instant). Thus, '"He understands" must have more in it than: the formula occurs to him' (PI §152).

Wittgenstein suggests, ironically, that what we do is try, 'to get hold of the mental process of understanding which seems to be hidden' (PI §153). Even if we found, however, some one thing that happened in all the specific examples of understanding, why should *that* be the understanding? Wittgenstein points out, too, that talk of understanding being *hidden* is odd, since I can say that I have understood when I have understood!

I might find *particular circumstances* that justify my saying 'Now I can go on'. I learn the meaning of a word under particular circumstances (Z §§114–16). Hence,

> Try not to think of understanding as a 'mental process' at all.—For *that* is the expression which confuses you. ... In the sense in which there are processes (including mental processes) which are characteristic of understanding, understanding is not a mental process. (PI §154)

It is important to notice that Wittgenstein does not here *deny* mental processes. He denies that there is a *particular* mental process meant by understanding. There may be various mental processes occurring during an act of understanding, but none constitutes it.

What it is to remember, therefore, is not fully given by reference to inner processes. Wittgenstein argues rather that remembering is something that takes place in particular circumstances and, moreover, that these external circumstances give us grounds for ascribing mental capabilities. It would follow that an account of acquired diffuse neurocognitive dysfunction that concentrates on internal, mental processes as a way to explain intentional psychological phenomena would be too narrow. Understanding dementia also requires reference to be made to circumstances, to the surround, and to the world. I shall return to discuss problems surrounding inner processes during my discussion, in Chapter 5, of cognitive neuropsychology.

(iii) Rules and causal processes

Similar thoughts are relevant to the suggestion that rule-following is a matter of causal processes. Such a view suggests that the normativity of intentional psychological phenomena is just a matter of certain things being caused. For instance, it can be argued (as in the disease model, which I shall discuss in Chapter 5) that my being able to recognize someone is a matter of particular physical processes going on in my brain. Similarly, in the case of reading, Wittgenstein mischievously considers the possibility that all we really need to be certain whether or not someone is reading is a better acquaintance with the nervous system (PI §158). These neurons cause me to remember a face or to read correctly and their absence means I forget. If intentional psychological phenomena are constituted by causal processes, a narrow conception of the disease model of dementia would be true. Wittgenstein's discussion, however, suggests that causal processes provide an inadequate construal of rule-following.

Wittgenstein discusses the topic of reading at some length, perhaps because it allows him to consider the possibility of a reading *machine* (PI §157). Such a machine would work along causal lines and it can be compared to the mechanistic processes that might go on in human readers. Written words can be regarded as imposing a rule on the reader.

Wittgenstein considers the possibility that, 'you *derive* the reproduction from the original' (PI §162). The notion of 'deriving' might help us to explain the psychological mechanism that constitutes being compelled by a rule, in this case the rule that causes us to move from printed letters to particular sounds. As with understanding, it appears we are looking for the essence of what it is to derive—something hidden—whereas the meaning of 'derive' is plain in its use. Still, deriving turns out not to get us any further than reading itself. There will be different circumstances in which we shall say that someone can read (PI §164). Wittgenstein puts to himself the objection that 'reading is a quite particular process' (PI §165). But he is unable then to identify any *particular* process, although it is clear that various different things occur when we read, as is shown by the difference between reading ordinary print and reading capitals. There is not one essential feature that occurs in all cases of reading (PI §168).

For both reading and understanding, the story is the same, as summarized by Anscombe thus:

> ... there are experiences connected with reading, but 'reading' is not the name of any of them. Similarly there is a variety of experiences connected with an occasion of understanding, but 'understanding' is not the name of any of them. (Anscombe, 1991: 7)

Following a rule, as exemplified either by reading or understanding, is not a particular experience and is defined neither by some characteristic mental accompaniment (it is not a mental process), nor by a set, causal sequence of events (it is not a particular causal process).

A sense of normative constraint is in evidence again when Wittgenstein discusses copying doodles on a piece of paper and the feeling that one is guided in so doing. We might say, 'I did it *because* ...', and that 'because' seems to have a special force; in other words, there was no other way. Wittgenstein called this experiencing the *'because'* (PI §176). He wishes to say, 'I experience the because' (PI §177), but he does not want to call any *phenomenon* the 'experience of the because' (PI §176). There is no *thing* in the external world, nor in my internal world, requiring that *that* line or stroke should produce from me *this* line or utterance. However, it remains true that I felt I had to do it this way. I wish to say, 'I experience the because', when I reflect on what I experience, since,

> I look at it through the medium of the concept 'because' (or 'influence' or 'cause' or 'connexion') (PI §177)

The notion of 'the medium' emphasizes the causal power that is being described. There is a hypothetical mechanism acting through the 'because', which thereby acquires the substantial status of a medium, to cause whatever it is that is caused (a copied doodle, or a spoken from a written word).

We can gain a better purchase on Wittgenstein's point by making a comparison with Hume. Their arguments share certain features, but are importantly different. The similarities include Hume saying that in single instances of mental or physical activity,

> ... there is nothing that produces any impression ... of power or necessary connexion. (Hume, 1975: 78 [Sect VII, Part II])

Both philosophers state that there is no phenomenon in the world to cause the feeling of compulsion. McGinn makes a similar comparison by suggesting that both philosophers demonstrate 'epistemological naturalism', in that they both note the importance of training, customs and practices in their attempts to understand (e.g.) causation (McGinn, 1984: 40–1).

On the other hand, there are important differences, in that Hume makes matters highly empirical: you just always have seen billiard balls react in this way when they hit each other; whereas Wittgenstein's point emphasizes language. Hence, for instance, his talk of 'the because'. Wittgenstein wishes to lead us back to ordinary language in which we use such concepts thus and so. For Wittgenstein, this use is intrinsically normative: our use of concepts is constrained and constraining. Hence, as Luntley (2003a) has convincingly argued, Wittgenstein is not encouraging the thought that we can get no further than describing ordinary language, as if it is totally transparent. What is required by Wittgenstein is an understanding of 'ordinary use' that is not transparent. According to Luntley, this comes in the notion of 'use as practice':

> Use as practice is opaque, for even if it is describable, what gets described are patterns of correct use immanent in ordinary language. (Luntley, 2003a: 63)

We might put this by saying that the ordinary use of language—even if it *is* 'ordinary' in the sense that it is everyday—contains within it something that is darkly mysterious. Somehow, embedded in our language, there is something that is powerfully constraining on the world. If we are to say it is a causal process, Wittgenstein's point is that there are lots of possible processes to point to, but they do not get to the heart of the issue, which is a constitutive one, where it shows a misunderstanding to think we have pinned down the notion of understanding by pointing to causal processes in the brain or even in our thoughts. These are contingent matters, which could be otherwise, whereas what it is 'to understand *x*' is only *one* thing. Moreover, this normativity is immanent in the sense that it is within the language use itself. It does not reside elsewhere.

Hume is merely making a descriptive epistemological point about regularly observed connections coming to be habitually expected. The contrast here is between the contingency of the epistemological point and the normativity of the conceptual point. In Hume's epistemology things might have been different, but in Wittgenstein's metaphysics, these concepts being thus and so, their use is constrained and constraining. This is not a contingent matter, but a constitutive and immanent one. Hume leads towards scepticism concerning causality, whereas Wittgenstein's discussion accepts causality but places it in a broader constitutive field. What is key for Wittgenstein is the thought that normativity is a constitutive and immanent feature of certain sorts of human practices, whereas Hume's account fails to sustain the normativity that a positive account of rule-following requires. If causal processes are also relevant, they cannot constitute everything that needs to be understood about intentional psychological states.

Summary

In this section, I have considered some of Wittgenstein's negative arguments concerning rule-following. His arguments demonstrate that rule-following is not adequately described by a metaphysical account, nor by inner or causal processes. Models of dementia that depend on such a construal of intentional psychological phenomena will, accordingly, run into problems too: acquired diffuse neurocognitive dysfunction is not metaphysical derailment; nor can it be understood solely by reference to inner abnormal processes in isolation from the external circumstances of the world; nor should it be considered merely in terms of an interruption to causal processes.

To return to Miss Breen, who is in many ways inaccessible (although we shall need to qualify this statement in due course), her inaccessibility (such as it may be) is not because she has lost herself at some sort of metaphysical level; nor is it that we have lost contact with the inner processes that she can no longer articulate; nor is it that—to understand her—we need to understand the causal connections that are now deficient. Her mental life is affected by her acquired diffuse neurocognitive dysfunction: she cannot read, remember, calculate, use language with much coherence, and so on. This failure in terms of intentional psychological phenomena is not, however, to be thought of in the terms that Wittgenstein has rejected in discussing these phenomena. None the less, Miss Breen does demonstrate a failure in terms of her ability to follow certain sorts of rules. Is this negative characterization all that we can say about Miss Breen? Well, so far we only have a negative account of what rule-following does *not* amount to. I shall return to the implications of the positive account for Miss Breen towards the end of the chapter.

Well, but is it then even possible to give an account of what constitutes rule-following, given the negative flavour of Wittgenstein's discussion? Is it possible that the negative arguments might prove overwhelming and lead to total scepticism concerning rule-following? On this view, intentional psychological states simply cannot constrain reality, since what has one meaning one day might have a different meaning the next. But this is problematic when we think of acquired diffuse neurocognitive dysfunction. For what was a sign of cognitive impairment yesterday or in one place, might today or in some other place be normal. It is to this sceptical interpretation that I now turn.

The sceptical challenge

Given the reality of acquired diffuse neurocognitive dysfunction, and the fact that we *do* operate in a normatively constrained world, the sceptical challenge must be met. As I shall come on to discuss, one response to such scepticism has been to appeal to the community as a way of securing normativity. On such a view, the norms that allow a diagnosis of dementia to be made inhere in the community. It is a short step, then, to consider the possibility, which I discuss in Chapter 5, that acquired diffuse neurocognitive dysfunction is a social construction. It is the sceptical challenge that motivates the community view, so here I shall demonstrate its power.

The charge that no constitutive account can be given of rule-following is made in connection with §198 of the *Philosophical Investigations*. That section starts by asking how a rule can show a person what to do at a particular point. Wittgenstein's interlocutor suggests that, on some interpretation, whatever I do is in accord with the rule. Wittgenstein prefers to say that interpretations of rules can be various, but hang in the air since, 'Interpretations by themselves do not determine meaning' (PI §198). Elsewhere Wittgenstein comments that the statement, 'Any sentence still stands in need of an interpretation', would have to mean, 'no sentence can be understood without a rider' (PG §47). This line of reasoning threatens to make language and communication impossible, because every statement would require an interpretation, ad infinitum.

The negative conclusion, with its suggestion of an infinite regression, lay behind Saul Kripke's now famous sceptical interpretation of Wittgenstein. Kripke argues that, whilst we suppose our language expresses concepts in such a way that, once grasped, all future applications of the concept are determined, in fact (whatever is in my mind), I remain free to interpret concepts differently (Kripke, 1982). This follows directly from Kripke's consideration of Wittgenstein stating:

> This was our paradox: no course of action could be determined by a rule, because every course of action can be made to accord with the rule. (PI §201)

Kripke maintains:

> [T]here is no fact about me that distinguishes between my meaning a definite function by '+' ... and my meaning nothing at all. (Kripke, *op. cit.*: 21)

Kripke's is a radically sceptical interpretation of Wittgenstein.[2] Since this sceptical challenge itself legitimizes recourse to the community view, and since that view has such influence, it is worth testing the strength of the scepticism. For instance, an exchange between Philip Pettit and Donna Summerfield demonstrates the thoroughgoing nature of Kripke's scepticism. In opposition to Kripke, Pettit (1990a) offers a non-sceptical conception of rules and rule-following according to which, he feels, the 'phenomenology of rule-following' could be saved. He argues that under appropriate circumstances an individual might develop an inclination to follow the correct determinate rule. A compelling response came, however, from Summerfield (1990), who stated: 'various interpretations of a linguistic sign are *always* possible'. Pettit fails in her view because: first, he ignores the sceptical point that we cannot say 'what determines *which* rule is *the* relevant rule?'; secondly, because he thinks an inclination or disposition might determine *which* rule is *the* relevant rule, ignoring that such inclinations themselves may be signs that can logically be interpreted in various ways. Thus:

> ... if rules are to guide our actions, and so on, the linguistic expressions by which we represent them to ourselves need to be interpreted, and we cannot fix the interpretation

merely by producing more linguistic signs that themselves require interpretation, or we launch the regress. (Summerfield, *op. cit.*)

This seems to me more cogent than the multiplicity of rules, which will yet be free (according to Pettit (1990b)) of problems of interpretation.

As Kripke realized, talk of inclinations (as used by Pettit) does not capture the sort of normativity that inheres in psychological concepts. Another thought, however, is that it might actually be *right* to say that the correct response to a demand for a constitutive account of rule-following is solely to point to examples of rule-governed practices. Over against Kripke, adverting to practices (as I shall discuss below) is by no means to be thoroughly sceptical, especially if practices themselves yield a normative account. Still, the whole point of Kripke's critique is that there is nothing to ensure normativity. This thought led Kripke to his form of the community view. Before considering communitarian views, however, I shall first consider the positive interpretation provided by an emphasis on practices.

Positive interpretations: accounts of practice

The way to avoid the sceptical trap is to focus on rule-following as practice. This needs to be fleshed out. So far I have suggested:

- intentional psychological states are normative;
- normativity can be thought of as rule-following.

I shall now add two further stages to the argument:

- rules and rule-following involve practices and customs;
- practices and customs are embedded in the world.

There are different ways of understanding practices. In this section, I shall consider two accounts: first, the community view, which implies that practices are a matter of community agreement; secondly, constructivism, which suggests that practices are a matter of people deciding as they go along. I shall reject both these approaches, but later in this chapter I shall set out alternative ways to think of practices, which provide richer accounts of our mental lives.

Just to relate this back to acquired diffuse neurocognitive dysfunction, if intentional psychological states really do demonstrate normativity (despite the sceptics), then our understanding of acquired diffuse neurocognitive dysfunction must similarly encompass a normative account of such mental states. A test that might be applied, therefore, to models of dementia is this: does this model allow an account of intentional psychological phenomena that shows normativity? Meanwhile, if normativity is akin to rule-following and rule-following is a matter of practice, in seeking to characterize normativity further, I need to consider how practices help at all.

Rule-following and practices

Wittgenstein uses the example of a pupil exclaiming 'Now I can go on' when trying to grasp an arithmetical series. He points out that this exclamation is not short for a description of all the circumstances that might surround such an utterance (PI §179).

My understanding and (say) a formula occurring to me are two different things (PI §154). It might be, for instance, that I can carry on the series without really understanding it, but just—as it were—by applying some rule. As so often, Wittgenstein points to the variety of things that might occur: there is no one essential thing, except that I can actually go on.

In the same way, understanding a musical theme is not one thing. In response to the question, 'so what do I actually experience when I hear this theme and understand what I hear?', Wittgenstein replies:

> – nothing occurs to me by way of reply except trivialities. Images, sensations of movement, recollections and such like. (CV: 70)

Another tactic to explain understanding, already discussed, is to point to some sort of inner mental process. But Wittgenstein is more interested in: '*the circumstances* under which' a person having such an experience is justified 'in saying ... that he understands, that he knows how to go on' (PI §§154–5). Concerning the exclamation, 'Now I can go on', Wittgenstein emphasizes: '*This is how these words are used*' (PI § 180). The exclamation is not a description of a mental state, nor a matter of noting a regular occurrence, which has now become habitual (as Hume might have suggested). It is a fallible expression indicating that one has mastered the norms, or normative patterns of use, that govern the practice of continuing the series and supply meaning to the notion of understanding. What is needed, as an antidote to the picture of the mental processes and states as merely internal goings-on, is an understanding of the role such expressions play in language (PI §182).

It is in worldly contexts that judgements are made about whether or not someone has really read or truly understood. Wittgenstein's remarks are intended to fracture the links, which seem to form habitually, between intentional mental states and the inner world and to forge instead links between intentional mental states and the outer world; that is, he wishes to draw our attention to the ways in which inner and outer are enmeshed. Hence the importance of looking, not just inwards, but at the *circumstances*, at the surround. For me to claim that I can read the Cyrillic alphabet or understand how to play chess is, therefore, importantly linked (whatever 'inner' things may or may not be happening) to external circumstances or contexts. It implies that I shall do certain things in the world under certain circumstances, not as a way of providing evidence that certain inner things are also occurring, but rather as a constitutive matter: this is simply what it is to read Cyrillic or understand chess.

The rule-following considerations focus on the intentionality of psychological verbs, the way in which 'the act of meaning can anticipate reality' (PI §188). Again, this is a recognition of the normativity of such concepts. Wittgenstein goes on to ask:

> ... what kind of super-strong connexion exists between the act of intending and the thing intended?—Where is the connexion effected between the sense of the expression 'Let's play a game of chess' and all the rules of the game? (PI §197)

His response is: 'Well, in the list of rules of the game, in the teaching of it, in the day-to-day practice of playing' (*ibid.*). This suggests that the understanding implicit in intending to play chess involves an acquaintance with the whole enterprise of chess-playing. There is a sense of immanence here: within the concept of intending to play chess—if the intention to play is genuine—since this implies a practice, there are already a whole set of things that must be the case. The world is constrained by the intention, but the normative constraint is inward: it does not lie elsewhere other than in the practice that surrounds the notion of intending to play chess. The point is that we should look to the full context of chess-playing to locate the connection between intending to play and actual playing, which involves the use of rules. This does not specifically answer the putative problem of intentionality, but it shows where the answer is to be found, namely within the day-to-day practices surrounding our use of psychological concepts. And this again makes the point that the answer does not lie in a metaphysical realm, nor in causal or inner processes.

Understanding the meaning of a word involves understanding its use. But another way to put this is to say that, as in the example of playing chess, to understand meaning is to participate in a practice. Part of what it is to understand is precisely to be able to take part in the practice; this is constitutive of the understanding. Again this is a reflection of the normative nature of understanding, which ensures that only certain things will count as true understanding and other things will not. As Wittgenstein puts it towards the end of the rule-following discussion:

> … there is a way of grasping a rule which … is exhibited in what we call 'obeying the rule' and 'going against it' in actual cases. (PI §201)

Thus, to be able to follow a rule and, more to the point, to understand something, are matters of grasping practices. But practices have a history, a context, or surround.

Intentional psychological phenomena, therefore, to be fully understood, require an external context. If anything is going to prevent the slide to scepticism it is likely to be found in the account of practices. Whether we are speaking of rule-following or the normativity that surrounds remembering, what makes the rule or the intentional mental state determinate is the constitutive practice of which the rule or the intentional mental state are instances. Practices involve external circumstances and contexts—the world no less—which should suggest a greater degree of resistance to scepticism than seemingly fragile inner processes and the like. What is needed, however, is a fuller account of such practices.

Kripke's sceptical interpretation of Wittgenstein is undercut by the appeal to 'actual cases' and by the realization that '"obeying a rule" is a practice' (PI §202). Nevertheless, however wrongheadedly, the sceptical challenge persists and the appeal to practice requires further unpacking. The community view and constructivism are ways of unpacking 'practice'. What is at issue, however, remains our understanding of acquired diffuse neurocognitive dysfunction. Could it be that, as social constructionism suggests, a diagnosis of dementia rests on judgements about intentional psychological states which amount to no more than social constructs? Or should we accept the constructivist view that what is normatively constrained is, as it were, made-up? There is instead an unfolding process of decision making. This would seem (rightly or wrongly) to threaten the notion of objectivity in diagnosis. Or is there, perhaps, an alternative view?

The community view

Kripke's (1982) 'sceptical solution' to the 'sceptical paradox' is a version of communitarianism. It is not just that individuals must interpret signs themselves; a communal practice sets a standard of rightness. So, here, the practice in which rule-following or normativity inhere is the practice of the community. My linguistic community sets checks on my use of concepts. Several responses to this view are possible. For instance, one response is to accept the sceptical point that nothing connects the meaning of a word to its correct use, but then to be sceptical about the community, and stress the ability of the individual to assign standards of correctness. The key thing is that 'rules are anchored in practice' (Blackburn, 1984). Alternatively, it can be argued that there is nothing in Wittgenstein's argument involving a commitment to a 'multiplicity of agents' (Baker & Hacker, 1984: 20).

> What is here crucial for Wittgenstein's account of the concept of following a rule is recurrent action in appropriate contexts, action which counts as following the rule. Whether others are involved is a further question. (*ibid.*: 20–1)

Wittgenstein might say that the grammar of 'rule-following' entails that a practice of rule-following must be *in principle* public, but this involves (according to Baker & Hacker [*op. cit.*]) no commitment to a social context.

Kripke is not alone in his recourse to the community view. Whilst not sharing Kripke's scepticism about meaning, Malcolm similarly writes that,

> … for Wittgenstein the concept of a rule presupposes a community within which a common agreement in actions fixes the meaning of a rule. (Malcolm, 1986: 175)

Baker and Hacker's view (*op.cit.*) is that it might be possible for a solitary person to follow a rule. McGinn agrees that rule-following is individualistic (McGinn, *op. cit.*: 198–200). Against this view, however, Malcolm (1989) emphasizes Wittgenstein's repeated insistence that there can be rules, 'only within a framework of overwhelming agreement'. The tenor of Malcolm's argument is captured by these quotations:

> A rule can exist only in a human practice, or in what is analogous to it. And what a rule requires and what following it is, presupposes the background of a social setting in which there is quiet agreement as to what 'going on in the same way' is. (*ibid.*)

similarly,

> Wittgenstein always puts emphasis on the fact that the words of language have meaning only because they are enmeshed in common patterns of human life. (*ibid.*)

The issue, for my purposes, is whether it is the case that normativity depends on some sort of community agreement. The general problem with Kripke's line is that if nothing connects a rule or the meaning of a word to its correct application, then all judgements lack factual truth (cf. Thornton, 1998: 76–9). In addition, there can be no such thing as the sort of normativity that the rule-following discussion picks out as being constitutive of such notions as understanding or reading. There is nothing to stop the sceptical turn once it has gained a purchase. In which case, as Blackburn (*op. cit.*) suggests, one can similarly be sceptical about the community. This means that one will have to be sceptical about any form of normativity whatsoever. Normativity, on this view, need not be normative, since rules are objectively indeterminate. The community merely dignifies something as a case of rule-following. This amounts to no more than 'a projectivist account of an ersatz version of normativity' (Thornton, *op. cit.*: 74).

Turning to the account given by Malcolm, according to which a word has meaning by virtue of its use by a community over time, even if this does not fall foul of the incoherence suggested by Kripke's scepticism, it nevertheless does mean that normativity inheres in the practices of the community. There is something laudable about the emphasis in Malcolm's account on enmeshment 'in common patterns of human life', a background social setting and 'human practice'. The emphasis on the *human* context is important, since it is this context that is intended to supply the possibility of going wrong (however the individual may judge matters).

Malcolm's communitarian account of normativity, however, veers away from the normativity of the Wittgensteinian account that I am commending. The possibility of going wrong implies that there is something external to the individual and, therefore, something that is potentially public. But the public (the community) does not provide, contrary to Malcolm's view, criteria for what it is to go wrong. Rather, the possibility of public scrutiny *results from* the normativity that constitutes what it is to follow (or go against) a rule. It remains true that rules (and the normativity of intentional psychological phenomena) are enmeshed in (and only properly understood within the context of) common patterns of human practice.

The view I have just commended is, however, subjected to considerable criticism by Williams (1999). Her support of the community view, which she derives from Wittgenstein, is expressed with great clarity.

> Wittgenstein's point is that a rule or master-pattern is such only from within a practice that is itself a kind of complex regularity, namely, community regularity as expressed in agreement in action and judgment.
>
> …
>
> The central point is that the very idea of normativity, and so the structure within which the distinction between correct and incorrect can be drawn, cannot get a foothold unless the practice is a social one. (Williams, *op. cit.*: 175)

Williams then highlights two important features of her account.

> First, it is the *social* practice that provides the structure within which individual understanding can obtain or individual judgment be made.
>
> …
>
> Second, community agreement does not constitute a justification for particular judgments. (*ibid.*: 176)

The first of these points is one that other philosophers (e.g. Baker & Hacker, 1984) have simply denied. They argue that a completely isolated individual, one who has never had an experience of community on which to draw, could still demonstrate rule-following. But, Williams asks, how could a radically solitary figure know the difference between correcting a practice to accord with a rule and changing the rule? The 'master-pattern' must come from somewhere else, and (she suggests) this depends on how *we* take the master-pattern (Williams, *op. cit.*: 172–7). The argument also depends on exegesis and Williams is able to point to the typical ways in which Wittgenstein talks (e.g. of rules being like orders), which seem to indicate that others would be around (Williams, *op. cit.*: 295, footnote 17). We have already adverted to some of the arguments against this view: even if others are typically involved, it does not follow that they need in principle to be involved. The key thing is that the practice has the requisite complexity to be established as setting the structure of which Williams speaks (*vide supra*). Luntley (2003a) is fairly dismissive of the community view. In considering the 'lone language user', he focuses on the sense of the 'use':

> If 'use' picks out a thin conception of use, mere empirical patterns of sign deployment, then it is utterly unclear how sign deployment gets policed by reference to what amounts to no more than more of the same; the sign deployment of the individual gets policed by being measured against the sign deployment of others. If there is a problem with what constitutes the policing of sign deployment as such, ... then simply throwing more signs into the picture offers no policing. (Luntley, 2003a: 16)

A thicker conception of 'use' is one in which normativity inheres in any case, so the community is not required to provide the 'policing'. This does seem, I think, to dismiss the first of the features highlighted by Williams (see also Luntley, 2003a: 123 footnote 24). What of the second feature? Williams fleshes this out thus:

> What we mean is not explained by an appeal to generalizations about what most people say. But that we mean what we do is because of what most people say and do. (Williams, *op. cit.*: 176)

This is interesting because it suggests that the community view is more about fitting into a practice, rather than pointing to the general use of signs. Just pointing to more and more signs falls foul of the criticisms made above. But embedding meaning in a practice sounds less like Luntley's 'thin' conception of 'use' and more like the 'thick' conception. Here is Luntley:

> Use as practice is opaque, for even if it is describable, what gets described are patterns of correct use immanent in ordinary language. (Luntley, *op. cit.*: 63);

and,

> The patterns are patterns of actions. If you think of grammar as a structure, then what we find at the nodes of this structure are not signs, but actions of agents as they use signs. (Luntley, *op. cit.*: 18)

Williams seems very close to this:

> Grammar, then, for Wittgenstein, is *immanent* in our practices, not the transcendental condition of our practices. It is not independent of our lived practices. These practices just are de facto agreement in action and judgment. (Williams, *op. cit.*: 177)

There do seem to be reasons for arguing that strong resistance to scepticism comes from the notion of *language use as practice* and that the number of people involved in the practice is not the deciding factor, but rather the nature of the practice. Whether the lone Robinson Crusoe language user is capable of developing practices of sufficient thickness and opacity to demonstrate immanent meaning is an empirical matter, but there does not seem to be a reason *in principle* why this should not be possible.

Before moving on, it is worth relating this to acquired diffuse neurocognitive dysfunction. If we wish to think through dementia, we must understand the normative nature of intentional psychological states. Normativity is a matter of being enmeshed in the practices of the community. On the communitarian reading, this suggests that the model I use to understand acquired diffuse neurocognitive dysfunction should regard the loss of psychological capacities as a matter decided, at some level, with reference to the community. It is not just that the community is in a position to say Miss Breen has lost her memory, but Miss Breen's loss of memory is, or (at any rate) amounts to, a decision made in connection with, or by reference to, the community. Put this way, it sounds as if a different community might lead to a different decision; and that sounds as if the loss of memory might not always be loss of memory, depending on the particular community. But this is to undermine the normative nature of such intentional psychological phenomena. This is also to undermine any commitment to realism, according to which the meaning of our words is independent of our use of words; indeed it starts to sound as if the community view creates reality, a sort of linguistic idealism, in which we create our meanings by our use of language (an idea to which I shall return). This is, then, a problem in connection with social constructionism, which I shall discuss again in Chapter 5.

Both sceptical and non-sceptical appeals to the community can only provide an ersatz notion of normativity. The normativity of intentional psychological states is *constitutive*. The community view makes it seem as if normativity is simply a *consequence* of public opinion, unless (of course) the notion of 'use' employed in spelling out the role of the community makes it plain that 'use' refers to Luntley's thicker conception. But at that point the account seems constitutive of normativity, as immanent in language and to the notion of 'use as practice':

> Use as practice is … a conception of the way in which uses of language are normatively connected. … The normative patterns of correct/incorrect use are found within use, they do not lie behind it. … It is not a conception in which we describe language and then look for something external to language with which to measure the correctness/incorrectness of use. (Luntley, *op. cit.*: 64)

In which case, neither do we need to look to the community to provide our policing of correct and incorrect usage.

Constructivism and practices

In this section I shall provide an alternative account of practices. This is another way of understanding how practices counter the sceptical challenge and, therefore, another way of understanding the normativity of intentional psychological phenomena. If true, this furnishes us with another account of how we might understand acquired diffuse neurocognitive dysfunction. According to this view, practices—which are constitutive of understanding, reading and remembering—are a matter of people deciding as they go along. This gives us a different picture of normativity as akin to a disposition. Wright says:

> All that I can effectively intend to do is to apply 'green' only when it *seems* to me that things are relevantly similar; but that is not a commitment to any regularity—it is merely an undertaking to apply 'green' only when I am disposed to apply 'green'. (Wright, 1981: 37)

We simply have sincere dispositions, but there is no guarantee that we succeed in always applying the word in the same way. Elsewhere, Wright suggests that the rule-following discussion in Wittgenstein has, 'objectivity of meaning as its general target' and he labels this view 'constructivism', according to which we are, 'the perennial creators of our concepts, not in the style of conscious architects but just by doing what comes naturally' (Wright, 1986: 294).[3]

Wright has not been alone in stressing natural dispositions. Budd emphasizes, in his discussion of the positive conclusion of the rule-following considerations, on a person's having a capacity or disposition to respond to a sign in a particular way (Budd, 1989: 38). Pettit (1990a, 1990b) attempts to counter Kripke's scepticism by appealing to inclinations in particular circumstances. McGinn, too, writes:

> What has to be recognised is that at some level meaning is fixed by our nature: meaning something is not an achievement of a transcendent mind divorced from our 'form of life'. The basis of the normative is the natural. (McGinn, *op. cit.*: 86)

Similarly, Bloor suggests—in a manner that is strikingly constructionist—that 'we create meaning as we move from case to case. (Bloor, 1997: 19). He continues:

> The real sources of constraint preventing our going anywhere and everywhere, as we move from case to case, are the social circumstances impinging upon us: our instincts, our biological nature, our sense experience, our interactions with other people, our immediate purposes, our training, our anticipation of and response to sanctions, and so on through the gamut of causes, starting with the psychological and ending with the sociological. (Bloor, *op. cit.*: 20)

Now, it is not that these authors agree in their interpretations of Wittgenstein. Indeed, McGinn prefers to talk of a *capacity* to mean something rather than a disposition (McGinn, *op. cit.*: 174); and Wright (1989) has been severe on McGinn's views. But McGinn also describes Wittgenstein's fundamental thesis as being, 'that meaning rests ultimately upon the bedrock of *our natural propensities*' (my emphasis) (McGinn, *op. cit.*: 138). And Wright (1989) interprets Wittgenstein as saying that,

> ... the requirements of rules exist only within the framework of institutional activities which depend upon *basic human propensities* to agree in judgement. (my emphasis)

So, in these various authors we find a common recourse to natural dispositions, propensities, or inclinations, with a greater or lesser emphasis on the social manifestations of such dispositions, as a way of explaining how it is that meaning-normativity is maintained. In other words, I am normatively constrained by my nature.

There is something reasonable (at first blush) about the appeal to natural dispositions, in the sense that this is how things actually appear to be. I use words with meaning, I intend things, I understand, and in doing so I do not feel constrained by the invisible rails of Platonism, over against which constructivism stands. I have freedom to be inventive in my use of words, so that new meanings might (naturally) emerge. But it is not so clear that normativity itself can simply be a matter of my doing what comes naturally. Normativity must provide a way to discriminate between what *is* right and what *seems* right. Of course, I naturally use words in a way that seems right and when I understand the arithmetical series, it naturally seems to me that 1004 should follow 1002. But what guarantees that these things *are* right and are *normatively* constrained?

Wright recognizes that there is more to normativity than is supplied simply by an appeal to human nature. Hence he notes that Wittgenstein reminds us that,

> ... the requirements of rules ... are also, in any particular case, independent of our judgements, supplying standards in terms of which it may be right to regard those judgements, even if they enjoy consensus, as incorrect. (*ibid.*)

As this makes plain, it is not just a matter of our deciding in each particular case how we should be constrained, otherwise normativity would be lost. McDowell (1984) certainly contends that Wright's view, relying on dispositions or reactions, abolishes normativity. The point about normativity (exploited by Kripke) is precisely that inclinations and dispositions cannot capture normativity since that concerns how I *ought* to behave, rather than just how I am inclined or disposed to behave. Wittgenstein's approach, on Wright's (1989) view, was 'analytical quietism' according to which, 'the phenomenon of actual, widespread human agreement in judgement' is simply noted. The question remains: is there more to normativity than human nature?

Criticism of Wright by McDowell pays attention to his anti-realism, according to which meaning is ratified by my ongoing use of words. (Realism, on the other hand, would be where ratification depended on something in the world, in other words, something independent of my use of words.) On Wright's view the ratification is dependent upon my use and, hence, the focus on my natural dispositions. But McDowell alleges that,

> ... the denial of ratification-independence, by Wright's own insistence, yields a picture of the relation between the communal language and the world in which norms are obliterated. (McDowell, 1984)

For McDowell, it is important to retain the picture, 'in which the openness of an individual to correction by his fellows means that he is subject to norms' (*ibid.*), but since this requires that we have norms in the first place, rather than that the norms are merely a function of the disposition of a particular fellow, it seems to be an argument (and a transcendental one, according to McDowell) against anti-realism. On McDowell's view (which was intended to steer between anti-realism and Platonism),

> Understanding is grasp of patterns that extend to new cases independently of our ratification, as required for meaning to be other than an illusion ...; but the constraints imposed by our concepts do not have the Platonistic autonomy with which they are credited ... (*ibid.*)

The community view makes normativity a consequence of practice and constructivism makes it a matter of ongoing practice constrained by human nature. Both accounts link normativity to practice, but a problem remains: from how we actually *do* act, it may seem that we cannot derive how we *ought* to act. From the fact that, when I say I understand the formula, I intend 1004 to follow 1002, it does not follow that this *must* be so for me the next time, nor for someone else who understands the formula. Practice *in itself* does not provide the forceful account of normativity required to understand intentional psychological states. Something more is required to make practice sufficiently robust to carry the normative commitments of intentional psychological phenomena.

Understanding normativity will provide support to the broader understanding of acquired diffuse neurocognitive dysfunction, which I commend. This *broad* understanding locates acquired diffuse neurocognitive dysfunction not only in the biological, psychological, and social realms, but also in the realm of norms. When Miss Breen cannot understand what is going on, her failure to understand is a loss of intentional abilities too. So acquired diffuse neurocognitive dysfunction involves normative concerns. And in our understanding of normativity the role of practices is—from my perspective—crucially important, because it leads to an understanding of what it is to be a person with dementia. It tends to show that, despite her deficits, judgements about Miss Breen must be based not on models that see her mental life purely in terms of inner or causal processes, nor in terms of some form of dualistic or metaphysical (platonistic) realm, but in terms of her actual standing in a surround in which her behaviour and reactions can be interpreted in the light of human practices.

The embedding of practices

I have been pursuing the normativity of intentional psychological states. In order to avoid utter scepticism about normativity (and, therefore, meaning) I have been led to the importance of practices.

- ◆ Rules and rule-following involve practices and customs.

Neither the communitarian, nor the constructivist reliance on practice can, however, provide the account of normativity that is required. To the notion of practice I shall here add the idea of worldly embedding.

- ◆ Practices and customs are embedded in the world.

The point of this is to give an account of the normativity of intentional mental states. We have already encountered Luntley's idea (*vide supra*) of a thick construal of practice as use, where the normative patterns of correct or incorrect use are immanent: we do not have to look elsewhere; we simply look at patterns of language use, which inherently contain the criteria for correct or incorrect use. But they do this by their immediate engagement with the world. Luntley makes the further point that this engagement is *an engagement by us* as language users, not with each other, but *with the world*; and it is an engagement that involves taking an attitude, having a perspective:

> We, as active users, are integral to the positive phase of the master argument. And what we are doing in using signs is, fundamentally, taking an attitude to the world, the attitude of a judge.
> …
> The fundamental condition for the possibility of judgement is we see things aright.
> (Luntley, 2003a: 18)

Embedded practices provide the requisite account of normativity and suggest an externalist construal of intentional mental content. I shall re-emphasize the point that normativity, once understood in terms of embedded practice, has to be regarded as immanent. That is, pointing to the embedding of practices is pointing to the way in which practices—and therefore normativity—are inherently part of the world. As I shall suggest, this way of describing the normativity of intentional mental states amounts to a form of quietism or minimalism and it accommodates, with caveats, talk of internal relations between mental states and the world. The whole account is, however, transcendental in that it is one that looks to the pre-conditions for the potency of normativity, that is, it searches for the prerequisites for the constraining power of intentional psychological states. The conditions for the possibility of correct and incorrect use are to be found in our engagements as language users with the world. In the rest of this section, therefore, I shall:

(i) establish and clarify the transcendental and immanent nature of normativity;

(ii) consider the implications for the theory of mind, which becomes externalist;

(iii) put forward the quietist approach to normativity, which is a way to stress the irreducibility of normative accounts.

(i) Transcendence and immanence

In this sub-section, I shall make a connection between the transcendental account of normativity and the nature of embedded practices. The connection is this: in order for practices to be normative, in order for them to be impervious even to a thoroughgoing scepticism, they just have to be a part of the world. These practices (which show normativity) are as worldly as rocks and rainbows. So, I want to say, the embedding of the practices that constitute intentional psychological states makes them simply a feature of the world. For the human world to *be* the human world it requires that the normativity, which is shown in practices, is already in place, as an embedded and immanent feature.

In Wittgenstein's discussion, the spectre of the sceptical infinite regression of interpretations, which (given the actual existence of languages used unproblematically day to day) acts as a *reductio ad absurdum*, is dismissed by the positive conclusion of the rule-following considerations:

> … there is a way of grasping a rule which is *not* an *interpretation*, but which is exhibited in what we call 'obeying the rule' and 'going against it' in actual cases. (PI §201)

Wittgenstein argues that 'following a rule' is a possible description of my behaviour under certain conditions precisely because there are norms embedded in practices and customs. Hence, interpretations are not needed and the danger of absurdity is avoided. Earlier, having suggested that interpretations do not determine meaning (PI §198), Wittgenstein talks about being trained to follow a signpost in a certain way. To the objection that this is simply a causal connection, he says:

> … a person goes by a sign-post only in so far as there exists a regular use of sign-posts, a custom. (*ibid.*)

He returns to this thought in §201 when he speaks of a way of grasping a rule that is not an interpretation.

Although §201 links the normativity of intentional psychological states, through their rule-governed nature, to particular practices and customs, it is not clear how these practices and customs resist a sceptical challenge. However, the last step of the argument, which is that practices and customs are embedded in the world, provides a defence. Wittgenstein considers an analogy between following a rule and obeying an order (PI §206). If two people with the same training react differently to the order, who is right? Wittgenstein immediately switches to consider an explorer in an unknown country and asks in what circumstances it could be said that orders were being given or acted upon. He then says:

> The common behaviour of mankind is the system of reference by means of which we interpret an unknown language. (*ibid.*)

The thought here is that, faced by different practices, it would not be possible to say which practice was right and which wrong. Once, however, practices are embedded in a context—and the human context is the human world—then what we should call 'obeying the rule' and 'going against it' become clearer. In some circumstances (say when I am afraid of the person giving the order),

> I act quickly, with perfect certainty, and the lack of reasons does not trouble me. (PI §212)

That is, the circumstances (the context or surround) mean that the question of interpretation does not arise. It is the external embedding of the practices that obviates the need for interpretation.

Kripke's scepticism questioned the basis of the justification of claims to normativity and it might be said that mere contingent circumstances do not provide the sort of certainty that is required to underpin meaning. Practices embedded in the world, however, are not simply practices. The embedding means that they are normatively constrained: this is part and parcel of being embedded. By 'being embedded', I mean that the practices are part of the world. But that world is multifarious: it occupies physical space and involves both biology and chemistry, and also geography; it involves history, cultural, and spiritual traditions; it is the human world of ethical concerns and artistic endeavours, from poetry to music, from follies to cathedrals.

To dig deeper than bedrock is futile (PI §217). For I cannot get below what is fundamental and these practices are fundamental features of the world. Given that the world is this way, I simply obey the rule. When I understand the series and continue it, 'I do not choose. I obey the rule *blindly*' (PI §219). To someone who wishes still to be sceptical about the world being this way, it is not clear that there could be any further argument, other than to show that the position was nonsensical. It would be nonsensical to adopt such a radical scepticism if it denied the possibility of meaningful language (which it would do, given that for language to be meaningful it must follow rules). The fact that practices are not just, as it were, free-standing, but are part and parcel of a world, means that they have a history, that they have a significance on account of their place in the world. Moreover, the more deeply embedded a practice, the more difficult for it to be any other way. Blue things just are blue (PI §238). Mathematical rules just are as they are: 'That is part of the framework on which the working of our language is based' (PI §240).

One way to put this, following Luntley (1991), is to say that up to the step that stresses the embedding of practices in the world, the argument could be regarded as 'contractualist'. The linking of rules to practices could be seen as no more than a contract and a mere contract could be questioned. We would then have to resort to an infinity of contracts. The effect of embedding practices in the world is that no contract is required. Normativity is not built-in through a contract, it is already a constitutive feature of the world. The role of practices in the argument is just that they are the way in which normativity shows itself. The key is that they are embedded practices, themselves already constituting part of the human world and already (as part of the world) normative. The normativity is immanent.

According to Luntley (1991), the rule-following considerations can 'be thought of as offering a transcendental argument for the existence of non-contractual norms' (*ibid.*: 171). Luntley goes on to press the thought that,

> … without the norms that constitutively shape our experience it would not be an experience of hearing someone say 'add 2'. The norms must already be present in the experience. And the 'must' here is a transcendental must, for unless we can say that such norms and obligations are already a part of that experience we will fail to describe it as an experience with content. (*ibid.*: 176)

The embedding of practices amounts to the recommendation of a non-contractual account of normativity. It can also be conceived as resulting from a transcendental argument. For, if normativity is to have the force that it requires to support meaning and the very possibility of language, it must pre-conditionally be a part of the human world, not something that may or may not be added on. It is a transcendental requirement in that it is a condition for the possibility of language, where this involves correct and incorrect usage, that there should be normativity. In turn, this can be described as a realist account, because correct and incorrect use are mind- and will-independent. Thus, according to Luntley, there is still realism about patterns of meaning:

> … but the condition for the possibility of patterns of correct use is not the existence of transcendent patterns, it is the existence of active language users, judges with a capacity to see similarities in things. (Luntley, 2003a: 84)

Luntley is here rejecting the idea that there are transcendent patterns (in the platonic heaven as it were) to be followed in order to maintain the distinction between correct and incorrect use of language. None the less, the account of normativity is transcendental. The link that is revealed by the transcendent account, by looking for the preconditions for (or the conditions for the possibility of) rightness and wrongness in our language use, is between normativity and the manner of being of people, who are characteristically in-the-world. Much more can be said about our manner of being-in-the-world, but we are certainly minded beings and, further to the discussion of Chapter 3, I shall now consider the implications of the account I am presenting of intentional mental states for the theory of mind generally.

But before moving on, there is something to pick up from the last quote from Luntley (2003a). The transcendent account of normativity highlights the importance of 'active language users'; but Luntley then goes on to describe these language users as, 'judges with a capacity to see similarities in things'. Thornton (2006) has criticized this aspect of Luntley's argument. Luntley has steered clear of Platonism, but has he inadvertently veered into a type of constructivism or constructionism? Thornton points out that Luntley regards the seeing of similarities as basic or primitive; elsewhere Luntley writes:

> … the normative patterns of correct use of words emerge from the activity of seeing similarities. (Luntley, 2002: 275)

Luntley suggests that the patterns emerge through the interactions of agents with the world. But Thornton counters that, '. . .we do not await subsequent judgement to determine the extension of concepts' (Thornton, 2006: 135). In other words, when I understand something in a flash, it is not clear how this amounts to seeing similarities unless it requires that I have seen at least two instances of whatever is at issue. And, if so, it almost sounds as if an empirical procedure is being described, which is clearly not what Luntley intends. Thornton elucidates thus:

> … we are not free to see just any similarity. (*ibid.*)

The point at issue is whether the normativity comes from something we do, by seeing the similarity, or whether the pattern has to be there already in order to determine what counts as a similarity. There may be a way to appease this conflict, but if there is it will surely require—in order to maintain the potency of the normative constraint—something that is independent of human will. Luntley himself recognizes that, in adopting an attitude to the world, which is how he understands the idea of grasping the meaning of a word in a flash, we demonstrate, '. . . . a way in which one attends and presents oneself to that which is independent of will' (Luntley, 2003a: 167). This characterization would seem to place the similarity in the world as something waiting to be attended to, otherwise the risk of idealism (where the similarity is dependent on the mind or will) seems great. But, in which case, it is hard to see how 'seeing similarities' is going to be the primitive, basic notion over against the idea that the similarities are embedded in the patterned normative practices that constitute language use as a brute fact.

(ii) An externalist account of mind

In Chapter 3, I referred to the externalist account of mental content, which now emerges again. Externalism about content suggests that: 'content is not characterizable independently of that (the environment) which it represents' (Luntley, 1999: 9). Externalism follows from the fact that, according to the transcendental account of normativity, which makes normativity a constitutive, immanent feature of embedded practices, intentional psychological phenomena cannot be conceived from a purely 'psychological', or internal, perspective. If they are part and parcel of the world, involving normatively constrained, embedded practices, intentional psychological states cannot be regarded as simply 'inner'. Instead, understanding is linked to the criteria in the world that allow one to say that one has understood. My understanding something, therefore, is a matter open to public scrutiny. This is not to suggest that it is the public who decide whether or not I have understood. But whether or not I have understood is not something that can be judged independently of the world. The externalism of intentional psychological states is a consequence of their normativity, because that normativity places them in practices embedded in the world (cf. Thornton, 1998: 123–37). Hence, there is no gap to be found between a psychological state and its instantiation, between my understanding something and the application of that understanding, between my ability to read and my actual reading. What is normatively constrained by the intentional psychological state (i.e. what is involved in my claiming to understand or to be able to read) is realized in the entailed practice (i.e. actual acts of understanding and reading).

This link between the psychological state and the world has been described as an 'internal relation', reflecting the internal relation between a rule and its application (Hacker, 1996: 128). The notion of an internal relation has also been used to explain the agreement between thought and reality, or between an expectation and its fulfilment (Arrington, 1991). The problem is that an emphasis is typically placed on the grammatical status of this internal relationship. This diverts attention from the external circumstances, the context in which practices are embedded. It might seem as if we can understand the relationship between a word and its meaning, a rule and its application, without a grasp of reality, but purely in terms of the intra-grammatical logic. However, this is not sufficient to account for the relationship between thought and reality. It is true that Wittgenstein wrote: 'Like everything metaphysical the harmony between thought and reality is to be found in the grammar of the language' (Z §55; PG §162). But if it were *just* a matter of grammar, it would appear to suggest something like linguistic idealism, according to which the realization of my thought would depend upon the articulation of the thought in language. What such an interpretation misses, however, is the crucial worldly background of practices, of what I actually do.

Consider, for instance, McDowell (1991):

> But suppose I form the intention to type a period. If that is my intention, it is settled that only my typing a period will count as executing it. Of course I am capable of forming that intention only because I am party to the practices that are constitutive of the relevant concepts. But if that is indeed the intention which—thus empowered—I form, nothing more than the intention itself is needed to determine what counts as conformity to it. ... So there is something for my intention to type a period ... to be: namely, precisely, my intention to type a period.

It is true that (in one sense) there is an internal relation between the intention and its fulfilment. That intention is realized in the actual practice of typing periods. Once that background (the human practice of typing periods) is in place, however, then the intention becomes (on its own, not in relation to anything else) contentful. There is a link, then, between intentional mental content and practices that is, essentially and constitutively, normative. The harmony between thought and reality is a grammatical matter. But linguistic content (the having of meaning) is a matter of embedded practice. The internal relationship involves an external context, in which the normativity of intentional psychological states is embedded and immanent in practices.

In short, the embedding of intentional psychological concepts as practices means, therefore, that such concepts just are part of the world. And the normativity of the intentional psychological states is accounted for by a transcendental argument, which locates it immanently in the world of embedded human practices. Mental states engage the world; the world penetrates the mind. The upshot is externalism.

Normativity is a condition for the possibility of meaning one thing rather than another. But the normativity is not itself transcendental: it does not inhabit some platonic other realm. It is immanent, indwelling in our practice of language use. Hence, McDowell's talk of a shared command of language in which we, 'hear someone else's meaning in his words' (*ibid.*). The meaning is not something different, it is part of the language, and,

> … a linguistic community is conceived as bound together … by a capacity for a meeting of minds. … The essential point is the way in which one person can know another's meaning without interpretation. (*ibid.*)

Much the same, incidentally, could be said about musical culture, especially since music is often regarded as akin to language, or at least as able to convey meaning (perhaps where words cease). Thus the composer Ralph Vaughan Williams (1872–1958), who set Walt Whitman (see Chapter 2) to music in his *Sea Symphony*, commented:

> Music *is* indeed in one sense the universal language, by which I do not mean that it is a cosmopolitan language but that it is, I believe, the only means of artistic expression which is natural to everybody. Music is above all things the art of the common man. (Vaughan Williams, 1934: 114–15)

If language enables 'a meeting of minds', as McDowell suggests (*vide supra*), music does so too. But there is a real question as to how far the analogy with language can be pushed. Roger Scruton clearly sees music as something to be understood and, therefore, as having content. He talks of 'intentional understanding' that,

> … uses the concepts through which we perceive the world, and makes no connections or observations that are not in some way already implicit in them. (Scruton, 2004: 449)

His analysis suggests that the ways we hear music, 'are based in concepts extended by metaphorical transference' (*ibid.*). This leads Scruton to conclude:

> Understanding music involves the active creation of an intentional world, in which inert sounds are transfigured into movements, harmonies, rhythms—metaphorical gestures in a metaphorical space. And into these metaphorical gestures a metaphorical soul is breathed by the sympathetic listener. (Scruton *op. cit.*: 461)

The commitment to the notion that understanding music means understanding in some sort of (albeit metaphorical) conceptual way is tempting, but is it necessary? In Scruton's paper it leads to a form of constructivism, in that meaning and understanding are actively created. But the interesting thing, in the case of music, is that we seem to have mental content (the meaning of music) without specific (linguistic) concepts.

Luntley (2003b) discusses the possibility of non-conceptual content specifically in connection with music. He suggests that concepts and their meaning, 'have the potential to figure in the subject's rational organization of their behaviour' (Luntley, 2003b).

To pursue his argument he suggests the possibility of 'nonconceptual representational content':

> Nonconceptual representations are ways in which we respond to the world that we are not able to rationally organise. They are representations that provide us with a response to X, but not a rational response; they are not responses that can figure in the rational organisation of behaviour. (*ibid.*)

The example that Luntley uses is that of a novice (i.e. someone with no particular musical or theoretical training) hearing a dominant seventh chord and responding to it with an expectation, which will be fulfilled by the return to the tonic chord, but without the understanding to conceptualize the response. Without wishing to pursue the musical argument further, the point here is that understanding—at least in principle—is partly to do with our responses in the external world, which are, however, not necessarily conceptual. Even so, whether or not music is conceptual, it strongly suggests language because it so clearly communicates. Hence, in discussing Finzi's work, Russell (1954) commented:

> The greatness of *Intimations* is not so much a musical greatness as one of 'communication' between musician and poet. ... It is a marriage of true minds. (p. 13)

In the same issue of *Tempo*, Boyd (1954) wrote:

> The immediate pleasure which many of us derive from Finzi's work no doubt comes from our recognition of exquisite taste, unpretentious charm, a high level of technical competence, and, for English listeners, a frank delight in the literary and musical culture we share with the composer. (p. 18)

Perhaps in this we can see something of what it is to understand a theme or the Englishness of a piece by Finzi or Vaughan Williams. For there is something that is shared: the background or surround that is presupposed. Like Wittgenstein writing:

> The common behaviour of mankind is the system of reference by means of which we interpret an unknown language. (PI: §206)

Whilst this background has to be presupposed—and thereby informs the transcendental account (the condition for the possibility of meaning)—it is not the *social* nature of the background that is important. It is rather locating the theme in a particular light, as part of a patterned practice, which allows us to perceive meaning in the sentence or in the musical theme. But this sense of 'locating' has to be something that occurs immediately and immanently, as part of our participating in the patterned practice.

Whilst rejecting the notion of communal dispositions as a way of maintaining normativity, McDowell (1991) still appeals to 'communal practices' as a way of providing a framework in which, 'to situate our conception of meaning and understanding'. The notion of practice is crucial, but to save the day it must be *situated* or *embedded* practice. I shall discuss the relevance of this to the person with acquired diffuse neurocognitive dysfunction in due course. It should already be apparent, however, that this account of what it is to be a being with intentional psychological states suggests that it has to be situated. Being part of the linguistic community is to share in this particular type of being-in-the-world. My suggestion is that some of what it is to be a person is simply to be situated in this surround.

(iii) The quietist approach to the world

One final point is that there might still be the temptation to ask for more of the transcendental account, to ask what constitutes normativity beyond the patterned practices in which it is immanent. The answer to this question would then seem to be relevant to what it is to be the type of being that has intentional psychological states. But this temptation is wrong. It represents a failure to recognize the extent to which normativity is irreducible: there is nothing else to it other than its instantiation in patterned practices. The transcendentalist account of normativity is a quietist account.

Quietism is suggested by: 'What we cannot speak about we must pass over in silence' (TLP §7); as it is, too, by the thought that the solution to a philosophical problem is 'something that looks as if it were only a preliminary to it …' (Z §314). As Wittgenstein went on to say, the difficulty is 'to stop' (*ibid.*). Quietism (or minimalism) is the notion that no philosophical explanation is possible, that the only correct response is to accept and describe what is given. At this point, normativity cannot be further understood in terms of dispositions, metaphysical tracks, inner processes, mental representations, or community agreement. Normativity is irreducible. So, for instance, Thornton (1997a) suggests:

> The moral of the rule following considerations is precisely that no substantial answer can be given to the question [how can something I grasp in a flash determine future events?] and that the phenomenon must simply be presupposed and described.

According to Thornton's account of minimalism, there is nothing that acts as an intermediary, say, between my understanding how to continue the series and my actually doing so (Thornton, 1998: 88–99). Similarly,

> When one comes to understand the meaning of a word, one acquires an ability to use it correctly which cannot be further explained. One simply masters a practice or technique. … Understanding a meaning is a piece of 'know-how', a practical ability. One way of putting this is to say that meanings and rules are individuated by practices and that understanding a meaning or a rule is thus individuated by the practice over which one has mastery. (*ibid.*: 90)

Quietism, or minimalism, suggests that there can be no substantive explanation of normativity. It simply is an irreducible feature of the world and of intentional psychological concepts. So, for instance, although Luntley (1991) feels there is still a good deal to be said about the metaphysics of thought, he accepts as true:

> … the fact that the norms of meaning exist is something about which no more can be said. That there is such a thing as meaning is a claim that properly falls within the province of silence. We cannot expect to explain the existence of meaning and its norms on the basis of anything more basic.

In *Wittgenstein: Meaning and Judgement*, Luntley seems, at first sight perhaps, to change his mind: 'The Wittgenstein presented herein is no quietist' (Luntley, 2003a: vii).

But a short while later, having argued that language users are active agents engaging in practices that amount to 'taking an attitude to the world' (*ibid.*: 18), he asserts of this attitude:

> It is not something capable of full articulation. It is something that has to be seen. ... The fundamental condition for the possibility of judgement is not capable of theoretical articulation. (*ibid.*)

Later still, however, Luntley explains the target of his critique of quietism. He is against the view that all we can finally rely on is, 'descriptivism about ordinary use' (*ibid.*: 99). The end of the argument is not simply a description that is, 'no more than a set of homely reminders of our common-sense account of ourselves, our language and our world' (*ibid.*). Luntley describes quietism as,

> ... the view that not only is there no philosophical theory to be given of how meaning is possible, but that in describing our linguistic practices we describe them in familiar terms drawn from our common-sense description of what we are doing with language. (*ibid.*)

Luntley's objection to this view is that the description of our language use and the characterization of language users that results,

> ... changes the structure of our common-sense self-conception—our conception of who and what we are *qua* language users, of how we are in the world and how the world relates to us in judgement. (*ibid.*)

The description of how we use language is 'revelatory': 'for it reveals the immanent hidden' (*ibid.*).

Given that, on Luntley's view, the key thing is the agent's engagement with the world, the revelation here is dramatic. What it is for me to assert correctly that I understand something is that I am engaged in a practice as an agent, where the practice may involve social scaffolding, but where in essence I (alone) am interacting with and acting in the world. It is not that I have acquired some sort of theoretical knowledge. Luntley (2003a) talks of: 'seeing the world aright', which implies the notion of an active agent.

> What will show that they see things aright will be in their practice, their going on right. ...
> Their correctness consists in their taking the right attitude to things, of setting their face to the world in the appropriate way. This is to take part in an engagement with things in which word use is directly calibrated against that which provides the standards of correctness; it is a practice. (Luntley, 2003a: 154)

One reason for accepting this as a positive conclusion is that nothing else remains after the destructive effects of the rule-following considerations. In order to understand what it is to follow a rule (following Wittgenstein's critique), no appeal can be made to internal things (neither to mental processes, nor to dispositions, whether those of individuals or those of communities), nor to metaphysical standards. Normativity, therefore, is an irreducible given in the world.

But how is it possible to move from an account of what I do (the practices in which I engage) to an account of what I *ought* to do (the norms I am constrained by)? How do we justify saying that *this* way is the correct way to follow the rule? It was at this point in the rule-following discussion that Wittgenstein wrote:

> If I have exhausted the justifications I have reached bedrock, and my spade is turned. Then I am inclined to say: 'This is simply what I do.' (PI §217)

One of the charges made by McDowell (1984) is that anti-realism tries to get below bedrock. The thought to which McDowell objected was that it could be possible for a consensus to be reached *without norms* on whether or not to call a newly encountered object 'yellow'. This consensus would be based upon 'resemblances in behaviour and phenomenology' (*ibid.*). A reliance on dispositions is sub-bedrock because it does not seek normative justifications, it is only concerned with what people actually do. In response to this, McDowell mobilized a number of quotations from Wittgenstein to support the idea that norms still operate at bedrock, for example: 'To use a word without a justification does not mean to use it without right' (PI §289); and, 'Following according to the rule is FUNDAMENTAL to our language-game' (RFM VI-28). The counter-thought, then, is simply that there is no getting away from normativity: it goes all the way down to bedrock (it is deeply embedded) and talk of a community somehow being beyond this is unrealistic:

> ... if we respect Wittgenstein's injunction not to dig below the ground, we must say that the community 'goes right or wrong' ... according to whether the object in question is, or is not, yellow; and nothing can make its being yellow, or not, dependent on our ratification of the judgement that that is how things are. (McDowell *op. cit.*)

Summary

Having arrived at the importance of the notion of practice as a way of understanding normativity, it looked as if practices were only a matter of human agreement or human disposition. But then the problem is that normativity seems either to be contingent upon practices or a consequence of them. The embedding of practices is a further move to flesh out the positive thought, derived from Wittgenstein, that the normativity of intentional mental states brings into play features of the (outer) world and not just inner states. The way the world *is* involves normativity as a transcendental feature—it just is required as a condition for the possibility of language use and meaning—and, moreover it is immanent, lying within the patterned practices of our language, including our music and our poetry. This is not to say, however, that normativity is explained by other (physical, chemical, historical, cultural, or spiritual etc.) features of the world; it simply is another fundamental facet of *our* world. Normativity is constitutive of intentional psychological phenomena on account of their being embedded as practices in the world. But, having already noted it to be transcendental and constitutive, normativity is also irreducible, in that there is no further account to be given. Quietism concerning intentional psychological states involves recognition, on the basis of the transcendental account, of their constitutive, immanent, and irreducible normativity.

The upshot of this is that any account of dementia must allow this sort of characterization of intentional psychological phenomena.

What is required is a thick description of practices, which show normativity as a constitutive feature. This is why, towards the start of the chapter, we saw Wittgenstein suggesting that meaning is explained by considering how we lead a person to comprehend a poem or a theme (PI §533). In 1948, Wittgenstein asked, 'So how do we explain to someone what "understanding music" means?' (CV: 70). His response is to note that we might do various things, such as pointing out expressions, gestures, images, and the like. But then he says:

> Someone who understands music will listen differently (e.g. with a different expression on his face), he will talk differently, from someone who does not. But he will show that he understands a particular theme not just in manifestations that accompany his hearing or playing that theme but in his understanding for music in general. (*ibid.*)

Seeing the whole picture, the surround, is the way to stop the questions. Quietism is a way of asserting that what counts here as normative cannot be further analyzed. But this is not to say that the descriptions of what we actually do will be thin and mundane. For these descriptions must capture our whole way of being-in-the-world.

> Appreciating music is a manifestation of the life of mankind. (*ibid.*)

Back to Miss Breen

So what difference does this make to our thoughts about Miss Breen? Earlier in the chapter we left Miss Breen characterized in a negative way: her mental life has been affected by her acquired diffuse neurocognitive dysfunction, so that she cannot read, remember, calculate, use language with much coherence, and so on. These failures are definitely failures in terms of her intentional psychological states. But now we can start to suggest a more positive light in which to regard her. The transcendental account emphasizes that what it is to have an intentional mental life is to be able to participate in patterns of human activity that show the immanence and irreducible nature of normativity as a constitutive feature of that mental life. One immediate effect of this account is that we cannot—we should not—think of Miss Breen as inhabiting a mental realm that is *in principle* inaccessible to us, even if it is *practically difficult* to gain access to her mental world. For the externalism of mind, which is a concomitant of the account of intentional psychological states that I am presenting, suggests that the distinction between the inner and outer is breached and that our mental lives, our subjectivities, are potentially and in principle shareable. This is because of the surround that someone such as Miss Breen inhabits; it is her situated being that counts. She is situated, of course, in a social surround, but the transcendental account does not rely on the context being social. It relies on patterns of activity that show meaning. Do we wish to say that Miss Breen no longer inhabits such a world? We might be inclined to say that she cannot remember; but there are numerous different types of memory and, in fact, Miss Breen does demonstrate familiarity with the staff who now look after her. We might be inclined to say that she does not understand; but there are numerous things that she clearly does understand: that it is time to eat, that this person is friendly, that she is being addressed, that someone is leaving, and so forth. She cannot speak with any coherence; but she can convey a sense of her distress and anxiety by the short snatches of language that she uses. So, Miss Breen does demonstrate intentional mental states.

Is all of this simply a matter of empirical observation, in which case there may be no point to the more substantial philosophical discussion? Of course, at a severer stage of dysfunction we shall wish to say, purely on empirical grounds, that intentionality—and with it the possibility of engaging with the world in a meaningful way—has finally gone. (After all, this is the fate of everyone who slips into a terminal coma.) As we saw in Chapter 2, Luntley has expressed the view that the self, '. . . is the condition for the possibility of keeping track of outer things', so that, 'When that goes, the self goes too' (Luntley, 2006: 106). I suggested that 'keeping track' might imply too cognitive a view of the self, which is clearly lots of other things as well.

The transcendental account I have now put forward goes further: what it is to have an intentional mental life is to be able to participate in patterns of human activity that show the immanence and irreducible nature of normativity. Hence, even when her acquired diffuse neurocognitive dysfunction has worsened, Miss Breen's ability to participate in the requisite patterns of human activity can depend on the surround. Again, this suggests the social; but *in principle* it need not do so: being embedded *qua* human agent in patterned practices is the only (in principle) requirement, even if other human beings typically provide the rational scaffolding to give the patterned practices the content and meaning they normally hold. The transcendental account provides the 'in principle' account. Looking for the conditions for the possibility of language being used correctly or incorrectly drives us to see the requirement, whatever else may or may not empirically be the case, for an immanent, irreducible normativity in the practices that constitute intentional mental activity. The constitutive nature of the normativity means that the mere possibility of engagement in patterned practices of the requisite type is enough in principle to support the claim that human life such as this, where there is the possibility of subjectivity even in severe disease, is characteristic of persons. I shall need to pursue this point in later chapters.

Conclusion

In this chapter, I have derived a transcendental account of the normativity of intentional psychological phenomena from Wittgenstein's rule-following discussion. It can be summarized thus:

- intentional psychological states are normative;
- normativity is a matter of being rule-governed;
- rules and rule-following involve practices and customs;
- practices and customs are embedded in the world.

I have then proceeded to discuss normativity and have accepted a quietist interpretation of the rule-following considerations, which stresses the givenness of normativity within an embedding human world. Normativity is seen as constitutive, immanent, and irreducible. The normativity of intentional psychological states involves an externalist construal of such states. In the chapters that follow, I shall apply this normative account of intentional psychological concepts to different models of dementia. Meanwhile, we have already glimpsed the extent to which an account of acquired diffuse neurocognitive dysfunction, which furnishes a sufficiently broad view, must have implications for our understanding of the person. The embedded nature of intentional mental states gestures in the direction of the situated, human-worldly context of persons.

Endnotes

[1] See also Thornton 1998: 30–48; and Luntley 2003a: especially pp. 1–20.

[2] Many have criticized Kripke's now famous account of the rule-following argument, e.g. Baker & Hacker (1984); McGinn (1984); Goldfarb (1985); Pears (1988): 456–8, 479–80, and 499–500; Boghossian (1989); Stern (1995): 178–9; Stroud (1996): 306–7; Thornton (1998): 70–9; Luntley (2003a): 69–71. None the less, few would doubt the usefulness of Kripke's extremely clear account in stimulating thought.

[3] The suggestion that Wittgenstein is a constructivist has a significant lineage. For instance, 'Intuitionists speak of mathematics in a highly anti-realist (anti-platonic) way: for them it is we who construct mathematics; it is not already there waiting for us to discover. An extreme form of such constructivism is found in Wittgenstein's Remarks on the Foundations of Mathematics' (Dummett, 1958–1959). Constructivism is certainly a thread that can be discerned in Wittgenstein. For instance, Hacker, in discussing the putative effect on Wittgenstein of the main proponent of the intuitionist philosophy of mathematics, L.E.J. Brouwer, whom Wittgenstein heard lecture in Vienna in 1928, described Wittgenstein subsequently as moving from 'realism in semantics to constructivism' (see Hacker, 1972: 104).

Part III

Models of dementia

Chapter 5

The problem: models of dementia and normativity

Yes. I remember Adlestrop—
The name, because one afternoon
Of heat the express-train drew up there
Unwontedly. It was late June.

The steam hissed. Someone cleared his throat.
No one left and no one came
On the bare platform. What I saw
Was Adlestrop—only the name.

(From *Adlestrop* by Edward Thomas;
Gardner, 1972: 847)

Introduction

Inasmuch as Englishness appeared as a *leitmotiv* in the last chapter, it re-emerges here by association with the work of the poet Edward Thomas (1878–1917). My use of the opening stanzas of the poem *Adlestrop* is, however, for a mundane purpose. I wish to ask: what is it to remember? What was it for Thomas to remember Adlestrop? Nevertheless, it would be possible to draw out a broader theme. Let me indulge in a mere sketch. The point is certainly nothing to do with any particular nationalism. It is to do with our relationships, with each other, and with the world. But these relationships are embedded in a context. Our understanding (of music, of language) is also embedded. This was the theme of the last chapter: the normativity of our intentional psychological states is a matter of embedded practices, where the transcendental account of normativity reveals it to be constitutive, immanent, and irreducible. The poetry of Edward Thomas links to that of the English Romantics, and to the music of Elgar and Finzi, through its Englishness; but our *understanding* of this, like our understanding of Flemish paintings (and unlike our *mis*understanding of the art of radically different cultures e.g. that of ancient Egypt), relies on potentially shared practices (whether or not they are actually shared). This understanding has to be characterized (because it must be normative) as constitutive, immanent, and irreducible. And it links neither solely to England, nor to Holland, nor Belgium—even if these provide the immediate surround—but to the world.

In the Introduction to his selection of Thomas's poems and prose, David Wright cites C. H. Sisson:

> It would be a shallow judgement ... to think of Thomas as the poet of country places ... He is touched to the quick by the human relationships he has known, and one function of the natural background is to reduce people to a tempo in which they can be observed. All passion for the truth is revolutionary and Thomas's work is a critique of what the world thinks of itself, and of its methods of thought. (Wright in Thomas, 1981: 25)

What was it, therefore, for Thomas to remember Adlestrop? The full-view answer must capture the constitutive, immanent, and irreducible nature of the normativity of the mental state of remembering. In this chapter, I shall consider three models of dementia in order to interrogate their conceptualization of what it is to remember. To do this I shall use the characterization of intentional mental states derived in the preceding chapter. In each case I shall find the models wanting. This is not to say that the models do not also capture something useful, which will emerge here and in the following chapter, where I place the models in a broader view. But the aim in this chapter is to present some standard 'models' of dementia and gesture at the extent to which they are inadequate at capturing what it means to remember Adlestrop. In which case, these models are—to this extent—deficient, because they are based on misguided or incomplete accounts of what it is to be minded as a human being (Hughes, 2008).

We have already come across different accounts of the mind in Chapter 3. Physicalist theories of the mind can easily be conceived as underpinning biomedical or disease models of dementia. I shall discuss these first. Then, secondly, I shall discuss cognitive neuropsychology models of dementia. As discussed in Chapter 3, Fodor's representational theories form a useful underpinning to this sort of cognitivist account, which makes use of computer analogies. But there are other ways of dealing with the notion of mental representations. Daniel Dennett talks of sub-personal units that allow sub-personal meaning. Bolton and Hill have suggested that meaning is encoded in the brain. I shall consider these views briefly. But on my view, neither the disease model nor the representationalism of cognitive neuropsychology allows room for the sort of normativity required by intentional mental content. The third model of dementia I shall consider is based on social constructionism. As I shall discuss, this model, although it pays more obvious attention to normative concerns, is deficient in different ways depending on whether it is intended to give a causal or constitutive account of intentional mental states such as remembering Adlestrop.

But I also wish to maintain my focus on the person with acquired diffuse neurocognitive dysfunction. To this end I shall continue to consider Miss Breen. In the description of Miss Breen at the start of Chapter 3, I ended by saying that she did not recognize me when I visited her, even though she had seen me before. This is not surprising given that she only see me every few months. But the sad thing is that she does not recognize people she has been quite familiar with in the past. She does not appear to recognize neighbours she has known for 30 years. More distant relatives are also no longer recognized. Initially she started to misidentify her brother, whom she referred to as her husband. Later she seemed not to know him at all. Failure to recognize familiar faces has been used as a test of cognitive function in people with acquired diffuse neurocognitive dysfunction. This cognitive dysfunction enjoys the name prosopagnosia.

In what follows I shall use this cognitive deficit as an example in my discussion of the various models of dementia.

I suggested that I would find the models of dementia wanting, because what is required is something more mysterious (in one sense) than any model can give us. I shall not be discussing dualist conceptions of the mind, such as was discussed in Chapter 3, which might underpin dementia because there is no obvious established candidate for such a model. And yet, as suggested by the quotation from Lewis (see p.62), talk of mental things seems to make some sense. It seemingly makes sense on the Clapham omnibus too, which partly explains the grip of a latent dualism, which in turn affects common or garden conceptions of dementia. We need to avoid the grip of dualism; but we need to capture its insights inasmuch as these express something that is regarded as rationally acceptable at some level, albeit difficult to pin down.

Dementia: the disease model

In this section, I shall present a picture of the disease model of dementia. There are two preliminary points.

Preliminary points

First, I have deliberately used the notion of a 'disease' model, rather than spoken of a 'medical' model. The notion of a 'medical' model is often used in a pejorative sense. Kitwood (1997), for instance, talking of dementia states:

> Overwhelmingly today it is framed as an 'organic mental disorder' and a medical model ... has held sway. ... it was as if the evidence of organicity was so overwhelming that a 'technical' way of approaching the problem was what was needed: essentially, to elucidate the pathological processes and then find ways of arresting or preventing them. (Kitwood, 1997: 1)

He later refers to the 'medical model' as 'problematic' and 'old-fashioned',

> ... with its assumption that the diagnostic categories are in some way real. (Kitwood, op. cit.: 30)

I have already discussed, in Chapter 1, the ways in which the diagnosis of Alzheimer's disease are underpinned by evaluative judgements. Kitwood's critique is in keeping with this view. And yet, it is unclear whether or not clinicians, in general, actually use such a model. It is difficult to think of clinicians (as opposed to pure neuroscientists) who would be inclined to think of the person with dementia solely in the technical terms of neuropathology (and even 'pure' neuroscientists, I suspect, do not think in such terms when they think of the *person* with dementia). On the other hand, clinicians will often think of conditions *as* diseases and use the different components of a 'disease' model. The point is that the standard 'medical' model nowadays, as I shall discuss in Chapter 7, is probably biopsychosocial (Engel, 1977) and not just limited to the pathological. But there is a 'disease' model, which is prone by its very nature to a limited view with an emphasis on pathological lesions. Downs, Clare, and Mackenzie (2006) described the 'diagnostic overshadowing' that can result from the explanatory model that views 'dementia' as a brain disease, where the person 'is viewed as a passive victim' and 'all actions and expressions are attributed to the labeled condition' (p. 240).

Secondly, the disease model fits Fulford's description of the conventional (or science-based) view of the conceptual structure of medicine (Fulford, 1989: 262–7). According to this view, dysfunction is the logical root notion. This gives rise to disease concepts and hence to our notions of illness. The reverse (ethics-based) view is that illness—itself derived from 'action failure'—is conceptually prior to disease concepts. The thought is that 'illness' links more readily to evaluative notions, including to notions concerning the person. It may seem, then, that by taking the conventional disease model as a paradigm, I have set up a straw-man for my philosophical analysis, since—according to Fulford's account—the notion of disease is conceptually misplaced in the conventional view.

Whilst, however, the conclusions I reach will be similar to Fulford's in effect, the route I have taken is different. Instead of an analysis of concepts such as 'illness' and 'disease', my focus is on psychological concepts. I confine myself to dementia, which is closer (in Fulford's view) to the physical illness paradigm than other mental illnesses (Fulford, *op. cit.*: 80–1). As I have discussed in Chapter 1, although this seems true, it is none the less equally true that a diagnosis of dementia is yet surrounded by evaluative concerns. Perhaps this should point us in the direction of taking a closer look at other 'physical' illnesses, on the grounds that they are likely to entail more value judgements than might at first blush appear. Still, my strategy is complementary to Fulford's. For I shall argue, from my analysis of intentional psychological concepts, that dementia must be understood within a broad context. This places it, even as a physical disease, in a field of evaluative concerns. It is noteworthy that both of our approaches have implications for the notion of personhood (cf. Fulford, *op. cit.*: 252).

Since I am again discussing diagnosis, it seems right at this point to reconsider in a critical fashion the preferred nomenclature that I have been using for dementia: acquired diffuse neurocognitive dysfunction. This certainly casts dementia in a bio-medical light, in keeping with a disease model. In a sense this is inevitable, because the aim was precisely to find a word or words to take the place of 'dementia' in such a classification as the ICD. There are then two further points to be made.

First, the discussion in Chapter 1 of values and facts should already have made it clear that my use of the word 'dysfunction' is not a pretence that dementia could be summed up in a way that is value-free. What counts as dysfunction in this context cannot amount to an objective statement. We can give 'criteria of rational acceptability' to explain our decisions (cf. Putnam, 1981: 130, as discussed in Chapter 1). Thus, we might say that a failure to score 24 or over on the MMSE in general indicates cognitive *dysfunction*. The criteria for rational acceptability may, in this case, be statistical or clinical; hence we reveal the values that drive our assessments. But there is still the possibility that someone scoring over the cut-off will have dysfunction (perhaps because he or she used to function at a much higher level than the average person) and that someone scoring under the cut-off will be functioning perfectly normally (perhaps because he or she has never done well at this sort of test). So the values go all the way down, i.e. from judgements at the personal level about illness, to judgements at the level of the organ or organism about disease and dysfunction. (As I have said, I am ignoring the richer literature that discusses conceptual issues around the notions of disease and illness in more depth, which are covered elsewhere, e.g. in Fulford et al., 2006.)

Secondly, acquired diffuse neurocognitive dysfunction was intended as an umbrella term, which would then need to be specified more precisely as, e.g., vascular or Lewy body disease according to the pathology, with the caveat that the pathology might be overlapping or difficult to be certain about. All of this is still to be moving, however, within the realms of clear-cut diagnoses and the possibility of distinct, scientific classifications. This has been termed a nomothetic approach, in the sense that it is intended to capture natural laws. It is contrasted with an individual, case-based, or idiographic approach to diagnosis. These distinctions and the conceptual and practical tensions that they lead to are clearly discussed by Thornton (2007, 2008). I only wish here to put down a marker that, whilst I think it is preferable to talk about acquired diffuse neurocognitive dysfunction rather than dementia, I would also wish to commend the idea of an individualized or narrative approach. How it is possible to work practically in a way that recognizes and allows both a scientific and a personal approach is an issue to which I shall return, in Chapter 7 and thereafter.

Five characteristics of a disease

But now I wish to establish the standing of acquired diffuse neurocognitive dysfunction as a disease. I think this point is relatively easily won. Rather than having to present different details for a variety of different conditions, I shall limit myself to a discussion of Alzheimer's disease, which is after all the commonest identified type of acquired diffuse neurocognitive dysfunction. I recognize that there are simplifying assumptions even in speaking of Alzheimer's as if it were one clear-cut condition. This should, however, help to clarify the account and it is, in any case, an implication of the disease model that it should be possible to identify clear pathology linked to particular symptoms and signs. The simplification helps to give the strongest possible support to the idea that there is a bona fide disease model. Again I would point to standard texts to support the argument (Jacoby et al., 2008; Weiner & Lipton, 2009; Jolley, 2010; Ames, Burns, and O'Brien, forthcoming).

Tyrer and Steinberg (1993) have suggested that a disease model describes four elements: clearly recognizable symptoms and signs; a scientific account of the putative aetiology; an established course and prognosis; and pathological evidence of the disease. To these can be added a fifth element: an established treatment that modifies the disease process in a scientifically understandable way. Using these five characteristics, I shall now describe how Alzheimer's disease conforms to this model.

The first characteristic of a disease is that there should be clearly recognizable symptoms and signs. This is certainly the case in Alzheimer's disease once it is beyond the mildest stages. The symptoms and signs do not always differentiate one form of dementia from another and diagnoses remain only probable until a post-mortem. Nevertheless, although mistakes occur, certain patterns of symptoms and signs, in the absence of other features, can lead to a diagnosis with considerable certainty (Thomas, 2008b). For instance, using standardized criteria, Joachim, Morris, and Selkoe (1988) confirmed a diagnosis of 'probable' or 'possible' Alzheimer's disease at autopsy in 87%

of cases. Even if precise diagnosis is sometimes difficult, it remains the case that there are clearly recognizable symptoms and signs of Alzheimer's disease.

The second characteristic of a disease is that there should be an account of its putative aetiology which makes scientific sense. In the case of Alzheimer's disease the evidence in favour of a genetic contribution to the aetiology is impressive. An early family study found a four-fold increase in the likelihood of a first-degree relative of someone with senile dementia developing the disease (Larsson, Sjogren, and Jacobsen, 1963). A meta-analysis by van Duijn et al. (1991) showed a 3.5-fold increase in risk in first-degree relatives of someone with Alzheimer's disease. More recent large studies have continued to find statistical associations with a variety of genetic loci, although these still do not allow prediction of who might develop Alzheimer's disease (Seshadri et al., 2010).

The most exciting developments have come from studies at the molecular level (Holmes, 2008). The neuropathology of Alzheimer's disease has as its most characteristic finding senile plaques. These are deposits outside the cells in the brain largely made up of amyloid (Aβ) protein. According to the 'amyloid cascade hypothesis', it is the incorrect deposition of amyloid which leads to plaques, cell death and hence Alzheimer's disease. The Aβ peptides, which make up the amyloid protein, are derived from a larger protein called the amyloid precursor protein (APP). APP is broken down into smaller units by proteases known as secretases. Whilst α- and β-secretase do not lead to the accumulation of Aβ, when APP is cleaved by γ-secretase, amyloid accumulation results. How these proteases work is linked to particular genes, some of which are known to be associated with Alzheimer's disease (Holmes, 2008).

Of course, there is more to the pathology of Alzheimer's than just amyloid plaques and the amyloid cascade hypothesis remains a debated aetiological explanation, but nevertheless it makes some scientific sense, which is what the second characteristic of the disease model requires.

About 20 years ago, a link between a protein which carries cholesterol and triglycerides in the blood (apolipoprotein E or APOE) and Alzheimer's disease with chromosome 19 was established (Pericak-Vance, Bebout, and Gaskell, 1991). It has further been established that the higher the dose of a particular type of this protein (coded for by the ε4 allele) the greater the chances of developing Alzheimer's in later life. For instance, in families having several members affected by Alzheimer's disease, having two alleles on chromosome 19 coding for the protein (being ε4/ε4 homozygotes), led to over 90% of the individuals developing the disorder by the age of 80 (Corder, Saunders, and, Strittmatter, 1993). The way in which APOE relates to Alzheimer's disease is not straightforward. For instance, a study using Magnetic Resonance Imaging (MRI) suggested that the ε4 allele might modify the risk for acquiring Alzheimer's, but not influence the pathological processes thereafter (Barber et al., 1999). The important point is that there seems to be suggestive evidence of a genetic basis to late-onset, non-dominantly inherited Alzheimer's disease. Research into the genetics of Alzheimer's disease is complex and controversial, but—whilst environmental factors must also contribute to the aetiology—the strength of the genetic contribution to Alzheimer's disease seems enough to satisfy the second characteristic of the disease model.

The third characteristic of the disease model was that it should have an established course and prognosis. In Alzheimer's disease, a steady deterioration in cognitive abilities, as shown by cognitive function tests, can be predicted (Thomas, 2008b). Generally, changes in behaviour in Alzheimer's disease show great individual variation, but some changes can show a recognizable sequence (Hope, Keene, Fairburn, Jacoby, and McShane, 1999).

Neuroimaging also helps to confirm the course and prognosis of Alzheimer's disease. Some years ago, Jobst, Hindley, King, and Smith (1994) suggested that the combination of computerized X-ray tomography (CT) and single photon emission computed tomography (SPECT) scans yield a sensitivity of 90% and specificity of 97%, which would enhance diagnostic accuracy. These researchers demonstrated, too, that the rate of medial temporal lobe atrophy in the Alzheimer's disease subjects was ten times that of age-matched controls (Smith & Jobst, 1996). Neuroimaging is able to make a link between the mental manifestations of the condition, as shown by cognitive testing, and the brain pathology, as revealed by post-mortem (O'Brien & Barber, 2000). Subsequently, it has been demonstrated that medial temporal lobe atrophy has excellent discriminatory power for Alzheimer's disease compared to dementia with Lewy bodies and vascular cognitive impairment in pathologically confirmed cases (Burton et al., 2009). Such findings, coupled with assessments of cognitive function, support the contention that Alzheimer's disease can appropriately be described *as a disease*, because it is amenable to mapping of its course and prognosis.

The fourth characteristic identified by the disease model was the need for a pathological lesion. Aloïs Alzheimer (1864–1915) first described the pathology of Alzheimer's disease (Alzheimer, 1907). The characteristic features of Alzheimer's disease are: numerous senile plaques in the cerebral cortex, the hippocampus and subcortical structures; neurofibrillary tangles in similar locations; amyloid deposits in blood vessels; and frequent granulovacuolar degeneration and Hirano bodies in the hippocampus (Nagy & Hubbard, 2008). Along with these changes goes a substantial loss of nerve cells. Pathological studies have been able to demonstrate differences between the brains of patients with dementia and those without, but only in those with severe pathology (Tomlinson, Blessed, and Roth, 1970). As discussed in Chapter 1 in connection with the Nun study (Snowdon, 2003), many 'normal' aged brains also contain features typical of dementia and there is no pathological change that is pathognomonic. Hence,

> The pathology of Alzheimer's disease defies precise definition at present. … The key distinction between changes that can be dismissed as normal ageing and those of Alzheimer's disease is that the changes are all more numerous and, for some of them, more widely distributed in Alzheimer's disease than in normal ageing. (Esiri, 1997)

Despite a degree of variation and lack of definition even at the level of histopathology, it remains true that there are pathological lesions in the brain that are associated with Alzheimer's disease. Hence, it seems credible to designate Alzheimer's disease a disease, even if evaluative judgements are required at every level.

The final characteristic of the disease model was the possibility of treatment. In Alzheimer's disease it is now possible to point to medications that can alleviate symptoms (Wilcock, 2008). Such drugs, which (e.g.) enhance the activity in Alzheimer's disease of the otherwise depleted neurotransmitter acetylcholine, work in a scientifically understandable way. Furthermore, there is the possibility that newer drugs will act specifically against the process of amyloid deposition. For instance, Siemers et al. (2006) have studied a γ-secretase inhibitor, which may reduce the formation of Aβ peptide. Wilcock (2008) also reports a study of a drug that modulates γ-secretase, reduces Aβ, and has been found beneficial in early studies in terms of cognitive function, activities of daily living, and global functioning.

Alzheimer's disease, therefore, satisfies the five characteristics of the disease model. The model does not preclude the possibility of environmental factors contributing to the disease process and its prevention. Alzheimer's can also be analysed, 'in biological rather than ethical terms' (even if we do not think this provides the whole picture); and it leads to abnormalities of functions that are 'typically performed within members of the species' (Boorse, 1975). Furthermore, regarding Alzheimer's disease from the perspective of the disease model has proven to be clinically and scientifically useful. Yet, there are concerns.

Motivations for concern

The disease model is so well described and so useful clinically that it might not be clear that it raises any real conceptual problems. Given its sureness of foot, is it possible that it will slip into philosophical quagmires and, indeed, if it sticks to its path of describing the pathological basis of disease, is it obvious that there will be any philosophical snares to be avoided?

Most of the literature relating to the aetiology, pathology, diagnosis, and treatment of dementia avoids discussion of philosophical (or even ethical) issues. There are, however, several reasons why the philosophical issues need to be raised. Concerns about the underpinning physicalism of the medical model are several.

First, neuropathology proceeds within a context that involves values and norms. As I explored in Chapter 1, a neuropathological diagnosis is not value-free. Moreover, there are legitimate philosophical questions about the whole context within which science operates. One of my motivations is a wish to see the disease model placed in a broader context.

Secondly, neuroscientists *do* make philosophical claims, as in the case of Smythies (1992), who opined that science and not philosophy would solve the problem of how the mind and brain relate. Similarly, Hacker (1987, 1993: 69–72) has found it necessary (on Wittgensteinian grounds) to castigate prominent neuroscientists for ascribing mental predicates to the brain.

Thirdly, in the literature concerning the concepts of disease and illness, there is a tendency to equate disease with bodily dysfunction. Szasz (1960), for instance, holds that disease or illnesses, strictly speaking, can only affect the body (and, hence, mental illness is a myth). For Boorse (*op. cit.*), 'disease' is best understood in functional terms. Wakefield (1992) argues, similarly, that a disorder is a 'harmful dysfunction'. He takes 'dysfunction' to be a scientific term referring to the failure of a mental mechanism to perform a natural function for which it was designed by evolution. Although, according to his view, disorder combines both value and scientific components, it is a point of contention whether or not 'dysfunction' itself can be expressed in value-free terms (Sadler & Agich, 1995; Wakefield, 1995; Thornton, 2007: 30–4). Those who lay emphasis on bodily dysfunction, particularly if they think this can be described in value-free terms, inevitably encourage a biological view in keeping with the disease model. My suggestion, alternatively, is that dementia, understood in the light of the Wittgensteinian analysis, involves a rational and normative realm as well as the realm of biological dysfunction.

Fourthly, some neuroscientists working in the field of dementia do, in fact, draw philosophical conclusions. For example, based on work using positron emission tomography (PET), Rapoport (1992) concluded that the human mind could be reduced to the human brain:

> … many aspects of higher cognitive function in humans can be reduced to (mapped to and related to algorithms of) the local structure and integrity of brain networks. These results are consistent with the neurophilosophical contention (Churchland 1986; …) that critical parameters of mind can be reduced to the structure and function of the brain. They also demonstrate that the relations between mind and brain are disrupted in the course of Alzheimer's disease.

This suggestion in itself legitimizes a philosophical discussion of the disease model in the context of thought about dementia. It is striking to see reference to the Churchlands, whose eliminativist materialism seemed otiose as a way to think of the real Miss Breen in Chapter 3. The tendency to take a reductive view of the mind and of mental functioning is always a possibility in neuroscientific discourse, as in this example:

> The cerebral cortex provides the biological substrate for human cognitive capacity and is, arguably, the part of the brain that distinguishes us from other species. Therefore, understanding the evolution and development of this complex structure is central to our understanding of human intelligence and creativity, as well as of disorders of cognitive functions. (Hoerder-Suabedissen & Molnár, 2008: 141)

The broader view suggests that our understanding of human intelligence, let alone human creativity, needs to look to the socio-historical, cultural, and ethical background against which intelligence and creativity are judged. Taking the transcendental approach, outlined in the last chapter, will reveal the constitutive, immanent, and irreducible nature of the normativity that surrounds such judgements. The cortex as a 'substrate' may be fine; but its centrality is dubious, especially given that judgements about its *central* importance are themselves based on normative and ethical decisions.

Fifthly, attempts have been made to give psychiatry itself a philosophical basis. For example, Eric Kandel (1998) asserted:

> All mental processes, even the most complex psychological processes, derive from operations of the brain. The central tenet of this view is that what we commonly call mind is a range of functions carried out by the brain. The actions of the brain underlie not only relatively

simple motor behaviors, such as walking and eating, but all of the complex cognitive actions, conscious and unconscious, that we associate with specifically human behavior.

The ambiguities involved in Kandel's assertion that mind *derives* from brain and that the brain *underlies* cognition need clarification. Later, having won the Nobel Prize in 2000, Kandel (2005) repeated that, 'what we call mind is a set of functions carried out by the brain', which he regards as, 'a computational organ made marvelously powerful not by its mystery but by its complexity'; and, he asserts:

> We find it difficult to accept that every mental process, from our most public action to our most private thought, is a reflection of biological processes in the brain. (Kandel, 2005: 380)

Once again, the ambiguity of 'reflection' needs clarifying, but the reduction of the mind to a set of brain functions is unambiguous.

> Finally, given the persuasive nature of the evidence supporting the disease model, it is natural to start to think of acquired diffuse neurocognitive dysfunction in very physical terms. To some extent this is beneficial: it can be useful to carers, clinicians, and neuroscientists. Awareness of such benefits lay behind the statement in a recent report on dementia by the Nuffield Council on Bioethics (2009):

> Dementia arises as a result of brain disorder, and people are harmed at some point by having dementia. (p. 23)

But my contention is that understanding dementia needs to be from the broadest possible view. Although the disease model provides a significant part of the picture, it does not provide the whole picture. Thus, for instance, the Nuffield Council report goes on to suggest that quality of life can be maintained in dementia and it recognizes that this relies not just on facts, but on evaluative judgements (cf. Nuffield Council on Bioethics, 2009: §§2.21–2.23); the report also makes important statements about personhood in dementia, which themselves move beyond a purely physical account (*ibid.*: 30–2). If carers, clinicians, or neuroscientists were to mistake the disease model for the whole picture, the effect would be clinically, socially, and ethically disastrous. My motivation is a concern to accommodate the physicalism of the disease model within the broadest possible understanding of dementia.

Causal accounts of prosopagnosia

The construal of intentional psychological states presented by the disease model is physicalist. I shall be asking what this suggests for our understanding of acquired diffuse neurocognitive dysfunction and I shall make use of the distinction between causal and constitutive accounts of intentional psychological phenomena. The worry is that the disease model tends towards a limited view of what it is to have dementia. Recognizing that the disease model (in itself) only offers a causal account of intentional psychological states, whilst the Wittgensteinian critique requires a constitutive account, allows the broader perspective.

To return to the important work of Kandel, who won the Nobel Prize for his contributions to our understanding of the physiological basis of memory, what sort of account might his work suggest we give for what it is to remember Adlestrop?

We know that the hippocampus is a key area as far as any causal account of the memory impairment in Alzheimer's disease is concerned. Medial temporal atrophy, which can be tracked by neuroimaging, involves the hippocampus. Declarative or episodic memory, our memories for events and places, such as Thomas's memory of Adlestrop, is impaired if there is damage to the hippocampus. As a causal explanation of this type of memory loss, this account seems unobjectionable. But Kandel (2005) goes further:

> This deficit in memory is detectable at the cellular level; it is evident in a weakening of a process called long-term potentiation, an intrinsic mechanism that is thought to be critical for learning-related strengthening of synaptic connections. (pp. 83–4)

The ambiguity, which I referred to above in discussing Kandel, may seem to be a mere quibble over wording. If he had written, 'The deficit in terms of the process of remembering is detectable at the cellular level', there would be no problem. As it is, however, it seems that my inability to remember Adlestrop is something that can be detected at the cellular level. But this is wrong: it goes beyond the science, because it may be that I could still recognize Adlestrop, both the name and the place, even if I cannot recall the episode when the express train stopped unwontedly—so it is only a deficit in terms of a certain type of memory; moreover, *a memory*—and, therefore, a deficit in memory—just is not something that inhabits the cellular level. What it is to have a memory of Adlestrop, the constitutive account, entails that we bring in normative concerns, which do not reside in the cell, but in the world. If there is doubt about how fair this is to Kandel, recall his unambiguous statement (with added emphasis) that the mind, '*is* a set of functions carried out by the brain' (Kandel, 2005: 380).

The fundamental stipulation of the disease model in connection with acquired diffuse neurocognitive dysfunction is that it is fully explained by physical defects, by the pathology that differentiates it from normal brain ageing. Hence, any particular intentional psychological state is given a *physicalist* construal because it will have a *physical*, pathological basis. It is worth noting, however, that the evidence concerning the physical causes of dementia precisely concern *causes*. I shall pursue this discussion using the specific example of face recognition.

Prosopagnosia is an inability to recognize familiar faces. It can occur in Alzheimer's disease (Mendez, Martin, Smyth, and Whitehouse, 1992) and other types of dementia, as well as in other forms of brain damage. An analysis of post-mortem and CT scan data implies that bilateral lesions of the central visual system, situated specifically in the medial occipitotemporal region, are critical for the development of prosopagnosia (Damasio, Damasio, and van Hoesen, 1982). More recent research has encouraged a return to the older view that prosopagnosia is predominantly associated with right hemisphere lesions (De Renzi et al., 1994). Either way, by inference, the ability to recognize faces (an intentional psychological phenomenon) is maintained by the integrity of functioning in a particular part of the brain. The brain areas involved might be more delicately dissected by considering fine-grained aspects of recognition (Kipps & Hodges, 2008).

As the case of prosopagnosia shows, the disease model construes intentional psychological phenomena in physical terms. I shall go on to argue that there is more to face recognition than simply right hemisphere or bilateral medial occipitotemporal damage. But this is not to argue that the way in which the disease model accounts for prosopagnosia is wrong. The disease model provides a perfectly acceptable (causal) account of what must be in place for face recognition to occur. There is nothing alarming in accepting that the integrity of the medial occipitotemporal lobes *is* a pre-condition for face recognition. These brain areas, in turn, must connect appropriately to other body parts in order for the person to see the face and confirm that it is recognized. So when someone cannot recognize a familiar face (in the absence of other peripheral—as opposed to central or brain—causes) there must be damage to these brain areas, either in terms of structure or of functioning; and this can be confirmed by the appropriate sort of scan, or at post-mortem. That is, damage to the medial occipitotemporal lobes (bilaterally or unilaterally) *causes* prosopagnosia.

Forgetting familiar faces: Miss Breen

We can, therefore, put together a reasonably coherent physical explanation for why Miss Breen does not recognize her younger brother any more. It is caused by the defi-ciencies in the parts of her brain to do with seeing (the occipital lobe) and the parts of her brain to do with remembering (the medial temporal lobe). We could, perhaps, perform a SPECT scan to show her brother the areas of poor functioning. This would amount to a causal explanation of the problem. But it comes nowhere near capturing what this dysfunction actually means. For that, we need not only *Erklären* (the expla-nation of natural sciences) discussed in Chapter 3, but also *Verstehen* (the understand-ing of human sciences) (cf. Jaspers, 1923: 27). For one thing, Miss Breen's failure to recognize her brother might lead to his decision not to visit as regularly, which would be an ethical consequence. Understanding her prosopagnosia entails, at a psychologi-cal level, appreciating what it is to be recognized by anyone and particularly by an older sister. This failure is not just a lesion, it is a profound loss of a human relation-ship, a social catastrophe, which has the potential to lead to all sorts of further human consequences. Prosopagnosia, as Miss Breen's case shows, is not just a biological matter, but at least an ethical and psychosocial issue too.

It might, however, be that her brother will recognize that there are other things going on: that his sister still derives comfort from his visits, that there seems to be some kind of emotional recognition when he comes to see her. These responses could be regarded as further concomitants of the role that recognition plays in our lives. It might also be that a neuroscientific explanation could be given for how face recogni-tion can be tied to affective components and how these ties can be broken in disease. This is fine; but (again) the causal explanation does not tell us *what it is* to recognize or fail to recognize someone, neither in cognitive terms nor in emotional or affective terms. Knowing about Miss Breen's medial occipitotemporal lobes does not tell us much about her world, only about her brain. And to know her is to know what things might mean for her, which entails normative concerns, where these are embedded—constitutively, immanently, and irreducibly—in the patterned practices of her life. We need a grip on all of this. A causal account gives us a perspective, but not the full view.

Cognitive neuropsychology: memory and representation

I shall now move on to present a cognitive neuropsychology model of dementia. Again I wish to present the model in as strong a way as possible, because it is important to see how powerful it is in terms of the information it can give us. I shall discuss potentially underpinning philosophical theories—I have already discussed Fodor's representationalism in Chapter 3—from sub-personal processing to encoded meaning, but will conclude that the accounts of what it might be to remember remain deficient when measured against the requirement for the account to demonstrate how intentional mental states are normative.

Introduction to cognitive neuropsychology

Cognitive neuropsychology,

> … is an approach which attempts to understand cognitive functions such as recognising, speaking or remembering through an analysis of the different ways those functions can be impaired following brain injury. (Ellis & Young, 1988: 23)

It attempts to explain normal and abnormal cognitive function, 'in terms of damage to one or more of the components of a theory or model of normal cognitive functioning' (*ibid.*). Separate modules are held to be responsible for different cognitive operations and the 'hypothesised organisation of these modules may … be expressed in terms of an "information processing" diagram' (*ibid.*). For my purposes, the most important assumption in cognitive neuropsychology is that of 'isomorphism':

> the cognitive structure of the mind is reflected in, and arises out of, the physiological organisation of the brain. (Ellis & Young, 1988: 24)

In order to illustrate the sort of model used by cognitive neuropsychologists, Figure 5.1 shows a (highly simplified) cognitive processing flow diagram which demonstrates how, from dictation, a word might be orally spelt or written. When a word is heard, it is first analysed either in terms of the separate sounds that constitute the word (route 1 in the diagram), or as a whole entity (routes 2 and 3). Following route 1, the heard sounds may be converted directly into phonemes or speech sounds that can then be spoken. If the heard word is to be written down, then the phonemes will need to be converted to graphemes (e.g. individual letters).

The alternative route from the level of auditory analysis involves the whole word being recognized within the auditory input lexicon. The generally accepted route thence (route 2) is that words are further processed in terms of their semantic properties. The meaning of the word directly determines its spelling, so semantic processing leads from the heard word in the auditory input lexicon to the written spelling in the graphemic (or orthographic) output lexicon.

There is some intuitive justification for postulating two routes. I cannot hope to spell 'there' and 'their' correctly by an analysis of their sounds alone, but only by knowing their meanings in a given context. I must use, therefore, the semantic route (2). On the other hand, having never previously heard the non-word 'garp', I can only

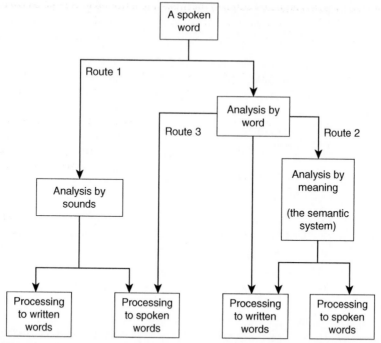

Fig. 5.1 A cognitive neuropsychology model to show how a spoken word is processed to be written or spelt out loud. Human Cognitive Neuropsychology, Ellis, A. W., and Young, A. W. 1998, Taylor and Francis. Reprinted with permission of the publisher.

hope to spell it by an analysis of its sounds, which I must convert to letters (graphemes) if I wish to write it down (route 1).

The validity of the distinction between two routes is based on the results of investigating patients with various forms of brain damage. For instance, some patients have particular difficulty in spelling words when there is an irregular correspondence between how they sound and how they look. Nevertheless, such patients may attempt phonologically plausible spellings, indicating they are using the sounds, for instance by spelling 'cough' as COFF. This error is taken to show that these patients have to use route 1. Alternatively, there are cases where patients cannot write unfamiliar non-words to dictation, whilst familiar words are managed well. This suggests they use the lexical route (2).

In addition to the two main routes just described, it has also been postulated that there are other routes from the auditory input lexicon to the speech or graphemic output lexicons (e.g. route 3). The suggestion is that some patients use a lexical route, but one which does not involve semantic processing. The cognitive neuropsychologist Karalyn Patterson, for instance, had a patient (GE), who was almost totally unable to speak following a stroke, but could still correctly spell words he did not understand (Patterson, 1986). However, GE could not spell non-words and he rarely made phonologically plausible spelling errors, so his spelling must have been lexical but non-semantic.

Patterson's closely argued account of the impairments found in GE—and how these impairments point to a particular model of cognitive processing—is convincing and impressive. It also suggests that what is at issue is a representational process. For example:

> It seems that for GE … proceeding from recognition of a spoken word to its orthography was not primarily based upon a *semantic representation*. … GE's spelling of large numbers of words, many of them very complicated, must certainly have derived from *representations* in the orthographic output lexicon. … My preferred interpretation is of course that these *representations* in the phonological output lexicon were, right from the beginning, sufficiently available to provide a mediating role between his virtually intact auditory input lexicon and his virtually intact orthographic output lexicon. (emphases largely added) (*ibid.*).

Thus, representations are (at least) spoken of as if they are entities that exist and mediate an internal process. The representations, according to the assumption of isomorphism, are reflected in and arise from the physiological organization of the brain. Whether neurophysiological or neuropsychological, however, what is postulated is a representation along with a process. This commitment to internal representations is similarly in evidence in cognitive neuropsychology's account of memory.

Memory

Memory can be divided into declarative memory (which allows me to recite a famous soliloquy by Hamlet) and procedural memory (which allows me to drive my car). In the recall of declarative information we require 'the activation of an internal representation' (for instance, if we are asked to name an object); whereas, 'the retrieval of procedural information requires a motor output' (Damasio & Damasio, 1992). Within declarative memory, a distinction is made between short-term (working) memory (which allows the storage of information for a few seconds only) and long-term memory. Tulving (1972) made the further distinction within the long-term system, based on empirical data, between episodic and semantic memory. Episodic memory stores events from a person's life. Semantic memory 'stores general knowledge about the world, concepts, and language'; it is 'impersonal and … independent of any time and place' (McKenna, 1991). Furthermore, many cognitive disorders can be construed as memory disorders:

> The anomic aphasic patient … appears to have lost conscious *access to the representations in memory* of the spoken forms of many words. … The patient with 'surface' dysgraphia has similarly lost conscious *access to the representations in memory* of the spellings of many words. (my emphasis) (Ellis & Young, *op. cit.*: 303)

It appears that semantic information is stored in a hierarchical and modality-specific manner. So, e.g. loss of the superordinate concept 'animal' might entail loss of the subordinate concept 'dog' (alternatively, presented with a picture of a dog a patient might say 'animal', showing that higher order concepts are preserved at the expense of lower order concepts). This apparent order within the semantic memory system is held to support the notion of processing within a representational system.

In Alzheimer's disease it is apparent that both episodic and semantic memory are affected. Hodges, Salmon, and Butters (1992) felt there was, 'compelling evidence of semantic memory loss in [Alzheimer's disease]', which in their terminology amounted to a 'breakdown of representational knowledge'. From a later study of face recognition and naming, they concluded: 'loss of semantic memory is a fundamental defect in [Alzheimer's disease]' (Hodges, Salmon, and Butters, 1993). The language of representation (as shown by the added emphasis) is fundamental to cognitive neuropsychology:

> Underlying the language impairment in [Alzheimer's disease] is a breakdown in the knowledge base, or what is termed 'semantic memory'. This refers to the *representation* of knowledge, including concepts and the knowledge of words and their meaning. (Morris, 1997: 55)

So far, I have presented an account of the sort of information-processing models that are used by cognitive neuropsychologists. Such models involve the positing of internal representations. I have also discussed the evidence for impairments in semantic memory, involving the loss of representations, in Alzheimer's disease. It is clear from the literature that representations are central to the cognitive neuropsychologist's information-processing model. I still need to secure the point that this model construes intentional psychological states as representational.

The representational construal of intentional psychological states

My suggestion is that intentional psychological phenomena are construed by cognitive neuropsychology in terms of representations. How strictly can the model be called representationalist? Does cognitive neuropsychology suggest, for instance, that to have memories is to possess entities or states, called representations, which can be characterized independently of that of which the memories are memories? Well, how would a cognitive neuropsychologist construe the remembering of Edward Thomas? It would have to be construed in terms of an inner representation of 'Adlestrop'. This name, according to the model I am considering, must be represented in a store of names. To remember 'Adlestrop', Thomas presumably must have gained access to a lexical store, part of the semantic memory, in which his knowledge of place names was represented. As he remembered, he must have retrieved from the store the representation of 'Adlestrop'. Remembering, therefore, according to this model, is a matter of accessing or retrieving representations, which do indeed sound like entities independent of the things they represent. Cognitive neuropsychology seems, therefore, to be based on a form of representationalism, according to which the content of mental states involves having *inner* mental representations. Thornton has suggested three aspects to the claim that mental representations are inner states:

> They are ontologically independent of the external world.
> They are the internal causal origins of action.
> Their existence is a matter of hypothesis. (Thornton, 1998: 20)

Each of these aspects is manifest in cognitive neuropsychology.

First, according to the cognitive neuropsychology principle of isomorphism, mind states are brain states. This suggests some sort of physicalist understanding. In discussing the disease model, I supported physicalism inasmuch as it provides *causal* explanations of intentional mental states, which are, however, embedded in the normatively constrained world. The mind is *not*, therefore, as suggested by the first aspect of representationalism, ontologically independent of the external world, but a part of it, as in the externalism of mind. According to cognitive neuropsychology, contrariwise, my mental representation of 'Adlestrop', in itself, is an internal feature (whether of the mind or brain) quite distinct from the external world.

Secondly, in cognitive neuropsychology, my mental representation of 'Adlestrop' is the necessary precondition for my being able to write or spell 'Adlestrop'. Nevertheless, thirdly, the existence of the mental representation can only be inferred. It explains my behaviour. For instance, if I were only able to give a phonologically plausible spelling of 'Adlestrop' (as, say, 'Adelstrop'), and my spelling of 'yacht' was 'yot', it would be hypothesized that I was using the phonological route for spelling, not the lexical route. It might be said that I was not able to gain access to the lexicon, or that the representations in the lexicon were degraded. These conjectures would have their basis in the inferred, underlying or hidden, causal explanation—which depends on the notion of inner processing of mental representations—of my spelling difficulties.

In each of these regards, therefore, this characterization of representationalism, which suggests that the content of mental states can be explained by the possession of inner mental representations, is one that fits with the cognitive neuropsychology model. My remembering 'Adlestrop', and the consequences of that memory, are explained by my possessing the mental representation of 'Adlestrop'. It seems reasonable to argue, therefore, that cognitive neuropsychology is representationalist. But how will the representationalist construal of psychological concepts in cognitive neuropsychology stand up to the challenge of the Wittgensteinian analysis? Does normativity figure in this construal as a constitutive, immanent, and irreducible feature? We can get to this by considering Miss Breen again.

Miss Breen and cognitive neuropsychology: from process to person

Miss Breen does not remember familiar faces. As I have suggested, this is a calamity in one sense—e.g. from her brother's perspective, he has lost something of his relationship with his older sister—whilst, in another sense, her prosopagnosia is not the defining feature of Miss Breen. As a person she still has emotional responses and volitions, even if her cognitive function is deficient in particular ways. The representationalism of cognitive neuropsychology suggests that Miss Breen has lost the internal representation of her brother. The memory of her brother's face must (as an intentional mental state) be given a normative construal. This must be constitutive, in the sense that it should be part and parcel of the memory that it is a memory solely of his face and not of someone else's face; it must be immanent, in that the normativity cannot come from elsewhere, it must just be part of the practice of having such memories (of *his* face) that the validity comes from within (as it were) the practice of remembering the face of a brother; and it must be irreducible, in that normativity cannot be defined away in terms of some other process or some other external criteria. But to understand prosopagnosia purely in terms of an internal computation involving internal representations is to ignore the need for an engagement with the world, where what constitutes veridical memory is a matter of public, worldly standards of correctness, that come neither from the internal process of access to representations nor from the store of knowledge that makes up semantic memory itself, but must have their legitimacy from elsewhere, unless they are to be susceptible to the sort of deep scepticism (discussed in Chapter 4) that normativity is intended to guard against.

To raise this doubt about the cognitive neuropsychologist's representationalism is to raise a doubt about the understanding of the *person* that goes along with the model's understanding of intentional mental states. In other words, if we cannot get our thoughts about her *thoughts* right, we cannot get our thoughts about *her* right. There are two ways (at least) in which this critique impinges on our thoughts about Miss Breen. First, our thoughts about her failure to remember familiar faces cannot now be regarded solely as a deficit. Thinking of her intentional mental states from the broader (Wittgensteinian) perspective gives them a surround. There is a broader engagement with the world at stake. We might, for specific purposes, wish to explain the failure in *causal* terms to her brother and we might choose to do this by referring to scans and by discussing how the brain, *metaphorically*, can be regarded as a computer. But the broader view is that she is not simply a broken machine.

The *constitutive* account, what it is to be Miss Breen and not be able to remember her brother, stresses that this failure (for such it is) involves normative concerns. Hence, we locate Miss Breen's failure in a realm of normative practices, which are not confined to a computer in the head. For—and this is the crucial point—to be located in the realm of patterned human practices is to be revealed in a context where other things matter. Miss Breen can also be surrounded by affective concern, by love and compassion, by careful approaches, and tender touch. The pattern of human practice that includes recognizing a brother's face for what it is also includes a recognition of warmth and friendship shown by tone and demeanour. So, the Wittgensteinian account of Chapter 4 helps to encourage us to look at the broader, patterned, surrounding fields in which Miss Breen's responses and behaviour can still be regarded as meaningful; and our responses to her can attempt to engage appropriately with this (her) world.

This does, of course, raise an important issue. For what if her responses and ability to engage with the world disappear even further? What if, at a severer degree of acquired diffuse neurocognitive dysfunction we can no longer find anything that is meaningful? I shall return to this issue in Chapter 8, but for now simply suggest, as a promissory note, that the crucial point will then be the nature of our situatedness and the breadth of the surround that we are willing to consider.

The second way in which the Wittgensteinian critique of the cognitive neuropsychology model might affect our thoughts about Miss Breen is linked to the first, because the issue is again to do with how we think of her and whether we think of her as an organ or as an organism: in her case, as a person. This takes us back to Fodor. One possible consequence of his representational theory of mind and cognition is that the involvement of the whole person is not crucially defining for intentional mental states. For Fodor, the distinction between organisms and organs, 'does not seem to be frightfully important' (Fodor, 1976: 53). He continues:

> … the states of the organism postulated in theories of cognition would not count as states of the organism for purposes of, say, a theory of legal or moral responsibility. But so what?

> What matters is that they should count as states of the organism for *some* useful purpose. In particular, what matters is that they should count as states of the organism for purposes of constructing psychological theories that are true. (*ibid.*)

So, it seems, the description of psychological states given by Fodor's account can be called 'states of the organism', even though this is vastly different from the sort of thing that counts as a state of the organism when we are considering law or morals. When the cognitive neuropsychologist explains what it is to remember 'Adlestrop' in terms of an information-processing diagram, this is what it is for the organism, the human being, to remember, or—as far as Fodor is concerned—it might as well be.

According to the Wittgensteinian analysis, however, this is simply wrong. In criticizing Fodor, Taylor observed: '... human and animal agents are beings for whom the question arises of what significance things have for them' (Taylor, 1985: 196). For Taylor, the crucial difference between humans and machines is that for the former, 'things *matter* for them', which is what he terms the 'significance feature' (Taylor, *op. cit.*: 197). Both for us and for animals (but not for machines) 'things have significance for us non-relatively' (Taylor, *op. cit.*: 201). Taylor goes on to argue that Fodor has made false analogies:

> When Fodor talks of the relation of psychology to physics, he is not talking about our account of ourselves as agents. His 'psychology' is an account of what we do in computational terms, and the reductive issue for him arises between an account at this level and one at the physical or neurological level. He is quite oblivious of the difference between an account in computational terms and one which characterizes us as agents with the significance feature. (Taylor, *op. cit.*: 209)

According to Fodor, whether or not something has significance must itself be a matter of certain computational states holding sway. For Taylor, however, the significance of things is a feature of the world grasped by us as agents. That things in the world have a significance for us establishes a link between the world and us. This is analogous to intentional mental states: for such states to have content an externalist account is required; that is, one which establishes a link between the inner mental world and the outer world of events and things. Fodor ignores this point. Instead, he suggests there are simply internal mental representations, which have meaning (semantics) purely on the basis of their syntactic 'shape', and which stand in causal relationships to other mental representations. In which case, these internal mental representations need make no reference at all to the external world. The problem with this view is that significance and meaning are attributes of the world of persons (who are agents and do not, therefore, take a passive view), whereas Fodor only points to a sub-personal realm of functioning. Fodor's view eliminates the relevance of the external world of meaning and significance in favour of internal functionings.

Wittgenstein's view is that wholes and not parts provide a reference for psychological concepts:

> An event leaves a trace in the memory: one sometimes imagines this as if it consisted in the event's having left a trace, an impression, a consequence, in the nervous system. As if one could say: even the nerves have a memory. But then when someone remembered an event, he would have to *infer* it from this impression, this trace. Whatever the event does leave behind in the organism, *it* isn't the memory. The organism compared with a dictaphone

spool; the impression, the trace, is the alteration in the spool that the voice leaves behind. Can one say that the dictaphone (or the spool) is remembering what was spoken all over again, when it reproduces what it took? (RPPi: §220)

Recall Kandel (2005) talking of the 'deficit in memory' being 'detectable at the cellular level' and compare this to Wittgenstein: 'As if one could say: even the nerves have a memory' (*vide supra*). Regarding this quotation from Wittgenstein, Schulte commented:

> Wittgenstein merely says that the traces in the organism—our 'records' or 'representations'—may be all kinds of things but are certainly not *memories*; the concept 'memory' must not be applied to them. ... we need more than mere traces in a memory store if we are to decide whether or not something is to count as a memory. (Schulte, 1993: 115–16)

What is needed is contextual embedding, which provides normativity to intentional psychological states. Unfortunately for representationalism (and Fodor), the result of such conceptual understanding, with its emphasis on normativity, undermines the notion that there can be vehicles of thought (representations) capable of being characterized independently of that which the thoughts concern. Linkage has to be made to the external world in which the thoughts are meaningfully embedded, which entails that mental states cannot be regarded as fully captured by internal, mental representations. Hence:

- The normativity of intentional mental states implies that such states should be given an externalist construal, so that meaning and understanding constitutively involve the world; in which case, an understanding of the whole person *is* crucial, because it is the whole person who acts and engages with the world.

Summary

The Wittgensteinian analysis, in stressing the preconditions for concepts having the meanings that they do, emphasizes abilities and human actions, which are constitutive of the intentional mental states to which the concepts refer. Abilities and actions are demonstrated in the world and cannot, therefore, solely be a matter of 'internal' representations and mechanistic processes. The Fodorians will perhaps respond that, whatever the outcome in the world, what is important for remembering is what happens internally, mechanically, in terms of representations and processes instantiated in the brain. But whatever the causal preconditions, remembering and meaning conceptually involve normatively constrained abilities, which are properly understood only in the context of their worldly embedding. Hence, these intentional psychological states cannot be characterized *purely* in terms of possessing inner states or entities, which are independent of that which they concern. The Fodorian model takes no account of the way in which the normativity of intentional mental states is a matter of such states being embedded in the world. Thus, Fodor's representationalist account fails. But are there alternatives? I shall discuss two further cognitivist models: the first relies on a distinction between personal and sub-personal levels; the second requires that meaning be encoded in the brain.

Sub-personal meaning or metaphorical representations?

Having established that cognitive neuropsychology models are representational, but that RTM as propounded by Fodor (which initially seemed to offer a promising paradigm) offers an account of psychological phenomena that is deficient with respect to normativity, I shall now consider (in this section and the next) the possibility that the normativity of meaning and intentional mental content could be brought into the sphere of inner representations. If this could be achieved, then representationalism might be salvaged. In the works of Dennett an attempt is made to import meaning and intentionality to the sub-personal level. The attempt fails because of a commitment (more or less acknowledged) to representationalism in the form of realism about mental states. What I shall suggest, contrariwise, is that representations are merely metaphorical. Hence, representations do not satisfy the requirements of representationalism. I shall go on to suggest that Dennett's personal and sub-personal levels form a useful model for cognitive neuropsychology.

Dennett insists that we should not conflate talk of persons with talk of bodies: the personal and sub-personal levels must not be confused. He goes on to say that this lesson, derived from Wittgenstein and Ryle,

> ... has often been misconstrued, however, as the lesson that the personal level of explanation is the *only* level of explanation when the subject matter is human minds and actions. In an important but narrow sense this is true, for as we see in the case of pain, to abandon the personal level is to stop talking about pain. In another important sense it is false, and it is this that is often missed. (Dennett, 1969: 95)

For Dennett, both levels of explanation have their place. He wishes to talk of pains as being something to do with whole persons, but he does not wish pains to be divorced from talk of nerves. For the pain in my head is something to do with things occurring in the stuff of my brain.

Dennett's attitude to representationalism is not completely clear, although he clearly accepts that there is a sense in which it is permissible to talk of representations in the brain:

> Somehow ... the way a brain represents hunger must differ, physically, from how it represents thirst. ... There must also ... be a difference between the way a particular adult brain represents Paris and Atlantis, for thinking of one is not thinking of the other. How can a particular state or event in the brain represent one feature of the world rather than another? (Dennett, 1991: 192)

Dennett's answer has involved his theory of 'multiple drafts', of how the brain's numerous units are simultaneously processing the plethora of information given to it by the senses, and incorporating information already stored (some of it innately in the brain's structure as it has evolved), without a central controller (or 'ghost in the machine'), but in a way which allows the emergence of a 'narrative'. This narrative is what emerges at the personal level, but it is nothing more or less than the operations of the numerous units, or homunculi—'a Pandemonium of Homunculi' (Dennett, 1991: 455)—that exist in the brain which act, in effect, as an enormous 'parallel distributed processor'. But it is in these units or homunculi that our mental states find their instantiation: this is where the thoughts and memories are represented.

The notion of homunculi seems to be crucial to Dennett's account, although these need not be taken as literal manikins in the brain, but rather as processing and sub-processing units. These units necessarily operate at the sub-personal level. It is they that affect the join (for Dennett) between the sub-personal and personal levels of explanation. The processing which the homunculi are required to perform, however, needs something to be processed and it is here that the representations make their appearance. The representation of 'Adlestrop', for instance, needs to be processed by the sub-personal units or homunculi.

There is a degree of ambiguity to Dennett's representationalism. He discusses, for instance, the data structures of Artificial Intelligence (AI) models in a sympathetic way. They can be regarded as models akin to those of cognitive neuropsychology. He discusses them in terms of homunculi interacting at different levels: 'each homunculus has representations that it uses to execute its functions' (Dennett, 1978: 124). He suggests then that there are two philosophical responses:

> One could grant that they are indeed self-understanding representations or one could cite the various disanalogies between them and prototypical or *real* representations (human statements, paintings, maps) and conclude that data structures are not really internal representations at all. (*ibid.*)

Dennett suggests, however, that this would undermine the well-established principle that 'psychology needs internal representations' (Dennett, 1978: 125). He goes on to indicate that he feels the AI models are on the right track. So the positing of internal representations would seem to be a natural concomitant.

Whilst Dennett is critical of Fodor, he is nevertheless overtly representationalist when he talks of 'sub-personal' cognitive psychology:

> ... it will be 'cognitive' in that it will describe processes of information-transformation among content-laden items—mental representations—but their style will not be 'computational'; the items will not look or behave like sentences manipulated in a language of thought. (Dennett, 1987: 235)

Dennett tries to show how a machine-like structure can behave as an intentional system and can thereby carry meaning. According to Dennett, having acknowledged that there are personal level intentionally characterized abilities and activities, a decompositional analysis must take place to reveal the sub-systems which themselves can be regarded as intentional systems. It is the interaction between these sub-systems or homunculi that explains the intentionally characterized abilities and activities at the personal level. But this is not to be taken as a reduction of the mental to the physical, because the sub-systems themselves (as well as the systems as wholes) are to be regarded as intentional. The decompositional analysis must persist, otherwise the question as to how we account for the intentionality of the homunculi is not answered. So we move to sub-homunculi and this will continue until an explanation of the interactions of the lowest levels of homunculi requires only 'problem or task descriptions that are obviously mechanistic' (Dennett, 1978: 80). At this point no further representations or homunculi need to be posited because the work has been reduced to a functional task and no further explanations of intentionality are required.

The worry for Dennett's account is the 'homunculus fallacy', which Kenny describes as the practice of taking predicates, 'whose normal application is to complete human beings or complete animals' and applying them 'to parts of animals, such as brains, or to electrical systems' (Kenny, 1984: 125). The whole notion of intentionality is tied to the personal level. Dennett allows that intentional ascriptions can be made of homunculi at the sub-personal level, but this just begs the question. For, if at this sub-personal level intentionality is the same as it is at the personal level, it is hard to see how that intentionality can be dissipated; or, if it is not the same sort of thing (and it is hard to see how it can be, given that it is a notion that marks out the distinction between personal level language and talk of mechanistic processes), then it will not meaningfully characterize—at the sub-personal level—that which is captured by the full-blown term at the personal level. In brief, intentionality at the sub-personal level seems to be merely metaphorical intentionality; i.e. not intentionality at all.

The problem Dennett highlights is that of bringing intentionality, including meaning (and, therefore, normativity), into the realm of the sub-personal. For, mental representations are either metaphorical or, if they really represent something, they do so by engaging at the personal level. It is only at this level that things either do or do not have meaning. Hence, if mental representations are said to exist at the sub-personal level, they cannot be the bearers of semantic content. And this is, of course, inimical to any representational theory of mind.

The problem with the sub-personal level is that it does not allow the world-involvingness of content and, therefore, it can accommodate neither intentionality nor normativity. According to McDowell:

> The 'sub-personal' account of a sensory system, which treats it as an information-processing device that transmits its informational results to something else inside an animal, cannot adequately characterize what its sensory systems are for the animal (as opposed to what they are, metaphorically speaking, for the internal parts that receive the results of the information-processing): namely, modes of sensitivity or openness to features of the environment—not processors of information, but collectors of it. (McDowell, 1994: 197)

Explanations at the sub-personal level do not equate to what is going on for the creature as a whole. For humans, this is because the sub-personal does not engage with the world in the way required for there to be meaning.

McDowell illustrates his point with the distinction, discussed by Dennett too (Dennett, 1978: 163), between what the frog's eye tells the frog's brain and what the frog's eye tells the frog. Whilst it is perfectly true that there are distinctions to be made within the distinction between the personal and sub-personal levels of explanation, if we accept talk of the frog's eye telling either the frog's brain or the frog anything, we have already accepted a particular picture of mental processes. It might be more illuminating to recognize that the frog's eye does not 'tell' anything, except by a metaphorical use of language, but a use that may tend us towards a representational account of psychological phenomena.

So, as Dennett acknowledges (Dennett, 1978: 123), talk of personal level attributes at the sub-personal level has to be metaphorical. Dennett attempts to make representations normative by stretching the normativity at the personal level down to the sub-personal level. There are two arguments against this strategy.

1. Normativity at the personal level—and this was part of the substantive conclusion of Chapter 4—is a matter of practices being embedded in the human world. The sub-personal level, which is the level at which (according to cognitive neuropsychology) 'Adlestrop' is represented and processed, is (by definition) not embedded in the (typically human) world of meaning and normativity. It can only have, therefore, metaphorical personal level attributes. So importing Dennett's analysis of sub-personal representations to cognitive neuropsychology models would not save them, inasmuch as it remains representationalist, because it does not deliver normativity.

2. Normativity cannot be discharged. Dennett's suggestion that a move can be made from norms to a causal account is a reduction. The Wittgensteinian analysis argues that we cannot *causally* say what it *is* to have a thought. Dennett suggests that the intentional can be reduced to the non-intentional, that normativity can be explained in non-normative terms. But the transcendental analysis of normativity as constitutive, immanent, and irreducible, denies this possibility.

At root, the divide between personal and sub-personal levels is precisely a divide between meaningfulness and its absence. If we are talking about meaning and intentionality we must *ipso facto* be talking about persons and not just about brains or cognitive processes. For there to be meaning, with its transcendental requirement for normativity, we require practices or uses to be embedded in the world of whole persons. This is a constitutive argument, since this is what it *is* to have intentional mental states, irrespective of the causal regularities underlying such mental states.

The encoding of meaning?

I turn now to a different attempt to argue, on the basis of a cognitive paradigm, that meaning (and normativity) reach the level of mechanistic processing, this time by being encoded in the brain. Bolton and Hill accept: 'the broadly Wittgensteinian view that meaning is grounded in social practices, embedded in culture' (Bolton & Hill, 1996: 113). But they also wish to hold to their 'encoding thesis', namely: 'neural states encode, and process, information' (*ibid.*: 76). Their concept of 'information',

> ... has to be a semantic one, linked to meaning, intentionality, representation, etc. ... the information processed by the brain has to be *about* something (it has to *represent* something), namely, actual or possible states of the environment, results of action, etc. When brain function is described in these terms, in terms of intentionality, it is in effect being regarded as functioning like the mind. (*ibid.*)

Bolton and Hill are keen to keep away from the idea that, 'there are signs (signs with syntactic structure) in the brain doing the representing' (*ibid.*: 114). In the place of language-like, syntactic, structures they wish to substitute, 'the view that meaning essentially pertains to rule-guided activity, or again, [to] intentional agent/environment interactions' (*ibid.*). They think it is appropriate that their theory is vague about how the brain encodes meaning, but their notion of meaning as being essentially involved with activity links their theory, they suggest, to the Wittgensteinian view. Hence,

> Rule-following activity ... is what warrants the attribution of meaning to the agent, or to the brain, which as a matter of fact is the material system most of all involved in the regulation of action. (*ibid.*)

But, they are also clear, 'it is not the brain in isolation which carries meaning, but the brain in its role as regulating action' (*ibid.*: 115). Otherwise, concerning the intrinsic, physical aspects of the brain, they would agree with Hacker (1987: 492) that it actually *does* very little.

Bolton and Hill offer a very direct answer to the question concerning how mental content has meaning. It has meaning because the brain has meaning. Elsewhere, Bolton (1997) makes it clear that the encoding thesis is meant as a way of showing how the causal properties of mental content are to be explained without relying on syntax (as Fodor does). For Fodor, it is syntax (i.e. sentence construction and the rules that govern this; hence the need for a *language* of thought) that provides the connection between the causal properties of a symbol and its meaning. But if, therefore, meaning is not itself regarded as being a part of the information that is passed around the brain, according to Bolton, '*there is no explanation of intentional (environment-directed) action*' (*ibid.*). Put simply, it just is the case that the encoding thesis,

> ... is what is required for the purpose of understanding the role of neural processes in the regulation of intentional activity. But the implication is that the language of neural encoding should not blind us into thinking that in some way everything semantic is in the brain. On the contrary, if meaning (representation, cognition) *is* anywhere, it is in the whole interaction between the living being and its natural and social milieu. (*ibid.*)

The Bolton and Hill line is similar to that of Dennett inasmuch as they, too, wish to ascribe intentionality within the sub-personal realm. Bolton and Hill, however, do not wish to do this because of advances in AI, but because otherwise (by their lights) it is difficult to explain how mental states with meaningful content can be causal. That is, meaning and normativity need to be imported to the neuronal level; hence, the encoding of meaning in the brain. Part of their aim is to obliterate the gap between the personal and sub-personal levels. Representations, then, must just be personal because they have personal level effects. If they are personal, they are rooted in the practices of the embedding world by being such. Yet, (contra Bolton and Hill) how there can be meaning in the brain, which is quite distinct from the assertion that meaning is in the whole interaction of the human being with a social milieu, remains mysterious. Given that it is the person who interacts, rather than the brain, the meaning and representations in the brain seem still to be metaphorical.

The admirable effect of Bolton and Hill's idea is that it allows an account of a condition, such as Alzheimer's disease, to be given which moves seamlessly from disruption of neural processes, to disruption of psychological processes, to disruption of action. Moreover, it allows an account of 'functional, meaningful, compensatory strategies' in response to such disruptions. However, it also begs some questions, because—having just stated it must be so (in order for there to be mental events which have causal properties through their meaningfulness)—the talk of encoding meaning implies some mechanism as well as some sort of code. If Bolton and Hill clearly reject the code (it is not a matter of syntax), they do not so clearly reject the notion of mechanism, which is required by their continuing commitment to a representational theory of mind (Thornton, 1997b). But with that commitment comes an adherence, whether they like it or not, to the problems of the dichotomy between personal and sub-personal levels. In short, in trying to force a Wittgensteinian account (which regards meaning as a matter of practice within a human context) onto a cognitive science account (with its commitment to representationalism and thereby to the personal/sub-personal dichotomy), Bolton and Hill have tried to have their cake and eat it: they want the (undoubted) causal efficacy of the brain to be not just a matter of brain events leading to action, but a matter of inner states giving reasons for and guiding action (cf. Thornton, 2007: 153–60). But this requires: '. . . the context of a broader interpretation of the agent which connects the agent to the world' (Thornton, 2007: 159). The endeavour fails because the personal/sub-personal divide is precisely a divide between meaningfulness and its absence. If we are talking about meaning and intentionality, we must *ipso facto* be talking about persons and not just about brains; so talk of brains encoding meaning must be metaphorical.

Adlestrop, Miss Breen, and sub-persons

The point about Edward Thomas's poem is not simply that he remembers something! Rather, the poem is evocative of a mood and time. There is something atavistic about it, as in the music of Elgar perhaps. Its evocation of nature connects it to the romanticism of Wordsworth:

> And willows, willow-herb, and grass,
> And meadowsweet, and haycocks dry,
> No whit less still and lonely fair
> Than the high cloudlets in the sky.

> (From *Adlestrop* by Edward Thomas; *vide supra*)

What it is, to remember Adlestrop, is to engage in the realm of human meaning and significance. The constitutive account, whatever the sub-personal causes, brings in a host of other surrounding concerns, from social history to emotional resonances. The meanings that are evoked can only be understood in the context of the broader human world, where they are embedded and can be interpreted correctly or incorrectly. That is, there is normative constraint. Not that different interpretations are impossible; and not that our interpretations are immutable. But not just anything will do. There must be some sort of coherence and engagement with our shared, public experiences of the world.

So, too, with Miss Breen. We can give an account of her behaviour, her lack of face recognition, in terms of causes. But the full meaning of her behaviour is only understood from a broader field of view. What is happening at the sub-personal level, whether this is regarded as something physiological or psychological, can explain her actions, in the sense that we can say what might have caused them. But what her actions amount to, what constitutes them, takes us back into the realm of meaning and significance. In this realm, there is more to Miss Breen than her deficits. But what will be required is an interpretation, which in turn requires as much information as possible about Miss Breen. What surrounds her current behaviour is her life as a whole. Our initial interpretation may not be correct: we shall need to know more about her *as a person* to understand what she is doing, even if we know the (sub-personal) causes. Some of this is already present for us: we already share certain responses and ways of being. But a hermeneutic approach may be required in order to understand her meaning-making more fully.

> 'People are continuously involved in processes of meaning-making. They interpret and try to make sense of what happens around them, so that they understand the world and know what to do. Processes of meaning-making are not the result of conscious calculations or decisions by the individual; they precede such activities and serve as their foundation. In dementia, meaning-making becomes problematic. Common ways of understanding often tend to break down. Perspectives, which used to be shared, may drift apart. From a hermeneutic perspective, the challenge is to find ways to reintegrate these perspectives once again. This requires a dialogical attitude, exemplifying both openness and preparedness to change. A fusion of horizons is not a conscious achievement brought about through the exchange of information. It is a realignment that occurs when people take part in joint movements and rituals and find themselves changing into a community. (Widdershoven & Berghmans, 2006: 190)

The need for dialogue and community impels us into a discussion of the social construction of dementia.

Social constructionism and dementia

It should already be apparent, from the discussion in Chapter 3, that social constuctionist theories have relevance to dementia. Any theory of mind will have implications for a condition in which the mind is apparently lost. Further, social constructionism's emphasis on discourse is relevant because acquired diffuse neurocognitive dysfunction often involves loss of language. Moreover, whilst any illness or disease occurs within a social context, acquired diffuse neurocognitive dysfunction inevitably has social consequences which often pose the main problems for carers: disturbed behaviour, for instance. So there are numerous ways in which social constructionist theories can be used relevantly in connection with dementia. I shall, first, briefly present some of the literature that makes such connections, chiefly from Kitwood and Harré, but from other authors too. Secondly, I shall apply the Wittgensteinian critique from Chapter 4.

Changing the view: the social construction of dementia

It is noteworthy that social constructionist approaches have brought about changes to practice and to our theorizing about dementia. Lyman (1989) provides a good example of how awareness of social constructionism has led to a different perspective on dementia:

> ... reliance upon the biomedical model to explain the experience of dementing illness overlooks the *social construction* of dementia and the impact of treatment contexts and caregiving relationships on disease progression. (emphasis added)

In part, Lyman bases her case simply on the recognition of the importance of relationships and social setting for people with dementia; but she also builds an assault against the 'medicalization of senility', in which the attempt to differentiate clearly between dementia and normal ageing is seen as 'a social construction to create order from the disorderly aspects of living with dementia' (*ibid.*). Her suggestion is that disturbed behaviour in dementia often results from disturbed care-giving relationships, which tend to be overlooked if behaviour is attributed to disease. Lyman's advocacy of the sociogenic perspective deserves respect:

> The sociogenic perspective recognizes that all human experience involves intentional social action and interaction, in socially structured environments, in the context of taken-for-granted socially constructed knowledge about aging, development, and disease. (*ibid.*)

Another link between social construction and dementia comes from the notion of narrative, which has also been used in connection with ethics. Thus Norberg's (1994) overview of ethical issues in dementia makes use of 'narrative relation ethics'. Narratology is recognized by Harré to be close to social constructionism, because it allows us to consider the stories that we construct of our lives. And, according to Norberg,

> ... we create and tell our stories within stories that others have already told. When we narrate we order actions into the past, the present and the future. ... People are simultaneously involved in many stories, that of their families, their countries, their professions, mankind and so on. There is also a personal story. The person tells and is told. (*ibid.*)

Such a view is clearly constructionist: the person is constructed by the various story lines in which he or she takes part and these stories are essentially public, so the construction is social. It has, according to Norberg, ethical implications:

> Being able to experience episodes of our lives as whole and meaningful stories is an important aspect of our narrative competence. The demented person gradually loses this competence. The caregiver then has an important task helping her or him experience wholeness and meaning. (*ibid.*)

It is clear, then, that social constructionist thought can play a role in some of the ethical issues that arise in connection with acquired diffuse neurocognitive dysfunction.

An ethical imperative to improve care for people with dementia also drove Tom Kitwood (1937–1998), whose work shows strong social constructionist tendencies.

Kitwood espoused the view that 'the problem' of dementia does not lie exclusively within the person with dementia, but, 'rather, in the interpersonal milieu' (Kitwood, 1993). At a time when inner security is vanishing, because of loss of memory and the decline of other cognitive faculties, 'personhood can only be guaranteed, replenished and sustained through what others provide' (*ibid.*). This sentiment reflects social constructionist thought, since it relies on the notion that personhood is constructed by others, whereas many would wish to stress the inner qualities (such as self-consciousness) or physical attributes (such as having an intact functioning human brain) necessary to confer personhood. Indeed, Kitwood (1989) gives a straightforward social constructionist avowal when he writes:

> ... virtually all the losses and difficulties of later life are socially constructed.

Kitwood famously defined personhood as:

> ... a standing or status that is bestowed upon one human being, by others, in the context of relationship and social being. (Kitwood, 1997: 8)

Personhood is, thus, according to Kitwood and Bredin (1992a), constructed by others in a social context:

> The core of our position is that personhood is essentially social; it refers to human beings in relation to others.

From Kitwood's (1990) perspective, 'the dementing illness is intricately woven into the pattern of life-history and social relationships'. On this view, dementia requires 'inter-subjective insight' and 'inter-subjective understanding' on the part of carers and health professionals (*ibid.*).

Kitwood's work, premised on social constructionist theory, has had a significant impact on theorizing concerning dementia, as well as on the actual practical business of providing 'person-centred care' (Baldwin & Capstick, 2007). Even if at a conceptual level Kitwood's theories can be criticized, the practical usefulness and humaneness of the perspective he has helped to create are undoubted.

Finally, in this sub-section, I wish to return to the work of Rom Harré, to show its applicability to acquired diffuse neurocognitive dysfunction. But first, I shall start with earlier work by Steve Sabat, who later co-authored papers with Rom Harré. (In the chapters that follow, I shall frequently draw upon Sabat's (2001) seminal work as a whole.) Sabat has recorded conversations with Alzheimer's disease patients for analysis. As a preface to this work, Sabat (1991) discusses Karl Ludwig Bühler (1879–1963), a philosopher and psychologist who,

> ... saw the elements of language as being social tools, the use of which was determined by the intentions of the user, with purposeful communication as the goal.

Interestingly, but as an aside, the theories of the Bühlers (Karl and his wife Charlotte [1893–1974], also a psychologist) are strongly evident in the work of Vygotsky (mentioned in Chapter 3), who provides some of the roots to social constructionism; moreover, Wittgenstein met the Bühlers and Toulmin (1969) conjectured that Wittgenstein might himself have been influenced by them.

Sabat (1991) convincingly musters evidence to show that, 'the social context of the conversation and the purposes of the interlocutors' are all-important. He proceeds to demonstrate that in two conversations with Alzheimer's disease patients,

> ... there was an exchange of ideas, information about the present and past, humor, sadness, concerns and advice; there were openness and compassion, there were changes of attitude.

> In short there was an experience, shared between two interlocutors, of some of the most fundamental human characteristics. (*ibid.*)

Although the conversations were disjointed, language was used as a social tool, in keeping with Bühler's theories, with the words having a purpose. This suggests that these were genuine conversations between persons. In social constructionist terms, extrapolating from Sabat, the personhood of the participants was constructed in part by the conversation. The conversation can certainly be seen to have contributed to their standing as persons in relation to one another.

In later studies, Sabat joined with Harré to argue for the preservation of self in dementia. This work was premised on the constructionist notion that,

> ... personhood is created primarily in the process of engaging in certain types of spoken discourse. (Sabat & Harré, 1992)

They make a distinction between self 1, which is the self of personal identity, 'experienced as the continuity of one's point of view in the world of objects in space and time', which is 'usually coupled with one's sense of personal agency' (*ibid.*); and selves 2, 'the selves that are publicly presented in the episodes of interpersonal interaction in the everyday world, the coherent clusters of traits we sometimes call "personae"' (*ibid.*). Alzheimer's, on this view, 'does not result in the loss of self 1 and only contributes indirectly to possible losses in selves 2' (*ibid.*). This is because self 1 requires that the person can index his or her discourse by the use of first person pronouns, an ability which endures into even severe dementia. And selves 2 will remain intact because any particular self 2 is not related to progression of the disease, but to 'the behaviour of those who are regularly involved in the social life of the sufferer' (*ibid.*). Sabat and Harré's conclusion here is much the same, therefore, as that of Kitwood. They state:

> ... if there is a loss of the capacity to present an appropriate self 2, in many cases the fundamental cause is to be found not in the neurofibrillary tangles and senile plaques in the brains of the sufferers, but in the character of the social interactions and their interpretation that follow in the wake of the symptoms. (*ibid.*)

Elsewhere, again using real conversations with Alzheimer's disease subjects, Sabat and Harré (1994) suggest that such patients remain 'semiotic subjects', by which they mean,

> ... people who can act intentionally in the light of their interpretations of the situations in which they find themselves, and who are capable of evaluating their actions and those of others according to public standards of propriety and rationality.

They suggest that the illocutionary force of discourse (i.e. what is done *in* saying something, rather than the actual words spoken), which can often still be felt in conversations with people with Alzheimer's disease (such as Miss Breen), is 'not diminished or obliterated by grammatical or phonetic errors, or by paraphasias' (*ibid.*). Just to emphasize again the utility of this work, its upshot is highly relevant to carers who find themselves with a duty to search 'for the meaning in the behavior of the afflicted when it is not readily apparent' (*ibid.*).

So far, the approach of social constructionism to dementia seems wholly bene-ficial, as well as appropriate. I shall now move on, however, to start the Wittgensteinian analysis of the social constructionist's handling of intentional psychological states.

Intentional psychological states as social constructions

In pursuing the Wittgensteinian analysis of social constructionism I shall, once again, ask how social constructionism construes intentional psychological states. The answer is clear: intentional psychological phenomena are social constructs. Inasmuch as this places an emphasis on the public following of rules in practices and customs, this sounds Wittgensteinian. Social constructionism is opposed to the view that the practices constitutive of psychological states must be *essentially private*. Instead, social construc-tionism opts for the position that regards the practices that underpin language and thought as *essentially public*. The Wittgensteinian analysis, however, suggests that such practices must be *potentially public*. If they have to be *essentially public* the account of intentional psychological states, on the view that I am suggesting, is circumscribed.

That said, it is still worth considering the degree to which the suggestion that inten-tional psychological states are social constructs accords with the Wittgensteinian analysis. Consider, for instance, Harré's assertion that,

> Insofar as psychological functioning is accomplished through the medium of speech-acts it must be both public and collective. (Harré, 1989a)

He also maintains that 'the discursive thesis entails a sociality thesis' (Harré, 1992). The emphasis is on the extent to which understanding psychological phenomena requires public display and agreement. For Harré, to be a psychologically functioning person is to be able to take part in public discourse. This immediately acts as a correc-tive to those models suggesting that psychological states are only understood in terms of the internal workings of the brain. Social constructionism, on this view, helps to broaden our notions of what it is to be a psychological person of this sort. To take another example, Coulter states:

> ... our interest need not be in 'underlying' rules or structures ... but in public displays of psychological phenomena and subjectivity-determinations as socially-organized accom-plishments. (Coulter, 1979: 61)

He later opined: '... the ascription and avowal of mental-conduct categories turn upon essentially *public* grounds ...' (Coulter *op. cit.*: 153). What is apparent is the rule-governed nature of psychological phenomena; but the rules are not internal, they are external, contained in practical, social accomplishments. Again there is a feeling of a corrective here, for instance to an overly biomedical view, which tends to look for internal explanations for problems in psychological functioning, rather than look to the social environment. The corrective can legitimately claim *some* support from the Wittgensteinian analysis, according to which intentional psychological states involve the public following of practices and customs. But there is no mention here of normativity. Just how social constructs can account for normativity will need to be made clear. As in the previous models of dementia, it is in its treatment of normativity that social constructionism will be found wanting by the Wittgensteinian analysis.

What is crucial is exactly what it means to construe such mental states in terms of social constructs. There are two alternatives:

- social institutions and practices *cause* intentional mental states to be the states they are;

- intentional mental states are *constituted* by social practices and institutions.

The ambiguity concerning these alternatives is deeply rooted in social constructionist literature. In the rest of this section I shall demonstrate this point.

I have already quoted: 'The core of our position is that personhood is essentially social: it refers to human beings in relation to others' (Kitwood & Bredin, *op. cit.*). Kitwood could be suggesting that personhood (which typically involves the possibility of ascribing intentional mental states) is *caused* by social relations; in this sense it is socially constructed. But the 'essentially' also implies that this is what personhood is *in essence*, namely a matter of social relations, which would be a *constitutive* claim.

Harré echoed Kitwood in writing: 'persons are discursively produced' (Harré, 1992), which sounds like a *causal* explanation of persons. Elsewhere he writes:

> Memories are created discursively … remembering is paradigmatically a social activity. (Harré, 1994)

Although the notion of memories being *created* by social activity sounds like a causal account of memories, the copula in 'remembering *is* … a social activity' could be taken as an indication as to the *nature* of remembering. Moreover, Davies and Harré (1990) state:

> An individual *emerges* through the processes of social interaction, … as one who is *constituted and reconstituted* through the various discursive practices in which they participate. (emphases added).

Whilst the emergence of the individual might be regarded as a *causal*, social process, the second half of the sentence implies the person is *constituted* by the social interaction. In which case, 'persons are discursively produced' might be given a constitutive interpretation too.

Similarly, Gergen's (1985) talk of the ontological basis of mind being 'within the sphere of social discourse', together with Coulter's (1979) suggestion that, 'the properties of mental-predicate ascriptions and avowals', should be attributed, 'to the culture, not to minds', equally show a tendency towards a *constitutive* account of mental states. But the *causal* tendency in social constructionism—for instance, Kitwood (1989) saying that 'virtually all the losses and difficulties of later life are socially constructed'—remains.

So too, concerning memory, Harré (1994) suggests:

> An entry in a diary is not a memory, nor is a molecular configuration in the brain. A memory is a representation. A representation is only a memory if it is an accurate or true representation of some past event ….

He goes on to say that a representation becomes a true representation through a 'public negotiation of authenticity'. This keeps in mind,

> ... the important observation that remembering is a task for people, and that the memory 'machines' in their heads are of no more and no less significance than the tape recorders and diaries they also use. (*ibid.*)

Harré had in his sights the cognitivist's account of memory, which I discussed above, but the point is thus, not only social, but constitutive: a memory is *constituted* as such by a public negotiation. Yet, the *causal*, constructionist line is strong: 'psychological phenomena are *created* in ... social encounters' (*ibid.*) (emphasis added).

So, even if the emphasis on public practices has a Wittgensteinian ring to it, the ambiguity concerning whether social constructionism offers a causal or constitutive account of intentional psychological states seems pervasive, which has implications for the account it gives of normativity.

So far, then, I have:

◆ offered, partly in Chapter 3, an account of social constructionism;

◆ shown that social constructionism construes psychological states as social constructs;

◆ highlighted an ambiguity concerning whether social constructionism offers a causal or constitutive account of intentional psychological states.

In Chapter 6 I shall pursue this ambiguity, which is for now left hanging. Nevertheless, the outline of the critique of social constructionism is becoming apparent. If the model only offers a causal account, in comparison with the other models of dementia it will be similarly limited. If it offers a constitutive account, it seems then to suggest that Thomas's remembering of Adlestrop has to be conceived as something that is *essentially public*; and yet, we might wish to hold that remembering is also something inward.

Conclusion

In this chapter, I have considered the disease model, the cognitive neuropsychology model, and the social constructionist model. I have interrogated these models of dementia in the light of the Wittgensteinian analysis of intentional mental states and asked, in particular, how they conceptualize remembering. In each case, although I have been able to acknowledge good points, I have found the models wanting. The disease model of dementia presents a perfectly reasonable causal account of what it is to remember (or forget) Adlestrop. But it does not speak of the constitutive account, of what remembering and forgetting actually mean. This model needs to be broadened. The cognitive neuropsychology model, with its reliance on inner representations and sub-personal processing, again gives us a form of causal explanation, but one that is metaphorical. It will need to be understood in a broader surround. The social constructionist model presents us with an ambiguity between a causal and a constitutive account. In the next two chapters I shall broaden the view of these models and confront the ambiguity of social constructionism.

There is then a hint that what it is to remember something, Adlestrop say, is difficult to pin down. Of course, there will be criteria of correctness—this is what normativity is all about. Remembering Slough is not the same as remembering Adlestrop. The transcendental account of normativity points to the conditions for the possibility of remembering, which are that the normativity is constitutive of the practice of remembering, immanent in it, and irreducible. Remembering Adlestrop is like nothing else. The poem captures for us a moment and an emotion.

> And for that minute a blackbird sang
> Close by, and around him, mistier,
> Farther and farther, all the birds
> Of Oxfordshire and Gloucestershire.

(From *Adlestrop* by Edward Thomas; *vide supra*)

What it is to remember, therefore, is clouded in some sort of mystery. In the end there are some things that cannot be said about it: our conception of our mental states points towards something other (the confusing impetus to dualism maybe), even though we are aware, darkly, that we cannot lay that conception bare. But it is also mundane: it is just what it is in the everyday world.

So, too, with Miss Breen: her forgetting is ordinary, with straightforward causal explanations; but is also extraordinary. It is a mundane fact of the world; but what we make of it shows our evaluative judgements. To forget the face of a loved one is to have lost a part of one's world; but it is not the whole of the human world. Our mental states reach out to the world and are constituted in part by it. Our embeddedness in the human world of practices is, therefore, part of what we are: these practices are constitutive; what is normative is immanent in them and cannot be reduced. Our understanding of what it is to remember Adlestrop—with all that normativity entails—means that our understanding of Miss Breen cannot be circumscribed. The text is always open to further interpretation.

Chapter 6

Moving towards a solution: dementia and the normative world

Introduction

The text is always open to further interpretation, but there are normative constraints on our understanding of what anything in particular might mean. There is, thus, a seeming tension that emerges from thinking through dementia. This chapter highlights the tension, but starts to suggest that the tension gestures at the solution. What is required is the right perspective, the right view. The surroundings need to be perspicuous, inasmuch as this is possible. But to get to the potential tension and the possibility of a solution, we need to work through what is already to hand, namely the models of dementia that we have considered so far.

The first aim of the chapter, therefore, is to complete the account of what is right and wrong with our models of acquired diffuse neurocognitive dysfunction.[1] The disease model presents a causal account of what it is to remember or to forget. But this is a *causal* not a *constitutive* account: it explains things but does not (on its own) increase our (empathic) understanding. This model needs to be broadened so that causal explanations have a framework rooted in our empathic understanding of humans in the world. The cognitive neuropsychology model provides further causal explanations using inner representations and sub-personal processing; but the explanatory model is metaphorical and needs to be understood in a broader surround. The social constructionist model is broad, but ambiguous: is it causal or constitutive? The initial work of this chapter is to broaden the view of these models and to confront the ambiguity of social constructionism.

The idea that we need to broaden the perspective is one that I shall then pick up in Chapter 8. We need to grasp that what we see is, indeed, a picture: one that can be viewed from a variety of angles; one that sits in different surroundings. The correct perspective, I shall argue, is the one that makes the surroundings obvious (or perspicuous), which does not lose sight of the contextual embedding. But the context is not just pictorial, it can also be narratively construed: it is the text that stands open to further interpretation.

What sense, however, does this talk make when we speak of healthcare in general and acquired diffuse neurocognitive dysfunction in particular, especially when we come back to the reality of treating real people such as Miss Breen? What does it actually mean in practice to speak of seeing her in a truly holistic fashion? Can we ever see everything at once? The answer, I think, is that we cannot understand individuals all at once from the perspective that we now occupy: one reading is not enough. What is required is a high degree of self-awareness and an openness to the possibility of further readings and to a broadening of the view, rather than the reverse. This is, after all, how we ordinarily get to know someone: we hear their stories, in chunks, bit by bit. It is, moreover, part of the joy of getting to know someone intimately. And at the most profound levels of intimacy there emerges a sense of mystery. I shall return to these thoughts in Chapter 7. But in this chapter, having suggested that our models need a broader perspective, the further aim is to gesture at a solution—in terms of maintaining the correct, broad, perspicuous view—to the tension that seems to emerge from the Wittgensteinian critique.

At the start of this chapter I have spoken of the potential tension in terms of, on the one hand, the possibility of further interpretations and, on the other, the normative constraints on understanding. Normative constraints seem to point to something objective, something that is non-individual, or perhaps mind-independent (realist in this sense): it is not open to me alone to decide that just anything counts as remembering Adlestrop. For Adlestrop is a real place in the world and not a place I have constructed in my mind. Being open to further interpretations does, none the less, suggest that I am at liberty to read more into the poem as a matter of subjective determination. In this sense, then, the further interpretation of the meaning of the poem is mind-dependent (idealism in the sense that the meanings can be created by me). So I might decide that remembering Adlestrop is something quite different from remembering a particular location at a particular time. It might be to do with a loss of innocence and of a world.

Indeed, the putative tension is to do with our worldview: it is a matter of keeping the broader perspective, of seeing the individual *and* the surround. My suggestion in this chapter is precisely that this is what is required of models of dementia and probably in medicine generally. So, the first aim of the chapter is to complete the critique of the models and the second is to confront the tensions that emerge in order, thirdly, to gesture at the solution that will underpin the discussion in the rest of the book.

In more detail, I shall start by reconsidering the account that the disease model presents of prosopagnosia. My conclusion will be that scientific explanations must involve some sort of reference to the broader world in which understanding is normatively constrained. I shall then discuss Fodor's model of internal mechanisms as a way to push home the point in connection with cognitive neuropsychology that the normativity of internal mental states has to be seen as embedded in the world. Internal mechanisms require external states to provide the appropriate criteria of correctness. In other words, we need externalism of mind and a focus on worldly practices. Inner representations on this view become meaningful only by connection with outer criteria of meaningfulness. Finally, social constructionism, if causal, is too narrow a view and certainly does not capture the normativity of the transcendental, constitutive account. Alternatively, if constitutive, social constructionism can either be regarded as idealist or realist; but neither reading is entirely satisfactory for the reasons that I shall consider. In the final part of my discussion, focusing on the work of Rom Harré, I shall show how we are impelled to a broader conception of the person by the move in social constructionist thought from inner to outer conceptions of the mind and selfhood.

The critique of these models of dementia moves us towards a different level of understanding, towards a solution to the supposed tensions that I have alluded to above. The solution comes from the perspicuous view: the view that shows us things clearly, but which is also an overview, so that we see not just the one thing, but also the surround that gives contextual meaning. This is to make use of Wittgenstein's notion of an overview, surview, or *übersicht*—a notion that was of crucial importance to his later thought.

> A main source of our failure to understand is that we do not *command a clear view* of the use of our words.—Our grammar is lacking in this sort of perspicuity. ...
>
> The concept of a perspicuous representation (*Übersichtlichen Darstellung*) is of fundamental significance for us. It earmarks the form of account we give, the way we look at things. (Is this a 'Weltanschauung'?) (PI §122)

Thus, however, we must go on to ask (in the next chapter) whether there is a better model (a better *Weltanschauung* perhaps) that captures the appropriate perspective and, if so, what comprises such a model.

The standing of the disease model

We should start by recalling the tremendous clinical and scientific usefulness of the disease model, as recorded in the previous chapter (and in Chapter 1). Its construal of psychological concepts in physical terms is reductive, in that psychological phenomena are only explained by digging deeper into their physical basis. The reductive impulse is, however, opposed by the Wittgensteinian analysis, which places psychological concepts within the broader context of normatively constrained human practices. This analysis, therefore, suggests perhaps that we should reject the disease model. In which case, however, we should be rejecting something that is clinically and scientifically useful.

The scientific tendency to move from macro-structure to micro-structure, or away from everyday language to explanations in terms of sub-structural mechanisms, is strong. This reductive impulse, however, seems to move medical science away from the concerns of ordinary people afflicted with disease.

Wittgenstein wrote:

> Philosophers constantly see the method of science before their eyes, and are irresistibly tempted to ask and answer questions in the way science does. ... I want to say here that it can never be our job to reduce anything into anything, or to explain anything. Philosophy really *is* 'purely descriptive'. (BB p. 18)

It is important to note that this is not a point about science, but about philosophy. Wittgenstein accepts that science is reductive, but insists that philosophy, which involves the analysis of concepts by looking at their uses, pulls us in another direction. A further point is that the use of the scientific model in the wrong field is deleterious. A philosophical critique of the disease model, therefore, should leave the model itself as it is—the science of it is not our concern—but it should be no surprise if such a critique placed the model, and our understanding, in a broader context.

One response, from the dementia scientist, to this point about philosophy could be to say that this is all very well, but the concern of the scientist is *solely* with causal mechanisms and processes. Thus, none of my philosophical points needs to be taken as relevant to the perfectly proper business of scientific research on acquired diffuse neurocognitive dysfunction. Indeed, I have myself already highlighted what is good about the disease model, namely its ability to give a useful *causal* account. The danger is, however, that the disease model facilitates a surreptitious move towards the errone- ous thought that it *alone* might tell us what dementia actually *is*, as if the disease model might tell us what *constitutes* dementia. This ignores the extent to which Alzheimer's disease, say, is a breakdown, not just of cholinergic pathways, but also within (what Sellars (1997) termed) the space of reason, where normativity holds sway. The purpose of my philosophical discussion, therefore, is to locate our under- standing of dementia in this broader field.

The analysis of intentional psychological concepts in the disease model of dementia provides us with a way of bridging the gap between scientific explanation and person- centred understanding. Scientific explanation generally, and the disease model in particular, must be located in the broader context of the normatively constrained human world. In this context people act according to historically and culturally embedded practices and customs. Indeed, McDonough (1991) suggests that at some level the explanatory power of scientific models will run out and the task will become purely descriptive, just as in philosophy; at which point,

> The real philosophical problem is to understand the meaning of statements about atoms by looking in the other direction, 'upwards', to the role of those statements in the embed- ding culture. (McDonough, 1991)

He states: '*the very meaning of mechanical models must be cashed in terms of their use in a culture*' (*ibid.*). He also suggests that it is Wittgenstein's view,

> … that scientific statements and models are meaningful … insofar as they do some cul- tural work. But this kind of work does not enable science to 'penetrate phenomena' (reduce them) to the mechanisms which are 'really there' (*ibid.*)

Our understanding of the disease model itself involves normatively constrained understandings, embedded in the world of practices and customs. The physical fea- tures and normativity of the world are part of the same world and are inevitably enmeshed. The scientific explanation of prosopagnosia in acquired diffuse neurocog- nitive dysfunction is understood in the context of meanings and concerns, in which face recognition plays a culturally, historically, and emotionally embedded role. Psychological concepts pick out aspects of the human world that are simultaneously both physical and mental: there is no dichotomy (cf. Z §§486–7). Similarly, prosopag- nosia is a matter both of brain pathology and psychological reality. The concept is itself understood as 'a phenomenon of human life' (PI §583). There is no real conflict between scientific explanation and human understanding, once both are seen as giving descriptions embedded in the context of the human world. This is a physical world, but it is at the same time one in which physical descriptions and models gain their meaning from their embeddedness in the broader 'stream of life' (LW ii p. 30). Thus, the disease model squares with the Wittgensteinian analysis of intentional psychological states.

The paradox of the disease model is solved in this way. There is nothing wrong with the scientific inclination to look for mechanistic and micro-structural explanations in a mechanical and physically structured world. This scientific inclination brings about clinically useful advances. The understanding of the scientific explanations (their meaning), however, must involve (and the 'must' is transcendental in the sense that it is a prerequisite of meaning) reference to the broader context of the human world in which understanding and meaning are normatively constrained. If this were not the case the scientific explanations, as McDonough suggests, would be meaningless. What the causal explanation of dementia is about, therefore, is only understood in the broader human context. If acquired diffuse neurocognitive dysfunction is a failure in the realm of neurophysiological functioning, it is a failure in the realm of norms too. In the normative context of the human world, looking *simply* at the micro-structure will inevitably miss something of the mental: precisely the normativity of intentional mental states, which are constituted not by underlying causal structures, but by relations between agents and things and events in the public world.

The disease model can only be articulated within the context of a range of inherently normative understandings and concerns. It is this human world in which the disease model is embedded and in which it can be used appropriately. This is the world of understanding and human meaning, where not to recognize a face signifies brain malfunction, but also a personal calamity.

Is it possible, then, for the physicalism of the disease model to lead to an account that is not just causal? This suggests the possibility of other ways of understanding physicalism and, therefore, other ways of taking the disease model.

Wittgenstein on face recognition

Face recognition carries normative commitments. To recognize a familiar face *just is* a matter of certain normative commitments holding sway. As I have suggested in Chapter 4, normativity is constitutive of, immanent in, and irreducible as practices embedded in the world. This led to the idea of quietism with respect to what might further constitute normativity. None the less, we *can* say more about what constitutes these practices *qua* practices embedded in the world. So, we can say that recognizing someone might carry social and ethical commitments. If recognition, normatively constrained, is embedded in the world, it is apt to involve those things that go to make up the world. We can say, therefore, that face recognition is, from one point of view, a physical matter. It is, of course, also a psychological matter. Likewise, from a different perspective, it is a social phenomenon. Hence, failure to recognize someone, in the way that Miss Breen no longer recognizes her brother, is similarly a physical, psychological, and social matter.

The constitutive account of face recognition, therefore, incorporates the causal account and a whole lot more besides. This follows directly from the Wittgensteinian analysis of face recognition as an intentional psychological phenomenon. For that analysis, with its emphasis on normativity, brings into play the reality of face recognition as an embedded practice in the world. This involves the physicalism of the disease model, *as well as* psychological and social aspects. These different aspects, moreover, are not different realities, but *different aspects of the same reality*, which is the reality of face recognition as a practice in the human world. So, if I am asked to say what constitutes face recognition, I must mention what it means to Miss Breen, *as well as* what occurs neuropsychologically in Miss Breen, *as well as* the physical basis of recognition in the brain (which will be a causal account), *as well as* the ethical and legal implications, *and so on*. The causal account is one aspect of the broader reality; and the broader reality (the constitutive account) tells us more about what dementia *is*.

In saying this, I have merely applied the analysis of intentional psychological phenomena to the disease model of dementia. What this analysis suggests is that Wittgenstein would have both accepted folksy ways of talking of mental states, whilst at the same time similarly accepting the physicalist description of the world. The emphasis on the embeddedness of intentional psychological phenomena *in the world* means that the dichotomy suggested by the mind–brain debate, at least as regards these phenomena, should seem chimerical. Hence Schulte's suggestion that, for Wittgenstein, 'many of the questions that have arisen in the context of discussions of the mind–brain problem are just confused or, at best, unanswerable' (Schulte, 1993: 166). So, inasmuch as we find statements relevant to the mind–brain problem in Wittgenstein, they cut this way and that. Indeed, commentators have accused Wittgenstein of being both a dualist (Hacking, 1982) and a physicalist (Hopkins, 1975). He does, however, make comments that appear profoundly inimical to physicalism:

> One of the most dangerous of ideas for a philosopher is ... that we think with our heads or in our heads. (Z §605);
>
> No supposition seems to me more natural than that there is no process in the brain correlated with associating or with thinking; so that it would be impossible to read off thought-processes from brain-processes. ... So an organism might come into being even out of something quite amorphous, as it were causelessly, and there is no reason why this should not really hold for our thoughts, and hence for our talking and writing. (Z §608);
>
> It is thus perfectly possible that certain psychological phenomena *cannot* be investigated physiologically, because physiologically nothing corresponds to them. ... Why should there not be a psychological regularity to which *no* physiological regularity corresponds? (Z §§609–10)

One apologia here would be to highlight the important insight concerning the differences between talk of thinking and talk of neurophysiological processes. Another defence would be to stress the need to take careful note of Wittgenstein's exact words. It is, for instance, a dangerous idea *for philosophers* to think that we think with our heads. Perhaps the point here is that philosophical confusion might follow from this idea even though it is an empirically useful notion. Or it could be suggested that the correlation of brain-processes and mind-processes is not a *natural* supposition, but a highly sophisticated one; and our thoughts *do* seem to appear causelessly. So too, it is (*logically*) perfectly possible for there to be no physiological underpinning to psychological states. Elsewhere he talks of brain mechanisms, which he thus clearly allows as a possibility, as being 'not our concern' (Z §304).

An alternative defence of these passages is to argue that they could be developed into the position adopted by Davidson. After all, Davidson's stricture that there are no psychophysical laws was anticipated by Wittgenstein's remark: 'Why should there not be a psychological lawlikeness to which *no* physiological lawlikeness corresponds?' (RPP i §905). If Wittgenstein were to be assimilated to Davidson, however, he would face similar problems: the lack of lawlikeness in the psychological realm would have to be grafted somehow onto the strict lawlikeness in the physiological sphere. But I think that the *Zettel* passages do *not* need to be interpreted with Davidson in mind. It is fairer to Wittgenstein to make an interpretation in the light of his other writings. Interestingly, this can still be done using the example of face recognition.

In *Zettel* Wittgenstein wrote:

> I saw this man years ago: now I have seen him again, I recognize him, I remember his name. And why does there have to be a cause of this remembering in my nervous system? Why must something or other, whatever it may be, be stored up there *in any form*? Why *must* a trace have been left behind? (Z §610)

Having asked why there needs to be a correspondence between psychological and physiological reality, Wittgenstein added, 'If this upsets our concepts of causality then it is high time they were upset' (*ibid.*).

Now, it would be natural to interpret this passage in the light of the remarks that surround it. For instance, Wittgenstein suggests that no process in the brain correlates with thinking. To illustrate this he considers the example of a seed and plant. He says: '. . . *nothing* in the seed corresponds to the plant which comes from it' (Z §608), and he adds that the properties and structure of the plant cannot be inferred from those of the seed, but '– this can only be done from the *history* of the seed' (*ibid.*). With these comments in mind, it might be suggested that, just as Wittgenstein did not know that the structure of DNA in the seed determines the structure of the plant, so he did not know that the workings of the medial occipitotemporal lobes control face recognition.

What should make this interpretation suspicious is that it fastens onto a solely causal account of the phenomena being considered. Part of my argument has been that Wittgenstein's analysis of intentional psychological concepts draws us to the constitutive, not the causal. Elsewhere there are enough comments by Wittgenstein to suggest that he was not primarily concerned with the scientific explanation of the problems he was considering. For instance, he wrote in connection with the study of psychology:

> The existence of the experimental method makes us think we have the means of solving the problems which trouble us; though problem and method pass one another by. (PI p. 232)

My suggestion, therefore, is that Wittgenstein was talking conceptually when he considered the seed and the lack of correspondence between recognizing someone and what might be going on in the brain.

Wittgenstein mentions face recognition elsewhere. In the midst of the rule-following considerations, he discusses how the experience of reading is as if the letters and sounds form an alloy or unity. He goes on:

> In the same way e.g. the faces of famous men and the sound of their names are fused together. This name strikes me as the only right one for this face. (PI §171)

He then criticizes this account as an account of what constitutes the process of reading. For reading cannot be defined in terms of some essential aspect or process. What constitutes reading has to be understood in terms of reading as an embedded, worldly custom and practice. The normativity, which involves *this* word meaning *this* and *that* face being *Churchill's*, cannot be further analysed in terms of what constitutes *it*. But this irreducible normativity is constitutive of the phenomenon of reading, immanent in it, and is a transcendental necessity, since without it there would be no such thing as reading. The same holds for face recognition.

This takes me back to the passage in *Zettel*. Does my recognizing someone have to have a cause in my nervous system? Wittgenstein's concern in these paragraphs is with the intentional psychological phenomena of recognizing, remembering, and thinking. If we take it that his concern was typically with the constitutive nature of such phenomena, not with their causal preconditions, then his comments no longer seem naïve or maverick. What it is to think, or recognize, or remember, is not straightforwardly explicable in causal terms if we are considering the phenomena themselves. My recognition of someone and recall of his name does seem, in terms of these phenomena, to come from 'something quite amorphous' (Z §608). The face and the name are fused *in a sense*, but what it is to recognize a familiar face is part of a practice, with a history. If my *mind* is to be compared to the seed, prior to the recognition there is nothing in it that can afterwards be correlated with the recognition, except that my mental *history* will include the elements that make the recognition possible, namely that I have seen pictures of Churchill before. There is nothing here that should deny the brain activity that is a condition for the possibility of this recognition. But that was not Wittgenstein's concern. His concern was with the conceptual and constitutive understanding of intentional psychological states.

McDonough (1989) has trenchantly argued, too, for a non-apologetic interpretation of these paragraphs. His argument is predicated on an holistic characterization of meaning in Wittgenstein's later philosophy, such that Wittgenstein denies the 'semantic correspondence thesis', which suggests that '*elements in the meaning* correspond with elements in the brain' (*ibid.*). McDonough also stresses that Wittgenstein's notion of use is, 'the notion of context embedded linguistic behaviour' (*ibid.*). He continues:

> This embeddedness is not constituted by causal connections between utterances and contexts, but by criterial or conventional connections between them. The description of the use of an utterance is, therefore, nothing like the description of a physical state. It is more like the description of *a criterial connection* between words and significant contexts. Even if use, in this sense, cannot be traced to the brain it does not follow that utterances physically characterized cannot be traced to the brain. Wittgenstein's view is not incompatible with moderate physicalism. (*ibid.*)

This interpretation allows that the brain, itself a structure, can instantiate structural phenomena such as spoken or written words, but cannot picture meaning which requires its embedding context. Furthermore,

> Instead of causally tracing the outer behaviour of the person to a semantical engine inside him, one must in a different sense (conceptually), *trace the criteria for the description of the*

neural centre to the semantical system outside them. The person is not semantically centred in their brain, but in their institutional and cultural context. (*ibid.*)

McDonough is concerned with the theory of meaning, which I am not. But his suggestion that Wittgenstein has brought about a Copernican revolution, whereby, 'the person's centre of thought and meaning (a) is not inside the person, and (b) is not their individual possession', is in keeping with the normative analysis of psychological concepts that I have described and with the idea of the externality of mind. So, for instance, McDonough speaks of, 'rules, procedures, norms', which are constitutive of the context in which use is embedded. He eschews a causal connection between the utterances and context, but plumps for a 'criterial or conventional' connection. This is still too weak for the transcendental account of normativity required of intentional psychological concepts, since it suggests that meaning is fixed by criteria or convention, rather than norms being a constitutive precondition of meaning. Nevertheless, McDonough's account allows a *rapprochement* between the sort of moderate physicalist, who might otherwise have been put off by Wittgenstein's talk of there being no correlation between the brain and thinking, and those who wish to maintain a notion of linguistic holism and avoid the sort of reductions that would threaten such holism.

From this discussion, it seems possible to defend the following view, which is in keeping with the Wittgensteinian analysis of psychological concepts. Prosopagnosia is the result of brain pathology. Recognizing, or not recognizing, a familiar face, however, involves normativity, because such recognition, or its absence, carries other commitments. These commitments can be characterized as constitutive of the act, or failure, of recognition. The normative commitments are a prerequisite for such concepts having the meanings that they do (and are thus transcendental). The normative commitments also mean that the concept of failure of face recognition cannot just be a matter of brain pathology (normativity is irreducible), even though brain pathology provides a causal explanation for the failure. Being able to recognize a familiar face is subject to certain rules—this is part of what the normativity consists in—and it forms part of a practice (the normativity of face recognition is immanent). Not only can we (in normal cases) instantly say whether or not someone has recognized a familiar face correctly, but such recognition forms part of what we ordinarily do everyday and places us *in a certain way* within a particular context. This embeddedness in the context of the human world is what ensures the normativity associated with face recognition.

At the same time, however, the embeddedness also allows the physicalist construal of face recognition that is required by the disease model. There is something for face recognition to be in the brain (there is a brain state), as is shown by the lesions that lead to prosopagnosia. But for face recognition actually to be face recognition, that is, for it not just to be a neuronal circuit of no consequence, reference has to be made to the broader context in which 'face recognition' plays the part that it does. The broader context, of rules and regularities of practice and custom, is the one in which normativity inheres. In this context, which is defined by the realities and concerns of human beings (i.e. it is cultural, historical, political, social, geographical, ethical, etc.), normativity is embedded as a constitutive, immanent, and irreducible reality. Face recognition, similarly, is located—and normatively constrained—within this context. But so too are the neuronal mechanisms that support face recognition; and so too are the lesions involving the medial occipitotemporal regions of the brain that cause prosopagnosia. Those mechanisms and lesions mean nothing outside this human context. The reductionist impulse, which moves towards micro-structure, must be reversed to look towards the macro-structure where the insights of science have meaning. For meaning is a function of embedded context.

Summary

Extreme physicalism does not allow room for normativity. It even does away with mentalistic talk and (rather nonsensically) meaning too. The attempt by Davidson to allow that psychological and physiological descriptions are radically different is helpful from the point of view of normativity. But, having allowed the dichotomy between mind and brain to appear, characterizing the relationship between the two is radically problematic. The Wittgensteinian analysis of intentional psychological states roots them from the start in the physical world. So that inner and outer, mental and physical, brain and mind are enmeshed and mutually-involving. As Wittgenstein wrote: 'What goes on within also has meaning only in the stream of life' (LW ii p. 30). There is, thus, no dichotomy, since the locus of intentional psychological phenomena is the human world, which is constituted by physical *and* psychological *and* social *and* ethical *and* spiritual aspects, *and so on*. This allows, therefore, both physicalism and normativity. The physicalism of the disease model does not preclude a broad understanding of what it is for Miss Breen to fail to recognize her brother, even if it explains the underlying causal preconditions for prosopagnosia. But failure of face recognition and the disease model as a whole are placed in the broad context of a constitutive account of intentional psychological states.

Representations in the normative world

Fodor's paradigm and normativity

The Fodorian model implies that intentional mental states amount to the functioning of internal, mechanistic, physical systems. It also suggests, as we saw in Chapter 5 (see pp 136–7), that the involvement of the whole person is not crucially defining. The overarching argument, which I shall now develop, is that the Fodorian model takes no account of the way in which the normativity of intentional mental states is a matter of such states being embedded in the world.

- Intentional mental states cannot just be a matter of the internal processing of representations, because the normativity of such states involves their external embedding in the world; it is constitutive of such states that they are normative, but this involves worldly embedding.

- The normativity of intentional mental states implies that such states should be given an externalist construal, so that meaning and understanding constitutively involve the world; in which case, an understanding of the whole person *is* crucial, because it is the whole person who acts and engages with the world.

Internal mechanisms and normativity

Fodor makes it quite plain that what he envisages can be thought of in mechanistic terms:

> … what happens when a person understands a sentence must be a translation process basically analogous to what happens when a machine 'understands' (viz., compiles) a sentence in its programming language. (Fodor, 1985: 67)

Thus, when I understand the name of something, I access its mental representation in my semantic memory store. This representation can be processed or transformed to produce an output in various modalities: I could spell the name, write it or point to its picture. Similarly, Fodor's talk of computation 'presupposes a medium in which to compute' (*op. cit.*: 33). The language of thought is instantiated in the physical structure of the brain. It is part of the make-up of the machine itself and is determined by its engineering (*op. cit.*: 66). As a matter of biological necessity, its computations are not random (*op. cit.*: 71). This is in keeping with cognitive neuropsychology's concept of isomorphism (see Chapter 5, pp. 131–33). For cognitive neuropsychologists, as for Fodor, information processing is something that occurs physically. Similarly, mental representations must be reflected in, and arise from, brain physiology.

But if this is how we are going to construe intentional mental states, whence will come the notion of normativity? Understanding and remembering, according to Fodor, are merely functional states of the mechanistic brain. This is not, however, consistent with the Wittgensteinian account. Elsewhere, discussing memory, Wittgenstein suggests that memory is not a matter of personal fiat. If I think I have captured the notion of memory by pointing to internal representations, I have missed the point that I shall have,

> … no criterion of correctness. … whatever is going to seem right to me is right. And that only means that here we can't talk about 'right'. (PI §258)

The concern here is not with the epistemological point, that I might not know whether or not my memory is correct, but is with the constitutive point, that memory is bound up with external states of affairs. This is because of the normativity involved in remembering. When I remember something I make a normative connection with the world; what it is to remember involves this externalist orientation as a constitutive feature.

So, internal mechanisms separated from external states of the world provide no criterion of correctness, because normativity is not a feature of internal mechanistic states. Such purely internal physical states are not normative since, according to the Wittgensteinian analysis, normativity is a feature of the embedding of intentional psychological states in the world. The Wittgensteinian position sets out a conceptually unavoidable, externalist account. It is unavoidable because the constitutive account makes the normativity of intentional mental states immanent and a feature of the world. Thereby intentional mental states cannot be considered in abstraction. Our whole understanding of such mental states is structured by our normatively shaped understanding of the world.

There is nothing in the Fodorian account to suggest that the psychological states instantiated in the physical goings-on of the computational brain *must* be embedded within the broader context of human life and thought. Indeed, the implication is that psychological phenomena are explained, on this view, merely in terms of mechanical engineering. The non-randomness of computations is a matter of biological necessity. Whereas, according to the Wittgensteinian analysis, the irreducible nature of normativity is a conceptual, rather than an empirical, point. Of course, there is a causal explanation for things being the way they are in the world. The Wittgensteinian analysis, however, establishes the plausibility of a broader conceptual enquiry within which empirical enquiries have meaning.

Elsewhere Wittgenstein considered someone writing down 'jottings' to remember what has been said. The jottings are not connected by rules to the text:

> ... if anything in it is altered, if part of it is destroyed, he sticks in his 'reading'or recites the text uncertainly or carelessly or cannot find the words at all ... The text would not be *stored up* in the jottings. And why should it be stored up in our nervous system? (Z §612)

The jottings specify the text and, so too, the configuration of molecules in the nervous system might specify the memory. Disturbing the molecules might disturb the memory, just as disturbing the jottings disturbs the text. But talk of the memory being *in* the molecules, or the text *in* the jottings, is merely metaphorical. Fodor talks of the computations, which are (for instance) what it is to remember, as being *in* a physical medium. There is an important sense, however, in which this cannot be where the memory resides, even if the molecules do provide the causal preconditions for memory. The normative constraints, which surround our use of the concept of memory, cannot be reduced to the causal constraints that operate in the functional states of the brain. For internal states in the Representational Theory of Mind (RTM) are precisely inner, whereas normativity is a feature of the external world in which intentional mental states are embedded.

It is clear that there is systematic thought that allows comparison (on the one hand) with a language and (on the other) with a computational machine. According to the 'Generality Constraint', the structuring of thought is a matter of thoughts being, 'a complex of the exercise of several distinct conceptual *abilities*' (Evans, 1982: 101). Grasping the meaning of an assertion or thought, *'Fa'* for instance, conceptually involves the generalizable ability to use the name *'a'*, as well as the generalizable ability to use the predicate *'F'*. This general structuring of thought is taken by Fodor to be an empirical matter, which can accordingly be represented in empirical models of cognitive processes. But the point is unavoidably and really a conceptual one too, about the normativity of meaning. Grasping a meaning commits one to its future use being thus and so. The Wittgensteinian analysis counters the idea that the systematic nature (or structuring) is solely a matter of computation and representation. Neither thought nor language can be conceived as merely computational or representational, for they both involve conceptual *abilities*, as Evans suggests. Normativity resides, therefore, beyond internal computations and representations, in the world of such abilities. In this sense, normativity cannot be reduced. Such a reduction, which is what Fodor offers, can only amount to a refusal to undertake the conceptual analysis that would reveal the transcendental nature of the normativity of meaning.

So, for instance, Wittgenstein asks how we should counter someone who argues that for him understanding is an inner process (PI §181). Wittgenstein responds by asking how we should counter him if he said that playing chess was an inner process.

> We should say that when we want to know if he can play chess we aren't interested in anything that goes on inside him.—And if he replies that this is in fact just what we are interested in, that is, we are interested in whether he can play chess—then we shall have to draw his attention to the criteria which would demonstrate his capacity, and on the other hand to the criteria for the 'inner states'. Even if someone had a particular capacity only when, and only as long as, he had a particular feeling, the feeling would not be the capacity. (*ibid.*)

Normativity is not reducible merely to physical processes (even if they are involved); it is a matter of structured accomplishments within the world. To reiterate, this is not a matter of empirical investigation, but the result of conceptual analysis concerning what it is to understand or remember something. Hence,

- ◆ Intentional mental states cannot just be a matter of the mechanistic, internal processing of representations, because the normativity of such states involves their external embedding in the world; it is constitutive of such states that they are normative, but this involves worldly embedding.

Is it possible, then, to allow talk of representations and also to accommodate meaning and normativity? I turn now, before summarizing the argument and re-examining the status of cognitive neuropsychology, to an account (with which I largely agree) of representations and of how mental content can have meaning. Whilst Fodor attempts, as it were, to eliminate personal level normativity (– it is all explained by causal processes at the sub-personal level –), whilst Dennett attempts to sequester normativity from the personal to the sub-personal (by analogy and reduction), and whilst Bolton and Hill attempt to insert meaning directly into the representational workings of the brain, Gillett allows that at both personal and sub-personal levels there might be some sense to talk of representations. However, whereas sub-personal representations can be thought of in structural terms, personal level mental representations, which require meaning-normativity, must be embedded in the world.

Meaningful representations

Gillett is not averse to talk of mental representations. He regards representations as intentional and thinks it: '. . . both natural and plausible to say that our concepts get organized into *mental representations* of things in the world' (Gillett, 1992: 101). However, Gillett notes different uses of the term 'representation' and he accuses Fodor of conflating different uses of the notion. He continues:

> The essence of 'representation' as it is used in epistemology involves rule-governed human activity which obeys identifiable but informal norms to do with the use of signs, and it is in this complex and structured milieu that we can understand what it means. By contrast, the cognitive scientist's use of 'representation' is tied to processing networks and states of excitation in information systems and these necessarily concern only one organism and what it is disposed to do in certain conditions. There are no formalizable symbol complexes involved and no norms to be obeyed dictating how the individual *should* react to a canonical sign. (Gillett, 1989)

Pertinent here is the distinction between 'thin' and 'thick' information. Thin information involves, 'analysis of causal transactions between spatio-temporally specifiable states and events and has no place for normative features linked to judgements' (Gillett, 1992: 110–11); whereas, 'thick information is conceptual and is therefore essentially tied to reasons, inferences, understanding, perceiving, knowledge, belief, and meaning' (*ibid.*; see also Kenny, 1984: 128–9). Thin information, for Gillett, relates to the cognitive scientist's use of the term 'representation'. The information processing, which is part of the cognitive neuropsychologist's paradigm, involves thin (technical) information and the representations based on it are correspondingly 'thin'. By contrast, on Gillett's view,

> … representation, both to oneself and to others, depends on what is public and on the shared norms which persons follow to regulate and articulate activity. (Gillett, 1992: 118)

To be clear, Gillett accepts the cognitive neuropsychologist's use of the term 'representation'. But he does not allow that this use has anything to do with the way in which our actual (non-metaphorical) mental representations (– and he is happy to call them such –) affect our human behaviour and thoughts. For Gillett, thought content is, '. . . tied to the grasping of concepts and thereby to a natural language' (Gillett, 1992: 119). A useful summary of his position is the following:

> If we seek to explain the character and role of a given thought and what it is for a thinker to act on that thought, then we must look to the patterns of information sensitivity that the thinker uses in acting as she does. These are elucidated by a study of the rule-governed practices in which she participates and are pervaded by the essential features of those practices. Asking neurophysiological questions about the brain as an information processor is a matter for empirical science and just puts the cart before the horse. The essential nature of information as it figures in the explanation of human action remains a matter for philosophy of mind. (Gillett, 1992: 75)

The importance of this point needs to be emphasized, for it counters those cognitivists (including Fodorians) who might argue that their concern was to give an account of how the brain actually works, irrespective of what might be true or false at the personal level. Their account discusses how the brain processes 'information'; but Gillett points out that the very concept of 'information'—if, say, we are talking about what it is to *remember* 'Adlestrop'—must have thick, embedded, connections, otherwise we simply are not talking about what it is to remember.

Sticking to the account of human actions as concerning the agent's thoughts, rather than in terms of causes, Gillett comments that thinking about actions as guided by thoughts appeals: '. . . to a far richer conception of persons and their relations than that found in … an impoverished [causal] model' (Gillett, 1992: 76). He states:

> Human agents are able to reason because their brains function in causally regular ways, but the nature of their reasoning, and thus the structure and content of mental explanation, only merge when we consider them as rational and social beings. Mental explanation tells us which concepts are being used to shape an action. Concepts involve rule-governed links between a subject's behaviour and the world and thus determine the way that an action is sensitive to that world. (Gillett, 1992: 75)

He emphasizes the normative characteristics of concept-use and the way in which the distinction between the inner and the outer is not clear-cut. Gillett feels that the conceptual analysis of 'mental representations' involves public criteria and significance within the normatively constrained field of human discourse. His inclination, whilst accepting the importance of physiological accounts, is nevertheless to tie all talk of an intentional nature tightly to the realm of persons. Physiological accounts may use language metaphorically, but will be in error if they start literally to apply personal level ascriptions to the sub-personal level.

So, for Gillett, there are the internal representations of representationalist theories such as cognitive neuropsychology, which are metaphorical; and there are the mental representations, which constitute the content of our mental lives. But the reality of these representations stems from their embeddedness in the world of rule-governed practice and agents.

Summary

As in the case of the disease model, cognitive neuropsychology offers a clinically useful and scientifically fruitful way of explaining acquired diffuse neurocognitive dysfunction. In this case, the construal of intentional psychological concepts is representational. In the most obvious philosophical paradigm, however, the Wittgensteinian analysis shows Fodor's functionalist account of RTM to be deficient from the point of view of normativity. The challenge, then, is to give an account of cognitive neuropsychology models that do justice to normativity. This can be couched in terms of the question: how does representational mental content have meaning in the world of persons? For Dennett, it is a question of meaning being stretched down to the lowest sub-personal level of homunculi where it is decomposed to functional mechanisms. But at this level nothing is constrained normatively, even if it is causally determined, because of the gap between the personal and sub-personal levels. For Bolton and Hill, there just must be meaning in the representational workings of the brain in order for mental states to be causal. Yet how this is achieved is somewhat mysterious and still seems to require mental mechanisms, which can only be regarded, however, as metaphorical. According to Gillett, representational mental content has meaning precisely because it is embedded and understood only in the context of rule-governed practices. Mental representations involve public criteria and have significance within the patterned and normatively constrained field of human discourse.

Such an account of mental representations, however, is not an account of a representationalist theory. If mental representations are to be regarded as public phenomena, in the sense that they are subject to shared normative constraints, which guide the patterned use of the concepts that describe them, they cannot then be thought of as entities or states that are characterizable independently of that which they represent. My representation of 'Adlestrop', albeit there is a distinct story to be told in terms of brain processes, is shaped by a patterned nexus of understandings within the world. Remembering Adlestrop is, after all, to evoke a pastoral world of innocence before the First World War. Such resonances give the poem its particular quality. But this quality is a public feature resting on shared understandings, so that what counts as remembering Adlestrop is normatively given, irrespective of the underlying causal processes. There is no internal vehicle of content here; the representation is shared and public in order for the poem to work. So, if cognitive neuropsychology wishes to speak of representations, these must be metaphorical. Representationalism, which suggests real, independent vehicles for mental content, cannot accommodate normativity and must, therefore, on the Wittgensteinian analysis of intentional psychological states, be discarded as a theory purporting to describe such states. None the less, the findings of cognitive dysfunction can lead the clinician to a greater understanding both of the underlying neuropathology and of the difficulties that face the person affected.

The social construction of normativity

Having outlined social constructionist thought in Chapter 5, I shall now offer two clarifications:

- first, if social constructionism offers a causal account, it is not broad enough;
- secondly, as a constitutive account, social constructionism is deficient in its treatment of normativity.

I shall then outline the upshot of these clarifications, in line with the Wittgensteinian analysis, by considering the treatment of mind in social constructionist writings.

Clarification 1: broadening the causal account

First, is it right to say that our intentional psychological states are *caused* by social customs or institutions? It is difficult to doubt the importance of the social in our thoughts and other intentional mental states. I shall take the example of calculation, bearing in mind this is a cognitive skill that can disappear in acquired diffuse neurocognitive dysfunction. Now, the sum '175+81' calls for the answer '256'. It is a fact that there are numerous causal explanations, which are social, of what it is to perform such calculations. For instance, it must reflect learning. If my teacher were a maverick, I might have been taught such that I always mean 7 when others mean 5 and vice versa. My answer to the sum would then correctly be '238'. That my teachers did *not* teach me in this way is itself a matter of social causality: they were taught the 'normal' way too. This much seems mundane, but it makes the point that there is an ordinary sense in which our calculations being as they are can be explained, causally, in social terms. There is little doubt, therefore, that public agreement plays some part in calculations having the results that they do. Consider, for instance, that before 1971 in the UK, '£1+£1= 480 pence' was true; whereas nowadays '£1+£1 = 200 pence' is true. Thus, social institutions and customs can correctly be said to *cause* calculations to be as they are (but I have *not* said that these customs and institutions *constitute* what calculations are).

The same holds for all intentional psychological states. My ability to remember things, for instance, partly depends upon my ability to share and recall things in conversation. I can work out, as it were, memories with others. There is a social element to remembering (or, at least, the social element is potentially present), but in old age the opportunity to recollect things with others decreases. Some memories dwindle, it might be surmised, owing to a failure in the social environment.

In a variety of ways, therefore, a causal account of intentional psychological phenomena seems unobjectionable. There are social causes contributing to our understanding and interpretation of intentional mental states. These states are typically manifest in social contexts, in which the context can shape the manifestation of the state. At root, these states are made shareable by our shared language. It would be easy here to slip into talk of normativity, but I am only making the more mundane point that language is a social phenomenon and our ability to share certain concepts depends on it in a causal way. In the absence of spoken language, I might have to use a sign language to tell you that my intention is to hunt today, but that is enough to suggest that without language of some sort there could be no communication concerning intentional mental states. There are numerous social causes at work in connection with such states.

The clarification I wish to offer, however, involves pointing out that we do not *just* share a language and certain other social institutions and customs. Intentional psychological states are not caused *solely* by social factors. We also, for instance, share a bodily existence; and, in particular, a human bodily existence. Typically this involves having certain ways of performing; other ways are just not possible. Thus, we have certain ways of communicating intimacy. If there are variations between different societies, these remain understandable between societies. But I cannot frighten off a territorial intruder by puffing up the size of my body. Our bodies provide both our possibilities and our limitations. Our bodily existence seems also to shape some of our psychological responses. Too much or too little food or sleep affects our mental states. Drugs have the effects that they do on our moods because of our physical configuration. Our physical construction plays some part in our emotional responses.

The first clarification, therefore, is simply to point out that, if social constructionism aims to supply a causal account of intentional psychological phenomena, there are other causes at work too. This first clarification can be broadened: not only are there physical and psychological causes as well as social causes of intentional mental states, but we can also delineate historical, geographical, economic, religious, and aesthetic causal accounts. Social constructionists might wish to claim that these accounts are all manifestations of the social, but that is to simplify. Clarity will come from seeing the complexity. Part of the reason that different peoples calculate in different ways, or have different concepts (albeit concepts that can be compared between cultures), is not just social (or not just a matter of discourse) but a matter of mountains and seas, traditions separated over time, or made diverse by the differing availability of certain resources.

The first clarification, like social constructionism itself, has an anthropological basis, in that it implies that diversity within the human species testifies to the variety of causal factors, which shape our thoughts and our ways of understanding ourselves. But in which case, social constructionism is *wrong* inasmuch as it suggests that intentional psychological concepts (and the states they stand for) are *caused* by social factors *alone*. It is just as sensible to speak of physical or geographical causes. There is nothing wrong with presenting a social, causal account of intentional mental states, but this is only one amongst many possible causal accounts. If this is what social constructionism amounts to, it is a circumscribed account. The second clarification, meanwhile, gets to the heart of the philosophical argument, because it considers the stronger constitutive claim and this brings in normativity.

Clarification 2(i): the constitutive account—a form of linguistic idealism?

Secondly, then, is it right to say that our intentional psychological states are *constituted* by the social? This would be the claim that calculation, as a feature of mathematics, is actually a social institution or custom. If you ask what it is to calculate (or to understand or remember), the answer is that it is to take part in a social practice and nothing else. I here draw upon a dispute in social constructionism between whether it is to be interpreted as idealist or realist. Social constructionism seems more obviously to be a form of idealism and I shall pursue the suggestion that it is a form of linguistic idealism (which is linked to the suggestion that linguistic idealism is to be found in Wittgenstein too). I shall argue that if this were the case, then the account of normativity is deficient when exposed to the Wittgensteinian analysis of Chapter 4. The Wittgensteinian account suggests that, whether or not the practice is *actually* public, the transcendental account of normativity implies that it is *potentially* so. The normativity is a transcendental conceptual feature of intentional psychological states and the actual, public instantiation of the practices that constitute normativity is a secondary issue.

In the next section, I shall turn to the possibility that social constructionism is a realist doctrine. This is much harder to defend. Nevertheless, the impulse towards realism is a natural reaction to the deficiencies of social constructionism. The second clarification I shall make, therefore, is to say that social practices and institutions cannot be constitutive of mental states, because of the consequences for normativity. And this means that social constructionism is, at root, incoherent.

The idealistic characterization of intentional mental states, suggested by social constructionism, implies that such states amount to no more than the social exchanges, the language or discourse, that constitute such states. For instance, Sabat and Harré (ironically, because it is Harré who criticizes idealism in social constructionism) state:

> From the discursive point of view, psychological phenomena are not inner or hidden properties or processes of mind which discourse merely expresses. The discursive expression is ... the psychological phenomenon itself. (Sabat & Harré, 1994)

This is both a constitutive claim (there is nothing more to the psychological phenomenon than the discursive expression) and an idealistic one (since the reality of discursive expression—which is constitutive of psychological phenomena—is mind-dependent). This seems, therefore, *pace* Harré, to be a form of linguistic idealism.

According to Anscombe (1976), the test for whether or not we have linguistic idealism is the question: 'Does this existence, or this truth, depend upon human linguistic practice?'. Clearly, there is a strong tendency for social constructionism to push us in this direction. Bloor (1996) regards Wittgenstein as a proponent of linguistic idealism and, moreover, he interprets this in social terms. According to Bloor,

> Ostensive learning by paradigms is enculturation or socialization into the local practices of reference;

and,

> The ultimate authority for what our paradigms shall be is our own shared practice. (Bloor, *op. cit.*: 369–70)

Bloor makes a direct link between social interaction and the concerns of the linguistic idealist; they both involve self-reference and self-creativity. He concludes:

> The truths and realities created by 'linguistic practices' are clearly social institutions ...
> (Bloor, *op. cit.*: 375)

So here is one commentator who interprets Wittgenstein as a linguistic idealist in order to commend (what amounts to) a social constructionist account. In particular, for Bloor, normativity is a matter of shared standards emerging from social interaction (Bloor, *op. cit.*: 371–4)

However, I think Bloor's interpretation of Anscombe (1976) and Wittgenstein is wrong. For, although Anscombe talks of finding '*a sort of* "linguistic idealism"' in Wittgenstein's treatment of rules, she finally concludes that he was able to avoid it, since he accepts that: '*That one knows something is not guaranteed by the language-game*'. Thus he attained 'realism without empiricism'. Further, as Bloor and Anscombe acknowledge, Wittgenstein said, '*Essence* is expressed by grammar' (PI §371). But he never said, 'Essence is created by grammar', which *would* be linguistic idealism.

Nevertheless, Bloor argues against realism. He also reaches a conclusion that is entirely in keeping with a social constructionist way of thinking:

> Mathematics and logic are collections of norms. The ontological status of logic and mathematics is the same as that of an institution. They are social in nature. (Bloor, 1973)

Bloor has subsequently used Wittgenstein to support the constitutive and idealistic line:

> Wittgenstein sometimes expressed himself by saying that consensus is a precondition of rule-following activities, e.g. of arithmetical calculation: 'This consensus belongs to the essence of *calculation*, so much is certain. I.e.: this consensus is part of the phenomenon of our calculating' (RFM III: 67). (Bloor, 1997: 16)

But in such an account, the notion of normativity becomes a matter of social norms and conventions. Normativity is constructed and a matter of consensus:

> Normative standards come from the consensus generated by a number of interacting rule followers, and it is maintained by collectively monitoring, controlling and sanctioning their individual tendencies. (Bloor, 1997: 17)

Such a form of normativity, however, runs counter to the requirement that it requires a transcendental account. Normativity is not, according to the transcendental account, a matter of social convention—although the concepts are used in language in social settings—but rather a condition for the possibility of the concepts having the meanings that they do. The transcendental account was emphasized by Luntley (as I discussed in Chapter 4) in his discussion of having the experience of hearing someone say 'add 2':

> ... the norms that shape our future experience must already be there as constitutive of the experience, for they shape that experience. (Luntley, 1991: 176)

Thus, an attempt to reconstruct normativity from norm-free data will inevitably fail. There is a consensus concerning calculation, as Wittgenstein says, but the important point, which Wittgenstein makes again and again (e.g. Z §299 ff.; PI pp. 225–7), is that normativity just is a constitutive feature of calculation.

It is a mistake, as I argued in Chapter 4, to try to go further and say what then constitutes normativity. In social constructionism, however, if discursive expression *is* the psychological phenomenon, then the normativity that is constitutive of the psychological phenomenon must be no more than the discursive expression. But that goes against transcendental account, which suggests that normativity is irreducible. It makes the normativity, as Bloor would have it, a socially constructed fact. It ignores the point that if normativity were not already there as part of what it is to calculate (as a constitutive feature of calculation), calculation would not be calculation. Normativity is simply a part of (immanent in) the form of life in which calculation makes sense.

The difference between social constructionism and the Wittgensteinian account is the difference to which I have already referred. The practices that underpin the normativity of intentional psychological states are either *essentially* or *potentially* public. Social constructionism makes them *essentially* so: normativity is solely a consequence of the public nature of practice. The Wittgensteinian analysis, contrariwise, holds that normativity is immanent: it inheres in the intentional psychological states as an irreducible and constitutive feature and must do so for these to be the states that they are. The practices underlying normativity are *potentially* public, but even if it should turn out that such a practice were not *actually* instantiated, it would remain *conceptually* true that the potential for shareability must have been present. The transcendental account of normativity, if taken seriously, ensures that the emphasis is on the *potential* for the underlying practices to be public.

The tendency towards linguistic idealism in social constructionism, which follows from the attempt to make social practices constitutive of intentional mental states, leads to an account of normativity that makes it the consequence of social consensus. This is opposed by the account of normativity suggested in Chapter 4, which characterizes the normativity of intentional mental states as constitutive, immanent, and irreducible.

Clarification 2(ii): the constitutive account—a realist reading?

An alternative tack for social constructionism is to suggest that discourse is not creating reality, but reflecting it in some sense. In Harré, we find an attempt to defend social constructionism as a doctrine of realism. He argues against the anti-realism of Gergen (1991), whom he accuses of taking on only, 'part of Wittgenstein's account of discursive practices, namely the thesis of the autonomy of grammar'. Gergen, 'misses the other part, namely the "riverbed" over which all action flows, the human form of life' (Harré, 1992).[2]

The later conception to which Harré refers is seen in *On Certainty*, in which Wittgenstein writes of: 'the inherited background against which I distinguish between true and false' (OC §94). He then writes:

> ... the river-bed of thoughts may shift. But I distinguish between the movement of the waters on the river-bed and the shift of the bed itself; though there is not a sharp division of the one from the other. ... And the bank of that river consists partly of hard rock,

subject to no alteration or only to an imperceptible one, partly of sand, which now in one place now in another gets washed away, or deposited. (OC §97 and §99)

The imagery here suggests that some things are fixed, but not utterly. Stern, however, warns that talk of a fixed background could also be misleading, since it suggests something very determinate, whereas Wittgenstein's later notion of a background,

> ... is not something apart from or prior to our lives; instead it is the pattern of those lives themselves, the 'praxis of language' in all its detail and complexity. (Stern, 1995: 191, with quotation from OC §501)

It is to this fixed background, in which we inevitably participate, that Harré refers in his advocacy of a realist interpretation of social constructionism. He states:

> The ontological basis of all psychology must be found in joint actions and the persons who perform them. These are the elementary beings or prime substances of the universe on which the ontology of a genuinely scientific psychology must be based. (Harré, 1992)

Talk of ontology here is suggestive of a constitutive account and elsewhere, Harré asserts:

> ... there is no mind-substance. As far as individual human beings are concerned there are only contingently organized conversational and other symbolic practices. (Harré, 1989b)

In other words, the mental is constituted by the social. But it is also intended to be a realist doctrine, for what is real for social constructionism,

> ... must be whatever is intransigent to individual human desires coupled with whatever is necessary for there to be a human world at all. The intransigent background to all human action is the human conversation, the elements of which are the acts produced by the joint actions of speakers. (Harré, 1992)

An initial point is that, whilst Harré is critical of Gergen's failure to emphasize the river-bed, his own foundation is human conversation or discourse, which (without further support) would seem to be far too biddable in response to the changing currents of mere opinion. When we turn to Harré's necessary conditions for the possibility of discursive practice, we still find that discourse is always primary. Thus, according to Harré, the existence of persons provides a necessary condition for discursive practices, but 'persons are discursively produced' (Harré, 1992), so discourse is primary. If his talk of persons and discourse is sometimes ambiguous as to which is primary, his statement (which I have quoted above) about the shared thesis of social constructionism is unambiguous:

> ... all psychological phenomena *and the beings in which they are realized* are produced discursively. (Harré, 1992)

In Harré, therefore, all the stress is on discourse, language, and conversation.

If Harré wishes, however, to tie his brand of social constructionism to something as concrete as the only gradually-changing river-bed, he needs to find something more robust than just mere discourse and conversation.[3] The problem with this account is that it is *not* very realistic. There is very little room here for mind-independence. If the mind is construed in terms of discourse, it is nevertheless the primary reality. Harré and

Gillett move towards something more solid when they describe their view of the mind: 'as dynamic and essentially embedded in historical, political, cultural, social, and interpersonal contexts' (Harré & Gillett, 1994: 25). They continue:

> It is not definable in isolation. And to be a psychological being at all, one must be in possession of some minimal repertoire of the cluster of skills necessary to the management of the discourses into which one may from time to time enter. (*op. cit.*: 25–6)

But whilst, on the one hand, being culturally and socially embedded—which all discourses and conversations must inevitably be—adds solidity to the understanding of the mind in social constructionism, on the other hand, there is nothing in the embedding context that amounts to the full account of psychological phenomena required by the Wittgensteinian analysis.

The problem again is that the normativity of intentional psychological phenomena can only be accounted for on this view by mention of conversations and discourse. Harré's theory tries to offer an account of normativity, just as it offers an account of intentional psychological phenomena, in terms of conversation. According to the Wittgensteinian analysis, however, whilst the normativity of intentional mental states will be shown in the 'praxis of language' (OC §501), normativity is not constructed, as it were, as language goes along. Normativity is rather a prerequisite for language: it is a constitutive feature of meaning and without meaning there could be no language. There must, similarly, be meaning-normativity as a prerequisite to discourse if discourse is to make sense. But normativity cannot be decided at the time, even if it is only in discourse that it shows itself, otherwise what has meaning and what does not must await revelation in actual discourse. Whereas, on the Wittgensteinian view, the meaning is already there—normatively constrained—as a transcendental feature (the ground for the possibility) of the concept, in order for it to be the concept that it is.

In addition, there is a subsidiary argument lurking in the emphasis on the skills necessary for discourses, which are regarded as, in turn, necessary for a being to be regarded as psychological. One consequence of the view that to be a person one must be able to enter into conversations would seem to be that if language is lost by people with acquired diffuse neurocognitive dysfunction, then those affected are no longer 'constituted as people'. The acquisition of skills for entering conversations is a question of 'attaining mindedness', which is construed as, 'constructing private miniaturized versions, microcosms, of the great conversations that constitute civilizations' (Harré, 1992). Again, the emphasis is on the ability to enter into conversation. This is a threat to the personhood of those with acquired diffuse neurocognitive dysfunction, which may explain why Sabat and Harré (1992) are keen to demonstrate the extent to which some dementia 'patients' *can* enter into conversation. A broader view of what it is to be a psychological being, however, obviates the need to insist on the ability to enter into conversation as constituting a defining feature of personhood. Harré (1992) concluded: 'Discourse and person are mutually constituted beings. They are internally related'. Yet it can readily be objected that discourse just is not a *being* in the concrete way that seems to be suggested. Furthermore, if there is an internal relationship it is grammatical, whereas the talk of beings makes it sound ontological. The relationship is better put, in my view, by saying that the precondition for human discourse is the human existent.

The constitutive account—summary

To summarize the argument of this section, whether pursuing an idealist or realist version of social constructionism, the emphasis is on an understanding of psychological concepts in terms of interaction and a social context. This is as opposed to trying to understand psychological phenomena as purely intra-subjective, which was the approach of both the disease and cognitive neuropsychology models. Parallel to this move, from the individual to the social, is an emphasis on discourse or conversation. This represents, in part, an appreciation of meaning as understandable in the context of use. Now the move from the individual to the social and the emphasis on contextualized meaning have support in Wittgenstein. For instance, Wittgenstein wrote:

– To obey a rule, to make a report, to give an order, to play a game of chess, are *customs* (uses, institutions). To understand a sentence means to understand a language. (PI §199)

This conveys both the tendency in Wittgenstein to emphasize the social custom or institution and the inclination to understand meaning as given within a broader context. Hence, too, 'Our talk gets its meaning from the rest of our proceedings' (OC §229).

Despite these laudable moves in social constructionism, however, constituting the mental as the social comes up against the need for a transcendental account of normativity. Whether the emphasis is on human conversation or human consensus, normativity is reduced by accounts that try to explain it further, rather than notice it as an irreducible, immanent, and constitutive feature of intentional psychological states. Social constructionism does not suggest that normativity shapes discourse, that it allows some things to be said meaningfully and disallows others; rather, the discourse is the psychological phenomenon and, therefore, normativity is reduced to discourse. Normativity seems to be a mere *consequence* of human discourse and activity, rather than an intransigent feature of intentional mental life.

It is a latent recognition of the fact that normativity is a feature of the world, not just an epiphenomenon of discourse, I suggest, that led Harré to talk so much of the person, despite his primary reality being discourse. Human existents, *pace* Harré, rather than conversations, are the 'intransigent background' and 'ontological basis' of our psychology. The benefit of this broader view, from the clinical perspective, is that this counts (rather than discounts) people with severe acquired diffuse neurocognitive dysfunction. Harré's inclination towards realism might be regarded as an inclination towards the sort of individualism that seems to stand over against social constructionist thought. The second clarification, derived from the Wittgensteinian analysis, asserts that social practices, customs, and institutions cannot be constitutive of mental states, because of the consequences for normativity. Calculation involves consensus, but the normativity that is a constitutive feature of calculation must be there as a prerequisite for calculation to be possible. The corrective of the second clarification is, therefore, fatal to the philosophical standing of social constructionism. For, as in the first clarification (which concerned causes), what it is to be normatively constrained in the having of intentional psychological states cannot be constituted *solely* by social practices or customs. Into the constitutive account must come the physical and psychological descriptions of what it is to be a human being of this sort. This is not to say that normativity is *caused* by physical or psychological dispositions, but rather to make the point that a broad perspective is required in order to encompass the embedding context of the practices that constitute normativity. To be subject to normativity in the having of intentional mental states *just is to be a person of this type in this world*. It might be other things for as-yet-undiscovered creatures, but this is what it is for *us*. We cannot, therefore, be reduced to a constitutive account that only encompasses the social.

The upshot of the clarifications and the elimination of the mind

Having offered an account of social constructionism in Chapter 5, in the sections above I have:

+ shown that social constructionism construes psychological phenomena as social constructs;

+ highlighted an ambiguity concerning whether social constructionism offers a causal or constitutive account of intentional psychological states;

+ suggested first, by way of clarification, that if it is a causal account, it is not broad enough;

+ and, secondly, argued that, as a constitutive account, it is deficient in its treatment of normativity. For it makes normativity a matter of *actual* public practices and no more than such practices: normativity is purely a social matter. Alternatively, a transcendental account of normativity involves *potentially* public practices and these, moreover, in order to be understood, require the perspective of their worldly embedding context. On this view, normativity cannot be constituted simply by the social.

The clarifications, which clarified by separating the causal and constitutive accounts, have ultimately acted as condemnations of social constructionism, by showing that it is deficient as a way of conceptualizing dementia. This is so because of social constructionism's construal of intentional psychological phenomena. But in the last section I hinted at the tendency in Harré to emphasize the person,—inevitably, because persons are necessary for conversations and discursive stances. In this section I shall pursue a little further Harré's construal of the mind as a way of expanding on the Wittgensteinian account of intentional mental states. My aim is to re-focus our attention on the correct view of mental states. That view sees them, in line with the Wittgensteinian analysis, as both inner and outer. Harré is right to move us away from an inner view of the mental; but something is lost if the view is simply outer. I have already quoted Harré (1989b): '… there is no mind-substance'. Gadenne (1989) criticizes this view:

> While some psychologists seem to think that all can be explained by or reduced to cognitive processes, Harré goes to the opposite extreme by trying to eliminate the mental. This seems to me hardly more convincing.

Gadenne finds it unconvincing partly because he accepts the representationalist account of cognitivism. This causes him to reject the emphasis placed by Harré on conversations and the rules of discourse. Whereas Harré stresses the rules that govern the use of language to do with the mental, Gadenne wishes to hold to the notion of causal cognitive mechanisms. He suggests, for instance, that:

> Global events like speech acts or other social actions presuppose cognitive mechanisms specified by general causal hypotheses. (*ibid.*)

Whilst in the previous chapter I have been critical of mental representationalism (and would accordingly find some of Gadenne's suggestions uncongenial), like Wittgenstein, I would not wish to deny that there are mental processes. For,

> To deny the mental process would mean to deny the remembering; to deny that anyone ever remembers anything. (PI §306)

So, an interesting question to ask is: does Harré deny that anyone ever remembers anything?

At one level he does not: 'remembering is a task for people' (Harré, 1994: 37). But at another level Harré regards memories as social representations: they are 'created discursively' and 'remembering is paradigmatically a social activity' (*op. cit.*: 36). Hence, willy-nilly, Harré's discursive psychology plays down the experience of remembering inwardly. Whatever the difficulties of construing 'remembering inwardly' in a philosophically robust way, it seems phenomenologically naïve just to plump for 'remembering outwardly'.

This tendency, to eliminate the inner in favour of the rule-governed outer, is evident too (for again very laudable reasons) in the work of Sabat and Harré (1994) with AD patients. Their intention is to show that people with AD are still agents acting with meaning. This they convincingly demonstrate in particular patients. However, it leads them to suggest that,

> … a person suffering from Alzheimer's condition is like someone … trying to play tennis with a racket with a warped frame. The basic intentions may be there, but the instrument for realizing them is defective. (Sabat & Harré, 1994)

This analogy was criticized by Hope on the grounds that AD, 'can damage the inner mental life as well as its expression—the player as well as the racket' (Hope, 1994a). The tendency to regard the mental as created by discourse underplays its reality within human life. That reality is shown in sharp relief in AD when it begins to disintegrate. This is not to underestimate the importance of social constructionism as a counterweight to the attitude that people exist independently of social norms. My 'self 1' may well be destroyed by AD, but (at the very least) I still exist as a person through my 'selves 2'. So too, my mind may be destroyed by the disease in a very real sense and this is not just a matter of discourse. If it is also not a matter of the destruction of some *thing*, it is similarly not a matter of the destruction of *no*-thing.

In response to, on the one hand, the tendency to look for inner processes, Wittgenstein points to their outer manifestations. But, on the other hand, when he accuses himself of denying mental processes, he responds by saying: 'naturally we don't want to deny them' (PI §308). For Wittgenstein, it is even misleading to conceive the outer and the inner as being cheek by jowl. They are just conceptually intertwined in psychological concepts and teasing them apart should be avoided lest the full meaning of such concepts is lost:

> 'I noticed that he was out of humour.' Is this a report about his behaviour or his state of mind? ... Both; not side-by-side, however, but about the one via the other. (PI p. 179)

Talk of the inner and the outer is potentially misleading. Psychological concepts, such as 'the mind', involve both outer and inner aspects. Social constructionism puts all the stress on the outer manifestations of mental concepts and, in particular, on discourse. In doing so it seems, as Gadenne suggests, to eliminate the mental. What is required is an understanding that does justice to the inner realities (both physical and psychological) and the outer manifestations of mental phenomena.

According to McDowell, one way to understand Wittgenstein is to place him, 'in the wider context of German philosophy after Kant' (McDowell, 1991: 156). Kant positioned himself between empiricism, involving what he called the faculty of intuitions, and rationalism, which emphasizes the concepts of the understanding. For Kant, a synthesis of intuitions and concepts was necessary:

> Without sensibility no object would be given to us, without understanding no object would be thought. Thoughts without content are empty, intuitions without concepts are blind. (Kant, 2007: 86 [B75, A51])

In Wittgenstein, the synthesis is between language (or thought) and the world. This is another way of putting the point about the inner and the outer. For me to remember inwardly, nevertheless involves certain outer things being the case. The phenomenon of remembering cannot be fully understood in isolation from the normativity that constrains what will, or will not, count as remembering. That normativity is a matter of embedded, shaping, worldly practices. So the inner and the outer are both constitutively involved.

About the 'inner' world, McDowell wrote:

> That it is inner consists in there being nothing to its states of affairs except the instantiation in consciousness of the relevant concepts; the instances of the concepts, unlike the instances of concepts of the outer, have no being independently of the fact that the concepts that they instantiate figure in the content of consciousness. ... But that is not to say that these states of affairs have no being. ... The concepts set up internal links between the states of affairs which are their instantiations and publicly accessible circumstances: circumstances linked 'normatively' to the states of affairs in one kind of case, circumstances linked to them as their normal expression in another. (McDowell, 1991: 160)

To recall Chapter 4, McDowell's interpretation amounts to quietism, a straightforward description of how the language actually works. What we see is that our 'internal' concepts make links between language and the world.

To return to social constructionism, there are links to be made between discourse and the world. Discourse and the social cannot be ignored, even when it comes to a discussion of the mind. Just as Kant argued that concepts require the world if they are to have content, so discourse requires that there are real things—such as mental phenomena on the one hand, and actual bodies on the other—for the discourse to be about.

Similarly, the world of bodily and mental things must be grasped by discourse to be understood. For example, Wittgenstein wrote:

> How do I know that this colour is red?—It would be an answer to say: 'I have learnt English' (PI §381)

Or again,

> You learned the *concept* 'pain' when you learned language. (PI §384)

So, discourse and social interaction are central to our understanding of the world and a part of it; but not its totality, which also includes neurons and the feeling of loneliness.

Memories (or calculations and other intentional mental states) are not created by discourse, but the concept of memory links internally both to the state of affairs described by my saying 'I remember ...', and to the essentially public circumstances to which my words refer. (Even if the circumstances are not *actually* public, they are *potentially* so.) But memories are mediated by discourse, since discourse makes the normative link between the inner and the outer. Similarly, loss of memory is not socially constructed. It is a matter of particular states of affairs (both psychological and physical) no longer holding, on the one hand, and certain words no longer having meaning to an individual on the other. But loss of memory is manifested socially, in that certain social interactions are not possible.

Conclusion: to the person from social constructionism

There is much to commend in social constructionism. It has been useful in clinical practice as a way of focusing attention on ethical issues, the practice of caring and the nature of the person. Its Wittgensteinian roots are seen in its discussion of rules and practices. But, as I have just described, the over-emphasis on discourse (at least in Harré) does not leave room for the transcendental account of normativity suggested by the Wittgensteinian analysis of intentional psychological concepts. It has to be said, too, that as regards psychological concepts, social constructionism does not embed them in the world in a way that allows easy reference to their psychological and physical correlates. They are embedded first and foremost in conversations, but this simply seems too narrow a view of psychological reality.

A further flaw in the model is that, stemming from the restricted view of psychological phenomena, the notion of the person is also made highly dependent upon discourse. Thus Harré (1992) asserts: '... persons are discursively produced'. I have already noted the upshot that people with severe acquired diffuse neurocognitive dysfunction, who cannot take part in conversations, might be denied personhood on that basis. But this assertion might be countered by saying that persons are produced bodily. Similarly, Harré and Gillett state:

> We will therefore identify a person as having a coherent mind or personality to the extent that individuals can be credited with adopting various positions within different discourses and fashioning for themselves, however intentionally or unintentionally, a unique complex of subjectivities (essentially private discourses) with some longitudinal integrity. In this sense, there is a psychological reality to each individual. (Harré & Gillett, 1994: 25)

Whether this allows someone with *severe* acquired diffuse neurocognitive dysfunction (who cannot adopt 'various positions within different discourses' and cannot have 'private discourses' with 'longitudinal integrity') to have a personality or psychological reality must be in doubt.

To be fair, Harré's agenda is to broaden the perspective:

> In the restoration of personal psychology, I want to bring back the study of endeavour, conatus, striving, trying and the like. In the conditions for the use of these concepts I feel the presence of persons as agents rather than as passive passengers on a mental vehicle directed and powered by sub-personal vectors (or information-processing modules) of various kinds. (Harré, 1983: 185)

As well as being agents, persons are embodied:

> … human bodies sustain persons. … People are aware of themselves as embodied. (Harré, *op. cit.*: 11)

And they are situated, or embedded, 'in historical, political, cultural, social, and interpersonal contexts' (Harré & Gillett, 1994: 25)

In conclusion, social constructionism is flawed because of its over-emphasis on social practices and discourse. It fails to give a correct account of intentional psychological phenomena, because it reduces normativity to that which is public. In this model, normativity appears as a mere consequence of discourse. Over against social constructionism, according to the Wittgensteinian analysis, normativity involves potentially public practices, embedded in the world of human existents. What is essential is that the normativity is given a transcendental account: it cannot be reduced solely to *social* practices and is constitutive of the conceptual understanding of what it is to think, to calculate, and the like, whilst also being immanent in such practices. Nevertheless, the broadening, corrective tendency of social constructionism (shown by the quotations from Harré above) impels us towards a broader account of the person as a situated embodied agent.

Moving towards a solution

At the start of this chapter I spoke of a tension between the possibility of always having a further interpretation and, contrariwise, the normative constraint on understanding. I have then highlighted the tensions that can be observed in the different models of dementia.

The disease model is committed to a type of physicalism. If the causal account offered by the disease model is regarded as the whole picture, there is then a tension between this account and the broader concerns that emerge when we consider what it actually *is* to recognize or fail to recognize a familiar face. But there is no requirement that the disease model must be viewed through such a narrow lens. Understanding the causal explanations of the disease model does not preclude the possibility of broader understandings of the significance of physical goings-on in the brain.

Similarly, the cognitive neuropsychology model, whilst at one level providing a reasoned explanatory account of cognitive dysfunction—one that can be translated into an account of neurophysiological deficits—none the less is at odds with the need to provide a broader view of the meaning of such dysfunction in terms, for instance, of the concepts suggested by Harré: '. . . endeavour, conatus, striving, trying and the like' (Harré, 1983: 185). But the broader picture is readily available once the underlying functionalism of the cognitive neuropsychology model is regarded as metaphorical. The cognitive neuropsychology model can then be seen much as the disease model is seen, as providing a perfectly valid, but circumscribed account. It will also have heuristic value, because it directs us towards a clearer view of the problem.

The tensions at the heart of the social constructionist model can be understood in terms of the alternative idealist and realist readings. Either, meaning is created by use, or the meaning is already embedded in the actual practice of language as a constitutive feature. The latter view has much more in common with the Wittgensteinian critique of intentional mental states, but seems less like a true form of social constructionism, in that meaning and so on are not *constructed* by discourse, but seem immanent in it. Hence, although there is a tension, the realist account of social constructionism gestures in the direction of a solution, for it picks out the requirement for normativity to be embedded in practice.

This might seem to take us back to the possibility of tension between normativity and an openness to interpretation. Just as, however, it is possible to suggest an overview (*übersicht*) of the individual models of dementia, which then provides perspicuity concerning how the models fit into a broader understanding, so too the tension around normativity and interpretation turns out (from the perspective of the perspicuous overview) to be chimerical. The transcendental account of normativity, where normativity must be constitutive of practice, immanent in it and irreducible, entails openness, attention to the details of actual practices, and a requirement that understanding is not closed down, but that alternative possibilities, other readings, are considered.

For instance, to understand what it is (constitutively) to remember Adlestrop, albeit there is a normative constraint not to remember Slough when we think we are remembering Adlestrop, is to appreciate that this mental state may be variously instantiated. There will be different levels (or versions) of understanding concerning what remembering Adlestrop means, from recall of certain picturesque buildings to an appreciation of culturally and historically embedded values. The immanence of the normative constraint, its rootedness in this particular practice, means that we must consider what this remembering actually amounts to: we must appreciate the practice from the inside, as it were,—from within. If we are unable to do this—e.g. because the culture of early twentieth century English poetry is as unfamiliar to us as that of ancient Egypt is to many twenty-first century Westerners—we will not fully understand what it is to remember Adlestrop. And the irreducibility of normativity means that remembering or forgetting Adlestrop (or Miss Breen recognizing or failing to recognize her brother) should not be reduced to a particular function or dysfunction of a particular pathway in the brain, nor to the efficacy or lack of efficacy of a computational inner cognitive process, nor solely to the ability or disability to construct the relevant social reality or relevant discourse.

Thus, the presumed tension evaporates, because the normative account broadens the view rather than the reverse. In this way it becomes possible for the transcendental account of normativity to provide the impetus to a truly holistic view. When we look at individuals in detail, can we at the same time gain the relevant whole sight (Hughes et al., 2006a)? And what would this mean in practice? Well, it may require a hermeneutic process (Widdershoven & Berghmans, 2006). It may well mean several attempts to interpret the person or their behaviour. This further interpretation occurs in the context of normative constraints: not just *any* account will amount to a valid interpretation. The validity will stem from the degree to which the account squares with our day-to-day experience of the practices in which we engage as people who remember, forget, think, recognize, fail to recognize, calculate, understand, and so forth. Memory, or any other intentional mental state, must be seen precisely as worldly practices, where what it is (constitutively) to remember is contained within (is immanent in) the practice of remembering and cannot be reduced to a physiological mechanism, a conceptual accomplishment, or a case of social construction.

Instead, we require a perspicuous view of our practices of remembering, understanding, intending, and the like. And to gain such a view we need a degree of openness to the possibility of different views. In a very practical way, this at least means a readiness to embrace a multidisciplinary approach; although to achieve the necessary coherence of view, this will be better conceived as an *inter*disciplinary approach, in which various perspectives or narratives can be knitted together to provide the required *übersicht*.

It might, then, be that I should concentrate in some particular case on the ageing brain and how to treat it. In other words, I might wish to avoid lumping together cases as dementia and see them instead as unique manifestations of brain ageing. But to achieve the perspicuous view of the individual, I need to see the brain in context. *This* brain is located in *this* surround. For Miss Breen to fail to recognize her brother is for a particular lesion in her brain to manifest itself in the context of this particular narrative. These lesions have a particular significance, which we shall come to understand by hearing the variety of accounts from the different actors, professional and nonprofessional, involved in Miss Breen's individual and particular narrative, which will be unique.

This sort of talk will, however, militate against the chances of a single model capturing the requisite perspicuity. A model can contribute, but it will not—as we have seen—give the overview we require, which comes from a degree of breadth. This will only be achieved, however, by a mindset that allows and embraces multiple views or narratives, often from a multidisciplinary team working in an interdisciplinary manner to give a perspicuous account based on openness, by which I mean an expansiveness that stems from the inclination to resist reductionism. This sort of understanding reflects a truly constitutive account, given by those who appreciate what it is to forget or to be confused, i.e. those who have the requisite experience; and an account that recognizes the normativity that is immanent in the practice, thereby allowing a degree of empathy, i.e. the possibility that an outsider can know such practices since they are, at least in principle (whether or not actually), shareable. The requisite experience is also the sort required to understand with empathy, to engage in the right sort of depth with the hermeneutic process of meaning-making (Widdershoven & Berghmans, 2006). This open mindset allows that it is possible to achieve the sort of *übersicht* required by the Wittgensteinian analysis.

Conclusion

The suggested solution to the problems that arise when we consider different models of dementia in the light of the Wittgensteinian critique turns out to be no more and no less than a call to a broader engagement through a broader view, a surview, one that looks with openness and clarity at particular cases or narratives. This broader view amounts to an engagement with the world as it is: the human world in which we live, in which we share normative concerns and constraints as a condition for the possibility of meaning, understanding, remembering, intending, and so on. It is the world of the transcendental account of normativity. It is in the everyday world, in which normativity quietly resides, that we shall find the solution to the problem of a poor fit between our models and the world. But this suggests the lingering question, which is whether we shall ever find a model that captures the realities of the normative world of dementia.

Endnotes

[1] Further discussion and critique of the cognitivist and social constructionist models can be found in Chapter 4 of Thornton (2007); relevant discussion of all three models can also be found in Fulford et al. (2006).

[2] A useful account of the riverbed analogy is given in Stern (1995) pp. 186–92. Of relevance is Wittgenstein's comment in Z §173: 'Only in the stream of thought and life do words have meaning'.

[3] Wren (1987), who is sympathetic to Harré, still points to the need for some 'deep sense of what is truly important', something that will place constraints on the availability and viability of: 'interpretations, moral orders, identity projects, etc.'.

Chapter 7

The consequence: beyond models to the thing itself

Introduction

It is a good time to summarize. In Chapter 1, by examining facts and values (and seeing that the 'bare' facts are value-laden) it became clear that we see the world according to different *versions* of reality. We always see the world from somewhere, with a particular background or surround. Discussion of pathology suggests that there is no clear line to be drawn between normal and abnormal *apart from evaluative judgements*. And values diversity means we are faced by different versions, different views, different backgrounds, different contexts from which will emerge different evaluative judgements. The idea that different views are required was at work in Chapter 2; and it led me to discuss the situated embodied agent view of the person, which encourages the notion that the person should be seen against an uncircumscribable surround. Chapter 3 involved giving an account of theories of mind and of how the mind and the brain might connect or be understood. But the aim of the chapter was to move us towards a greater understanding of mental phenomena in the human context in order to understand at some level what it is to be a human person. Intentionality is a key concept in the link between the 'inner' world of the mind and the 'outer' world of things and action. Intentionality gestures at the inevitability of a link between thoughts and the world. The externality of mind makes the point overt: the mind is constituted by the world. In Chapter 4, I pursued the point by suggesting that the normativity of intentional psychological states involves an externalist construal of such states. I derived a transcendental account of the normativity of intentional psychological phenomena from Wittgenstein's rule-following discussion, according to which normativity must be regarded as constitutive, immanent, and irreducible. I accepted a quietist interpretation, which stresses the givenness of normativity within an embedding human world. In Chapter 5, I interrogated the disease model, the cognitive neuropsychology model, and social constructionist models in the light of the Wittgensteinian analysis of intentional mental states and, although I have acknowledged their good points, I have found them wanting. I ended that chapter by pointing in the direction of something mysterious about what it might be, ultimately (in some sense), to grasp what it is to remember. This comes from and contributes to the sense that we cannot ever *ultimately* know a person. Part of the intention of Chapter 6 was to explain that conclusion, because in it I suggested the way in which a broader view was always possible through engagement with the world as it is. In other words, despite the normative constraints on meaning, understanding, and remembering, we have to acknowledge the possibility of further perspectives, further accounts. All we can do is try to integrate these accounts to provide some sort of clarity, a perspicuous surview. But what we are considering is the complexity of the surroundings of the human world, which we can never *ultimately* perceive.

This chapter has three broad aims. First, I shall briefly discuss the role of models in general. They always simplify reality. For instance, they can simplify the relationship between the mind and the brain. We find models that suggest two different types of stuff: mental and material; or models that reduce mental stuff to material stuff. The simplifying tendencies of models can seem to be pervasive. Even the classification of diseases entails modelling, according to which particular types of condition fit under a single heading. Part of the work of Chapter 1 was to show how this approach can seem to be artificial once the details are considered. The model of classification clumps, whereas the reality is that individuals frequently defy clumping. In the next chapter I shall consider quality of life and how this can also be approached according to simplifying models; there is even something about the 'model' of person-centred care that is simplifying, which I shall come to. Perhaps, then, human encounters should be *without* models,—if they are to be true reflections of life *as it is actually lived* by people. I shall consider in this chapter the models that might be used to shape clinical practice. To a degree, I advocate the use of a supportive care model, but in the end even this might be a misunderstanding. I want to suggest that wherever we use models we are in danger of missing the rawness of the human (ethical) encounter, which must always be (in a situated, bodily, and agentive way) person to person.

Secondly, in pursuing the point about models, I wish to look beyond human embodiment to the phenomenon itself. That is, I shall take a phenomenological approach to the sort of ethical encounters I am considering. This is where I pursue my earlier gestures in the direction of the mystery that seems to lurk around the notion of mind, which (perhaps) gives some sense of purchase to the otherwise seemingly outmoded and otiose notion of dualism. The subject matter here is gossamer, requiring the 'negative capability' of Keats (mentioned in Chapter 1): '. . . when man is capable of being in uncertainties, Mysteries, doubts, without any irritable reaching after fact & reason . . .' (Keats, 1990: 370). It is not that I wish to commend dualism, but I do wish to capture from it a sense of subjectivity, albeit one that is situated. It is 'embodied subjectivity', to use Grant Gillett's (2008) terminology, which partly means that the human subject must be located in a narrative.

> Our view of human subjectivity should therefore reflect the many discourses (biological, social, personal, and moral) that articulate our understanding of human identity yielding a situated, holistic, indeed almost textual, view of what it is to be a person whereby the narrative structure of human life grounds the individuation of the human subject ... (Gillett, 2008: 14)

The third general aim of the chapter is to introduce the notion of dementia-in-the-world. This requires further explication, but it derives from the standing of the person with dementia as a being-in-the-world and the understanding that, as a corollary, dementia itself must be seen as a situated phenomenon. Thus, dementia-in-the-world is a matter of acquired diffuse neurocognitive dysfunction, of 'malignant positioning'

(Sabat, 2006a), of the need for care and solicitude, of the possibility of humour, of spiritual growth, or of deficits in acetylcholine, cognition, meaningful engagement, person-centred care, and so on. In short, dementia-in-the-world is the realization of any and all versions of the stories that might be told—good and bad—about people with dementia. But, as I shall argue, dementia-in-the-world should be a mere stepping-stone. For once we have seen dementia in this light (as dementia-in-the-world), which helps to emphasize the full breadth of the phenomenon, we shall have a perspective on the person as a being-in-the-world with the vulnerabilities of humankind, making his or her way (navigating and negotiating), surrounded by more or less solicitude and care.

In pursuing these themes, however, I wish again to be rooted in the reality of dementia. So I shall start by using particular elements from the real story of Malcolm Pointon, very kindly provided by his wife, Barbara. This will lead me to consider models that we might use to understand or deal with dementia. I shall reflect further on the story of Malcolm as told by Barbara in the course of the chapter in order to raise issues about the phenomenology of dementia-in-the-world and the need for solicitude.

Drawing and writing

At the age of 51, Malcolm Pointon received the diagnosis of Alzheimer's disease (Pointon, 2010). His wife, Barbara, has told the story with moving honesty, as well as compassion and critical thought (Pointon, 2007, 2010). In the UK, she has become a leader in terms of her advocacy on behalf of people with dementia and their carers. Malcolm was an intelligent and creative man:

> Most people saw him first and foremost as the complete musician. He lectured in music at Homerton College, Cambridge, his talents manifold. As a performer ... he could turn his hand effortlessly to fiendish classical pieces, jazz or pop and also improvise ... His many compositions ranged from simple children's songs to film music and complex avant-garde pieces ...
> ... he could speak several foreign languages and was also into astronomy, religions, philosophy, poetry, painting, history, physics and theatre. ... he could take on DIY, car maintenance and tough gardening ... (Pointon, 2007: 115)

Despite his knowledge and many talents, 'Malcolm wore his learning lightly' (*ibid.*): he was self-effacing, modest and had a good sense of humour. Nevertheless,

> ... very gradually, but inexorably, Malcolm lost everything the world values, which in normal circumstances would define who he was. (*ibid.*)

As his intellectual capabilities failed, so too his writing and drawing skills diminished and then disappeared. Figure 7.1 shows the last example of a sketch and writing that Barbara found some years later in a notepad they used to chronicle work done on the house. She puts the date at 1996, which was about four and a half years after his diagnosis, but at least six and a half years after signs and symptoms had started to appear (Barbara Pointon: personal communication).

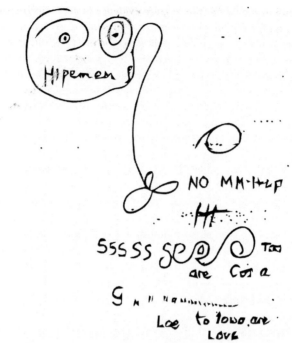

Fig. 7.1 Malcolm Pointon's sketch. Kindly supplied by and reproduced with the permission of Barbara Pointon.

What are we to make of Malcolm's sketch? It clearly requires interpretation. My initial use of the sketch is to raise questions about our standard models of dementia: how would the sketch be interpreted? What does the sketch tell us about these models? I do this both to show the usefulness of models and to show their deficiencies. I shall discuss the sketch in more detail later in the chapter.

Models and understanding

In this sub-section I shall, first, consider the three explanatory models discussed in the last two chapters; this will lead me, secondly, to discuss in more detail some theoretical considerations to do with the background that supports our models; thirdly, I shall outline models used in clinical practice; before, fourthly, considering the possibility of a world without models.

Explanatory models

Malcolm's sketch allows us to make the point again that the models used to explain the symptoms and signs of acquired diffuse neurocognitive dysfunction are useful and productive. One worry about the disease and cognitive neuropsychology models is that they might emphasize deficits and deficiency. In fact, looking at Malcolm's sketch we might wish to use these models to point out the skills that he clearly retained at this point. The well-executed curves and circles and the general structure of the sketch, with the caricature of the face at the top, are evidence of good visuo-spatial skills, which require good functioning of the parietal lobes. The general artistry of the sketch would tend to suggest that the right parietal lobe was functioning well. The left parietal lobe comes into play in the production of letters and writing. The frontal lobe of the brain is important for the overall execution and planning of the sketch and the visual coordination would be achieved in part by using the visual cortex in the occipital lobe. The possibility of perseveration, the repetition of certain marks, letters or words ('too', 'to', and 'towo'), may also indicate a frontal lobe problem. But cognitive neuropsychological explanations of the retained functioning would help to confirm the presumed anatomical areas of good functioning.

Alternatively, the explanations of cognitive neuropsychology could help to focus our attention on particular areas of the brain where functioning might seem deficient and, if we wished, we could use sophisticated neuroimaging to demonstrate exactly where the neuropathophysiological deficits were located. In all of this, the models of dementia seem to have explanatory strength. Although there is evidence of good functioning, there is also evidence of difficulties. The ability to write whole words with meaning seems to have been lost. Letter construction, on the whole, seems good. But it would be reasonable to suggest that semantic memory (the store of knowledge, including the store of words and their meaning—where the notion of 'store' is being used metaphorically!), located in the temporal lobes, has been affected and that this lies behind the loss of the ability to construct whole words. The loss of semantic memory and the effects on writing have been well documented in Alzheimer's disease (Hughes, Graham, Patterson, and Hodges, 1997). At some point it could be that peripheral factors (i.e. to do with movement of the limbs and not a direct result of central brain dysfunction) might affect the ability to draw or write, but the quality of the sketch argues against this possibility at the time it was drawn. The deficits in semantic memory would also at this stage have been likely to have shown themselves in terms of speech: difficulty finding the right words (i.e. expressive dysphasia—often associated with Broca's area near the front of the brain) is very common as acquired diffuse neurocognitive dysfunction progresses; and gradually the comprehension of language is also likely to be affected (i.e. receptive dysphasia—associated with Wernicke's area in the posterior of the brain).

In short, Malcolm's sketch can usefully be discussed using both the disease and cognitive neuropsychology models. Experts in these areas would undoubtedly have more to say about the sketch. I suggested that the models would also be productive and this might be in a number of ways. For instance, they allow us to say that Malcolm's deficits are global, that they affect various different parts of his brain, and, therefore, this sketch on its own, interpreted by the models, would help to make a diagnosis of dementia. Given the history and other findings a more specific diagnosis could be made and this could lead to symptomatic (i.e. non-curative) treatment, e.g. with acetylcholinesterase inhibitors. The cognitive neuropsychologist could use the information contained in the sketch both to demonstrate Malcolm's retained abilities at this stage of his illness and to suggest ways for the family to attempt to understand and perhaps compensate for some of his difficulties. For instance, recognizing the loss of words, it might have been possible sometimes to use pictures to help with some aspects of communication. Or the family might have used the technique of 'indirect repair' to help Malcolm's speech (Sabat, 2001: 38–9). This involves suggesting words and re-phrasings, with checks to see if the right meaning has been arrived at, in a facilitating manner. In a number of ways, therefore, we can see how these models are both useful in terms of the explanations they give and potentially productive in terms of their practical utility.

But there are also dangers. Downs et al. (2006) discuss various explanatory models of dementia in terms of normal ageing, spiritual explanations, neuropsychiatry, a dialectical process. They state:

> The explanatory models of dementia, which we as individuals and societies adopt, will affect both the experience of living with dementia and how we support people and their families living with these conditions. (Downs et al., 2006: 235)

Their description of the model that regards dementia as a neuropsychiatric condition most closely matches the disease and cognitive neuropsychology models I have been discussing. When they discuss the implications of this explanatory model they say that according to it:

> The person is viewed as a passive victim of a condition over which they have no control, thus inevitably as a 'sufferer'. An explanatory model of dementia which attributes the person's experience entirely to a neuropsychiatric illness means that the person experiences the stigmatizing and depersonalizing effects commonly experienced by older people with mental disorders ...
>
> Furthermore, a process of diagnostic overshadowing can result where all actions and expressions are attributed to the labelled condition. (Downs op. cit.: 240)

The worry is that the disease model (especially) has such a pull on people's thoughts that there is inevitably a degree of labelling, the effect of which is to increase the person's problems because they tend to be seen in a negative light. This is what Sabat (2006a) also refers to as 'malignant positioning':

> The diagnosis itself sets the stage: actions taken by the person with dementia will usually be attributed to their disposition (in this case, the disease) rather than to the situation they are facing. (Sabat, 2006a: 289)

Sabat (2001, 2006a) records numerous ways in which 'malignant positioning' might operate in terms of the interpretation of behaviour in response to testing, of behaviour that challenges others, of day-to-day responses to caring relatives who undermine the person's standing as someone with retained skills and understanding, and so on.

Seeing the person through the lenses of pathology, which is the worry whether the pathology is thought of as physical or in terms of cognitive processing, is to adopt a particular view of the person. It is, in any case, to see the person as a patient and as a physical or computational machine. It is not to see the person in a more dynamic way against the broader surround. Thus, in the case of Malcolm's sketch, all the focus from these models is on the inner workings of his brain, what it can and cannot do (and the worry is that the effect of labelling means the focus is more on what cannot be done), and there is no movement to consider how the sketch links to anything else. Indeed, there is little need, with *solely* these models in mind, to try to consider the significance of the sketch. For that would move us away from the pathophysiology and away from the cognitive neuropsychological deficits to the world (Malcolm's shared world) in which they are situated.

This is, of course, the world of social constructionism. In discussing Vygotsky (whom I have mentioned in Chapters 3 and 5), whose thought has inspired social constructionism, Williams asserts:

> ... where cognitivist theories move to the interior of the mind ... Vygotskian theory moves to the context of the behavior, to the social situation within which the action takes place. (Williams, 1999: 262)

As a reminder, we need to recall the basis of social constructionist thought in Harré's discursive psychology:

> We must really stop thinking of psychology as the science of what happens in and around individual people. We must turn to the most tantalizing and difficult aspect of human action, namely conversing, to find the empirical basis of our studies. (Harré, 1989a)

And there is also Kitwood's formulation, according to which personhood is constructed by others in a social context:

> The core of our position is that personhood is essentially social; it refers to human beings in relation to others. (Kitwood & Bredin, 1992a)

Returning to Malcolm Pointon's sketch, therefore, with the social constructionist model in mind, we should be inclined to ask: what was the social situation in which the sketch was made? What sort of conversation was Malcolm having? What is the connection between this document (Figure 7.1) and his relationship with others?

Well, we might not know the answer to any of these questions. Even so, I cannot escape the fact that *I* (and *you*) now interact with the sketch. Moreover, we cannot escape the context in which we are privileged to see the sketch: we know some of its history, we know its provenance. So we cannot escape the relationship in which we stand to it. Whether the meaning we attach to the sketch is correct, it emerges from a 'social situation', from a discourse in which we are now engaged. The 'eyes' of the sketch seem somewhat sad, but there is also an undertone of humour, or is it frustration? Although its literal meaning is not conveyed, it conveys some sort of, albeit nebulous, emotion. There is a sense of creativity in the almost coquettish doodling; but also a sense of anguish or perplexity. And the word 'Love' appears clearly, conveying a heightened emotional content that puts this above a mere doodle. There is no doubt that the sketch carries meaning and evokes a response. All of this has occurred in the context of our social encounter with it.

We do, however, have a little more information. This comes from Barbara Pointon and immediately we have to acknowledge that the extra information and Barbara's viewpoint are crucial elements to the social context in which Malcolm's sketch can have meaning. Barbara, too, says she 'can only guess at the full meaning', but she suggests (in a personal communication):

> Help me. No mum. Help.
> sssss (sh?) too (two?) are cos a (because of) G ...... (1st letter of
> brother's name?). Love to two are love.

Crucial to our understanding of the sketch might well be the date. Because of the position of the sketch in the notebook, and on the basis of other evidence to do with writing and painting, Barbara puts the date at 1996. But 1996 was also the year in which Malcolm's mother died. This piece of information immediately places our understanding of the sketch in a new light. If it is correct that Malcolm sought out a familiar old notebook to write something at the time of the death of his mother, when he had not written in his diary for several years (but where his last entries in the diary were entirely legible and coherent), the 'doodle' starts to seem much more significant. It is still difficult to know exactly what was in his mind, but there seems undoubtedly to be a strong emotional content and a wish to put something into words at a difficult time. Are the marks in the middle of the writing crosses to symbolize death? Perhaps not, but the cry for help seems real; and what I have regarded as eyes could be seen—at least in the context of Malcolm's history—as reminiscent of the eyes of the subject of Edvard Munch's (1863–1944) *The Scream*.

Whatever the interpretation, the important point to note is that none of these social circumstances seemed relevant to the explanation offered by the disease or cognitive neuropsychology models. Their interpretations of the sketch could be made without the embedding social context, without even any reference to Barbara (although it is (almost!) inconceivable that anyone would attempt to diagnose or interpret in the context of acquired diffuse neurocognitive dysfunction without reference to the broader history). The social constructionist view immediately deepens our account and the explanations that might be forthcoming. One aspect of this is that Malcolm is placed centre stage: our concern is now to understand *him*—which means his context, discourses, and relationships—not just his brain, and not simply his cognitive processing.

This is the dialectical process that Downs et al. (2006) also considered as an explanatory model. They were considering the theory suggested by Kitwood, according to which dementia is viewed, '. . . as a dialectical interplay between biology, psychology, and the environment, particularly the social environment' (Downs et al., 2006: 248). This model has different therapeutic implications:

> While relatively little can be done to arrest the underlying brain disease, much can be done to promote health and well-being. It prompts the development of supports and services that address the many facets of a person's life that might hasten or delay the onset, or ameliorate or exacerbate the effects, of neurological disease. (*ibid.*)

This sort of approach,

> … keeps the person at the centre of all our efforts to help. It focuses on the person's abilities and strengths and suggests a citizenship model of inclusion. (Downs et al., 2006: 252)

Although the dialectical model described by Downs et al. (*op. cit.*) takes into account the biological and psychological components, it should none the less be noted that this is not required by the social constructionist model when considered in its purer forms. One criticism, then, is that social constructionism does not in itself give any account of the brain and of brain functioning. Talk of the conversations that might surround Malcolm's sketch do not need to include conversations about his brain pathology, nor about his ability to access or manipulate the inner mental processes. This might be a mistake if, as I suggested above, there are therapeutic possibilities that follow from the accounts of the disease and cognitive neuropsychology models. But the whole matter might be solved if we simply do away with the conception that we should (or even could) operate using a single *pure* model of any type. In this light, the description of a dialectical person-centred model looks highly promising precisely because it allows interplay between all of the models we are considering. Before moving on to discuss other clinical models in more detail, including the model of person-centred care, I shall pause to draw out some further (more theoretical) thoughts derived from consideration of social constructionism and Malcolm's sketch.

The background and the individual

One thing we have seen is the importance of the background—what I am inclined to call the surround—that enables us to gain a richer understanding of the sketch and, by implication, of any other facet of a person's life. In his book, *The Construction of Social Reality*, John Searle discusses the notion of the Background. He presents the thesis of the Background as follows:

> ... the literal meaning of any sentence can only determine its truth conditions or other conditions of satisfaction against a Background of capacities, dispositions, know-how, etc., which are not themselves part of the semantic content of the sentence. (Searle, 1995: 130)

Searle recognizes that his concept of the Background draws on the work of Wittgenstein. This is the transcendental account according to which the normativity of intentional states resides, constitutively, immanently, and irreducibly in the practices that instantiate those states. In other words, the condition for the possibility of there being criteria of correctness in our use of language, i.e. for there to be meaning, understanding and the like, is that the practices that make up language and instances of meaning or understanding must just contain within themselves, as part of their make-up, the appropriate criteria, without appeal to some other source of correctness. And these practices are the hurly-burly of the world, which form the background to our judgements and meanings.

> Not what *one* person is doing *now*, but the whole hurly-burly, is the background against which we see an action, and it determines our judgement, our concepts, and our reactions. (RPP II §629)

But Searle also refers to Pierre Bourdieu (1930–2002) and his concept of 'habitus', which Searle equates to his own notion of Background. In Chapter 2, I made use of the work of Pia Kontos and some of her comments on Merleau-Ponty (cf. Ch 2: pp. 39–41). Kontos meanwhile also uses the work of Bourdieu to understand her observations in the Orthodox Jewish long-term care facility where she watched the day-to-day goings-on as part of an ethnographic study. She tells the story of a man called Jacob who had profound speech problems and would readily get into a rage if there were any disturbances in the synagogue. But his rages could be quickly calmed by the ritual of the ceremonies in which he would participate with energy and spirit. According to Kontos,

> Habitus consists in dispositions, schemata, forms of know-how and competence, all of which function below the threshold of consciousness, enacted at a prereflective level. (Kontos, 2006: 207)

Referring to Jacob's participation in prayer, Kontos states:

> Following the logic of the concept of habitus, these rituals underscore the *active presence of the past in the body itself.* (Kontos, 2006: 209)

The idea inspiring the notion of habitus is that the social rituals have become embodied, part of the make-up of the person. Bordieu talks of 'embodied history', which Kontos takes to suggest,

> ... that past experiences persist in the body in the form of transposable dispositions that collectively function as a matrix of perceptions and actions. (*ibid.*)

To return to Searle, he describes intentionality as 'aspectual':

> ... and the possibility of perceiving, that is, the possibility of experiencing under aspects requires a familiarity with the set of categories under which one experiences those aspects. (Searle, 1995: 133)

Or we could say that to see things in a particular way, which would include seeing how to continue a mathematical series, or seeing a face in one way rather than another, is to grasp a background—the background hurly-burly—that becomes ingrained and a matter of bodily know-how: simply the patterned practice that it is to see things thus and so; the sort of habitus—a deeply ingrained bodily disposition—that was reflected in the praying of Jacob. This is to turn again to the Wittgensteinian account of Chapter 4, where Wittgenstein's central insight, according to Luntley, 'is to make a shift to a perceptual account of the conditions for the possibility of judgement' (Luntley, 2003a: 152).

> The conditions for judgement consist not in a body of theoretical knowledge possession of which grants the subject with the capacity for using language, it consists in the subject seeing the world aright. (*ibid.*)

Thus, given that 'seeing the world aright' is a matter of having the appropriate background, we find Searle arguing that,

> ... the understanding of utterances and the experiencing of ordinary conscious states require Background capacities. (Searle *op. cit.*: 135)

It was, after all, by an appeal to shared background abilities and ways of seeing the world that it was possible to form some judgements about Malcolm's sketch. The ability to convey emotional tone and content apparent in the sketch results from shared background understandings, which allow our (reasonable) attempts at interpretation. The shared background is not something that is easily lost.

> Notice the sheer intellectual effort it takes to break with our Background. Surrealist painters tried to do this, but even in a surrealist painting, the three-headed woman is still a woman, and the drooping watch is still a watch, and those crazy objects are still objects against a horizon, with a sky and a foreground. (*ibid.*)

To bring the strands of this discussion together, on the one hand we have philosophical reasons to accept the idea that there is a background, a habitus, which informs our understanding, which is deeply ingrained and embodied, and which is implicated in the transcendental account of normativity: it provides the grounds for the possibility of meaning and correctness in our interpretations. On the other hand, we have Malcolm's sketch, which calls out for some form of interpretation, which seems to convey meaning, and which—even if elements of it can be explained in a causal way by disease and cognitive neuropsychology models—is best understood (in a constitutive sense) by locating it in its proper social context.

Now we can also see that the philosophical strand of the discussion should inform our more general (human) understanding of Malcolm's sketch. Take Searle's talk above of the Surrealists. We might also wish to point to the forms of Malcolm's sketch and note that my sense that he was sketching two eyes might be taken to demonstrate Searle's point. Even as his powers were declining, Malcolm's (bodily and emotional) disposition—perhaps as a reflection of habitus, of all the social and cultural influences that he had so strongly imbibed—was to convey something of the human form. There is at least, in the shapes and in the words, something in which we can share and of which we can grasp some sense. For, to a greater or lesser extent, we share Malcolm's habitus and the practices that might have shaped his intentions and meanings at the time of the sketch.

There is a further theoretical point thrown up by Malcolm's sketch.

When Malcolm made his sketch it was not seen by anyone and was only found some time later by Barbara. In Chapter 4 (cf. pp 34–7), I have already discussed the philosophical issue concerning whether it is possible for only one person (the lone Robinson Crusoe) to establish a meaningful practice. Remember that it is of importance to social constructionism that meaning is a product of discourse *with others*, of our standing *in relationships*, of the *social* situation. Social constructionists draw inspiration from Wittgenstein, especially quotes such as that given above from RPP II §629, which also appears in Z §567, which suggest that it is not what *one* person is doing that matters, it is the whole hurly-burly. Meaning, therefore, is created with others. But, as I outlined in Chapter 4, this is problematic. For, as Luntley argues,

> ... the fundamental problem with all such collectivist accounts is that it remains profoundly unclear why a collective display is any better at delivering normativity than an individual display. (Luntley, 2003a: 98)

Luntley goes on to discuss the issue by considering the question Wittgenstein poses:

> Is what we call 'obeying a rule' something that it would be possible for only *one* man to do, and to do only *once* in his life? (PI §199)

Wittgenstein answers:

> It is not possible that there should have been only one occasion on which someone obeyed a rule. It is not possible that there should have been only one occasion on which a report was made, an order given or understood; and so on.—To obey a rule, to make a report, to give an order, to play a game of chess, are *customs* (uses, institutions). (*ibid.*)

Luntley's exegetical argument is that the priority is placed on the notion of repeated occasions over time, not on the involvement of other subjects. He notes that Wittgenstein more or less ignores the first part of the question in §199, about whether it would be possible for just *one* man to obey a rule. The implication is that for this to gain the status of a practice, it must be repeated over time (whether or not by more than one person). According to Luntley (2003a: 106–7) it is only the word 'institutions' that suggests a social meaning. This may be harsh exegesis, since the notions of making a report, giving an order, and playing chess, although they can be conceived as involving only one person, make more sense in terms of at least two people being involved. Luntley's line is in opposition to that of Williams, already quoted in Chapter 4:

> The central point is that the very idea of normativity, and so the structure within which the distinction between correct and incorrect can be drawn, cannot get a foothold unless the practice is a social one. (Williams, 1999: 175)

It will be recalled that Williams was herself combating the assertions of Baker and Hacker who say, in connection with these passages in Wittgenstein:

> Note that nothing in this discussion involves any commitment to a multiplicity of *agents*. All the emphasis is on the regularity, the multiple *occasions*, of action (cf. §199). (Baker & Hacker, 1984: 20)

Setting aside the exegesis, for it may be that the problem at issue simply did not occur to Wittgenstein (otherwise he might have confronted it more openly), there is a real distinction, which I have already highlighted, between whether a practice is *potentially* or *actually* public. Wittgenstein clearly makes the case that it must at least be potentially public. But why should there be a need to go further than this, especially given Luntley's point above—and the argument of Chapter 4—that the community view does nothing to stop the form of radical, sceptical questioning that otherwise undermines normativity? What is necessary is the transcendental requirement that normativity is constitutively, immanently and irreducibly a part of the practice under consideration:

> ... the notion of practice picked out here cannot be something that is merely descriptively characterized; it must be intrinsically normative. It is not an empirical concept; it is a transcendental concept. (Luntley, *op. cit.*: 97)

Now, in one sense, this is irrelevant to Malcolm's sketch. Malcolm is not the sort of lone practitioner that the argument concerns, because he *has* been embedded in social practices (he is not naïve with respect to the embedding practices) and the meaning in his sketch can be properly regarded as a more or less healthy remnant of his engagement with the relevant sort of practices. As soon as the sketch was found, it was located in his narrative, in the context of his relationships with his mother, his brother, and with Barbara. In this context, it has meaning of various sorts. But what if it had *not* been found and the history was not known? In a sense the question is too hypothetical to be of relevance. We might as well ask: in the absence of the embedding historical and cultural context, what are we to make of the aboriginal art of Australia? If we see rock art in the caves of Uluru, but we are completely ignorant of the stories of the Dreamtime,[1] in what sense (despite our ignorance) can we say that the art contains meaning? Are we committed to some platonic realm in which Malcolm's sketch resides with meaning, to which, however, we do not have access? To use the obvious extreme example: what if a man were born in an isolated place (on an island say), where there was no human contact, and his mother died at the moment of childbirth, but he was then brought up by the local animals, and what if he produced a sketch that looked something like Malcolm's (but perhaps without the letters and words), would the sketch have meaning even if it were never seen by another living soul? What if he did not even socialize with animals, but was kept alive by some form of artificial means but without any social interaction of any sort?

My inclination in each of these cases is to say that we would have to ascribe meaning to the sketch without recourse to the platonic heaven. This is partly because even to conceive of the extreme situation is to create a social space in which any sketch would inevitably acquire meaning. If, say, we could bracket off any social context—there is simply the sketch in limbo—there would still be the *potential* for the sketch to fall under the description of a practice in which it will then be embedded so as to allow ascriptions of correctness and incorrectness in terms of potential understandings or interpretations. But this is partly predicated on the thought that this being will still be a human being with a human brain of this sort (and the ability to draw the sketch itself starts to show us the level of sophistication of the workings of this particular human brain). My suggestion is that once there is a human being *of this sort* in existence then, even in the absence of social contexts, there is a habitus, as shown by potential dispositions and the potential acquisition of know-how, that will make itself known through the person. That is, any human person *of this sort* potentially occupies a space and shapes it according to individual perspectival judgements. The result is the possibility of normatively constrained practices as a transcendental feature. And the relevance of this is that a person with acquired diffuse neurocognitive dysfunction will be a human person *of this sort*, as an inevitable consequence of his or her life history and habitus. Therefore, a person with dementia will always deserve the dignity that we would wish to see bestowed on any other human being by virtue of the individual's standing precisely qua human person. Thus, Malcolm's sketch is important for this reason: to be a human person is to have the potential to produce such a work and such a work locates the person as a being-in-the-world, where this carries a whole set of ethical and conceptual commitments. To have produced such a sketch is for Malcolm to have re-affirmed his standing as a person, but without any *necessity* for him to have done so. For his standing as a person in the world was already assured by his narrative and the habitus—the background or surround—in which he was embedded.

In a sense, my use of Malcolm's sketch is a deceit, for it is a means to make a broader point. The whole question of the normativity of meaning is a way to approach the larger question of how thought interacts with the world. The account I have been giving, based on the Wittgensteinian critique of Chapter 4, is a transcendental one. The broader point is that to be a being of this kind—a human being—is to have the potential to engage in practices, where these are understood in a transcendental manner, in which normativity is embedded as a constitutive, immanent, and irreducible feature. Any human being, as a person in the world, characteristically has this potential, for we are meaningful creatures for whom, as Charles Taylor puts it, things have a significance:

> What I am as a self, my identity, is essentially defined by the way things have significance for me. (Taylor, 1989: 34)

This is an important idea, but for now I turn to consider the models that might be used in clinical practice.

Models of practice

A view is always from somewhere. We cannot help approaching the world with some sort of framework, or set of expectations, dispositions, habitus, or background. Our models shape our practice and, therefore, it seems sensible to consider the clinical models that might be used by those looking after people with acquired diffuse neuro-cognitive dysfunction. I shall outline four models—the biomedical, person-centred care, palliative care, and supportive care models—and offer a brief commentary on them before raising the question, in the next sub-section, whether, in fact, we need any models whatsoever.

The biomedical model is almost the disease model by another name and I do not intend to discuss this much further, since it is covered in Chapters 1, 5, and 6. The theoretical critique of the disease model centres on its inability to provide anything beyond a causal account of acquired diffuse neurocognitive dysfunction. It cannot suggest, and seemingly takes little notice of, what it *is* for a person to have acquired diffuse neurocognitive dysfunction. As suggested in Chapter 5 (see p. 121), the 'medical' model is nowadays usually thought of in terms of a biopsychosocial approach (Engel, 1980). Hence the 'bio*medical*' model can be thought of as being broader than just the biological notion of a disease: psychosocial elements inevitably (in clinical practice) come into play. As I have already discussed, however, the biomedical approach tends to be reductionist, with too heavy an emphasis on biological approaches. It certainly suggests little room for a spiritual approach to illness and disease. Nevertheless, as we have seen, the model is undoubtedly beneficial in numerous clinical ways, especially when it is open to broader frameworks in addition to its focus on biology and, in particular, on pathology.

A broader and widely adopted model of care for people with dementia is that of person-centred care. This is the model of care adopted and encouraged by Tom Kitwood (1997). Kitwood, with the Bradford Dementia Group, developed a detailed understanding of what person-centred care might mean (Baldwin & Capstick, 2007). This was then further developed, with Kathleen Bredin and others, to produce the observational tool called Dementia Care Mapping (Kitwood & Bredin, 1992b). Having a broad, social view of what it is to be a person, which includes taking note of the person's relationships, and then trying to put oneself in the shoes of the person, are integral to person-centred care. Person-centred care is the result of the dialectical process discussed by Downs et al. (2006), who state:

> The development of a person-centred approach in dementia care is based on the argument that people with dementia, far from being passive victims, are active agents in their lives, actively seeking meaning, responding, and attempting to act on their world … (p. 245)

Dawn Brooker (2008) suggests that the term 'person-centred care',

> … was intended to be a direct reference to Rogerian psychotherapy with its emphasis on authentic contact and communication. (p. 229)

She has also usefully summarized its main components with the acronym VIPS:

V: asserts the absolute value of all human lives;
I : stresses the individualized approach;
P: encourages the perspective of the individual;
S: promotes the notion of a positive social milieu (Brooker, 2004)

There can be little doubt that the notion of person-centred care has had a profound effect on the ways in which people think of care in this field. There are, however, two difficulties.

First, the term has become ubiquitous, so that almost any institution providing care for people with acquired diffuse neurocognitive dysfuntion is likely to bill itself as person-centred. But, in a study conducted in the UK of respite and short-break services for people with dementia, we found the assumption that 'person-centred care' as a concept was widely understood was unwarranted, particularly because there was evidence of unacceptable variation in services, with even basic physical and personal needs not always being met (Bamford et al., 2009). In its report, *Dementia: Ethical Issues,* the working party of the Nuffield Council on Bioethics also recorded the concern from other sources that,

... the term [person-centred care] may have become debased and used to describe almost any care, regardless of the extent to which it is based on a genuine relationship with, and concern for, the individual, and that therefore the term may have lost much of its original value as a guiding principle. (Nuffield Council on Bioethics, 2009: 40 [§3.6])

Secondly, there may be a tendency for person-centred care to neglect the importance of the biomedical approach, or to see itself as an alternative to that approach (as opposed to complementary). This is unfair because Kitwood wrote: 'Maintaining personhood is both a psychological and a neurological task' (Kitwood, 1997: 19). He also wrote:

It is vital ... that close attention be given to all aspects of the physical well-being of a person who has dementia. In the eagerness to provide person-centred care, there can be a danger of neglecting this issue. (Kitwood, *op. cit.*: 34)

This seems balanced, but the attention that Kitwood actually gives to neuroscience usually emphasizes its weaknesses and the state of 'disarray' of the biomedical paradigm. Kitwood also mentions neuroscience more frequently when he is describing pathology. But the emphasis is on the impact of 'malignant social psychology'. And when he turns to consider improving care, the possibility of the biomedical approach proving helpful seems simply to be ignored. My comments might still appear unfair in that it would, perhaps, be too much to expect that Kitwood (who was many things, but not a neuroscientist) should have presented as much detail concerning the biomedical approach to acquired diffuse neurocognitive dysfunction as he did concerning the psychosocial. His comments show he was not unaware of the importance of physical care, but his work was (and is) a necessary corrective to the over-emphasis on bio-medical neuroscience in connection with dementia. Nevertheless, personhood as, 'a standing or status that is bestowed upon one human being, by others, in the context of relationship and social being' (Kitwood *op. cit.*: 8), is not a definition that mentions the relevance of embodiment and, therefore, not one to encourage the importance of a biological approach to care. And the 'new culture of dementia care', encouraged by Kitwood (cf. Table 9.1 in Kitwood, *op. cit.*: 136), places almost no emphasis on the biological and neurological sciences. The new culture is almost entirely psychosocial.

The problem here, therefore, is one of emphasis. For instance, there is minimal recognition of the importance of general practice and general (geriatric) medicine in Kitwood's discussion: the main targets for his (usually critical) comments are neurology and psychiatry. Yet, the physical health of people with acquired diffuse neurocognitive dysfunction (the treatment of pain for instance) is not just an extremely important part of their well-being, which Kitwood clearly recognized, but is also quotidian, especially as the condition worsens. Furthermore, although Kitwood was aware of the importance of spirituality (he was ordained a priest in 1962)—as shown by his fondness for Buber's (2004) talk of *I-Thou* as opposed to *I-It* relations—he did not overplay its importance in his general writings (but cf. Kitwood, 1970). In connection with this and the previous point about physical health (especially in the later stages), he did not confront the palliative care needs of people with acquired diffuse neurocognitive dysfunction. Indeed, he went so far as to suggest that the 'new culture of dementia care'—i.e. person-centred care where all the emphasis is away from the biomedical model—might lead to 'rementing' and, as care improves,

> We may reasonably expect to find far less vegetation—possibly none at all. (Kitwood, 1997: 101)

The need for attention to palliative care and to spirituality, along with a proper weighting to general medical care, including pain relief, takes us on to consider the model of palliative care as it is applied to acquired diffuse neurocognitive dysfunction.

There has been a steady rise in interest in the model of palliative care in connection with dementia (Volicer & Hurley, 1998; Hughes, 2006b; Hughes, Jolley, Jordan, and Sampson, 2007). It is worth noting that direct comparisons have been made between palliative care and person-centred care: in a number of ways they aim at exactly the same concerns (Hughes, Hedley, and Harris, 2006; Small, Downs, and Froggatt, 2006). The juxtaposition of person-centred and palliative care also suggests the ways in which (what Small, Froggatt, and Downs (2008) refer to as) 'life-world narratives' and 'professional discourses' might intersect. This is the broader view that tries to see things from different perspectives to gain more of a surview and thereby a greater understanding.

If, however, there are some advantages to the model of palliative care in comparison with person-centred care—in that it places greater weight on physical care as part of holistic care (where this implies not only a biopsychosocial approach and concern for spiritual issues, but also inclusion of the family)—there are disadvantages too. These are partly summed up by its association with cancer care, where there has tended to be a dichotomy between cure and care, with the feeling (which is not, however, as legitimate as it once was) that palliative care only starts when attempts at cure have failed. The trajectory (although it can be similar to other long-term conditions that require palliative care) and different types of acquired diffuse neurocognitive dysfunction mean that palliative care is not the same here and, whilst the broad palliative care approach can easily be modified to suit different diseases, perhaps the suitability of the palliative care model for acquired diffuse neurocognitive dysfunction is vitiated. If nothing else, in circumstances where the emphasis should be on living well (and not on dying), the natural link that is made between palliative care and end-of-life (or terminal) care can be off-putting to people with acquired diffuse neurocognitive dysfunction and their carers. We have argued elsewhere that what is called for is a broader approach to accommodate all of the management options that might arise in dealing with different types of acquired diffuse neurocognitive dysfunction:

> The notion of palliative care would need to expand to accommodate prevention, direct treatment of pathophysiology, rehabilitation, and even cure or 'restorative care'. Expanding the concept of palliative care in this way cannot be prohibited, but it seems to be stretching a point. No doubt palliative care can have an impact throughout the course of dementia, but perhaps it should be seen as just one component—of tremendous importance—in an approach that, at best, should include a good deal of flexibility and, over time, might include attempts to prevent the underlying pathological processes (e.g. by treating cardiovascular risk factors), to cure the condition (e.g. by inserting shunts for hydrocephalus), to rehabilitate (e.g. following an in-patient stay for delirium), and so on. (Hughes, Lloyd-Williams, and Sachs, 2010: 6)

Our favoured option, therefore, was to plump for a supportive care model. We characterized the vision of supportive care in the following way:

> The aspiration here is no more than that there should be a complete mixture of biomedical dementia care, with good quality, person-centred, psychosocial, and spiritual care under the broad umbrella of holistic palliative care throughout the course of the person's experience of dementia. … There should be no dichotomies between which we should have to choose: no division between the need to cure and the need to care, no battle concerning whether the care is high or low tech, no tension between whether the care is biological or social, no concern over whether it is patient- or carer-centred, no debate about whether dementia care is mostly about 'being with' or 'doing to.' The supportive care model allows us to say that people with dementia deserve all of these approaches whenever and wherever they are applicable, from the time of diagnosis to the moment of death. (Hughes et al., 2010: 7)

In the final chapter of *Supportive Care for the Person with Dementia*, we added the important point that:

> … the *appropriate application* of aggressive biomedical treatments (at the right stage of disease and consistent with the goals of care of specific patients and families) is a component of supportive care for patients with dementia of all aetiologies. (Hughes et al., 2010: 302)

And we reiterated the point that what was required was a broad view:

> Supportive care represents a broad view; it is a broad view of the person with dementia …, who must be seen in all of his or her biological, psychological, social, and spiritual complexity, where care is aimed broadly, holistically, impeccably, and with enthusiasm, but also with clinical judgement. (Hughes et al., 2010: 306–7)

I do not intend to try to lay out in any more detail here what constitutes supportive care in this context. It was, however, a notion of care that was picked up and emphasized by the working party of the Nuffield Council:

> The concept of supportive care appears to be particularly helpful in dementia, in that it emphasises the need to support both the person with dementia and their family, from the

moment of diagnosis, regardless of the availability or appropriateness of treatment for the underlying brain disorder. In terms of our ethical framework, such supportive care recognises the value of the person with dementia and is concerned to promote the well-being and autonomy of that person while also paying attention to the interests of carers. (Nuffield Council on Bioethics 2009: 41 [§3.10])

Now, the good thing about the supportive care model is that it will accommodate almost anything, as long as it is aimed at helping the patient and his or her carers. In other words, it does not matter whether the treatment is usually used in a curative manner or simply for palliation, if it might help now, it should (if possible) be tried. But in allowing supportive care such a large scope, it is possible to raise a question about the need to refer to the type of care by any particular name. The Nuffield Council spotted the point:

> However, we note that the 'label' attached to care is less important than the beliefs and attitudes underpinning that label. If care is provided on the basis that the person with dementia is valued as a person and supported to 'live well' with dementia, within the context of their own family and other relationships, then the label becomes immaterial. (*ibid.*)

A further point to note is that, in arguing for supportive care, it becomes necessary to say that other models are in one way or another deficient. This can be done, but as was apparent in my discussion of Kitwood and palliative care above, the deficiencies are more often in terms of emphasis, rather than radical differences of content.

It is, indeed, possible to demonstrate this point from the literature. For instance, we reviewed the literature concerning different types of centredness, in an attempt to elucidate the essential components of person-centred care (Hughes, Bamford, and May, 2008). We looked at family-centred, relationship-centred, client-centred, patient-centred and person-centred care and undertook a thematic review of the reviews of the literature. We found ten themes that were common to all the different types of centredness (see Table 7.1).

At a conceptual level we could not identify thematic differences between the types of centredness. The literature on the different types of centredness all said the same sort of thing! We concluded that different types of centredness are required in different contexts where they have differing practical utilities.

> Meanwhile, the notion of centredness itself, which ... emerges in the unifying common themes, reflects a movement in health and social care, away from the narrower biomedical view, in favour of the broader view, which involves increasing the social, psychological, cultural and ethical sensitivities of our human encounters. (Hughes et al., *op. cit.*)

Much the same could be said of the various models of dementia. They all work in certain contexts and have their good points. It may be that they miss some aspects of care because they emphasize others. I have wished to promote the model of supportive care, but even this might potentially be misleading at some point. Models all have the capacity to make us think too rigidly—in line with the model. It will often seem better to have a flexible and eclectic approach. Part of the appeal of supportive care is that it seems to stipulate very little in a way that prohibits or is critical of any other model. Whatever might work should, on this view, be tried. But looking for a model that allows such breadth of action and vision raises the inevitable question, which we have been approaching, namely why we need a model at all. Why do we not follow the

Table 7.1 Summary descriptions of themes from literature on different types of centredness

Theme	Description
Respect for individuality and values	Recognizes the importance of valuing people as individuals with awareness of differences, values, culture, their unique strengths, needs and rights, including the right to dignity and privacy.
Meaning	Accepts the unique perspective, reflecting the phenomenological and subjective nature of the person's experience, with self-defined goals and a potentially shared understanding of the meaning of illness.
Therapeutic alliance	Involves the possibility of genuine empathy and unconditional positive regard. Therapeutic alliance is based on respect for personhood, with warmth, trust, openness, care, honesty, the instillation of hope and confidence. Non-judgemental relationships should encourage competency, belonging and a shared language, where the professional is a facilitator.
Social context and relationships	Attends to our social nature as people, with an emphasis on relationships, on our situated context of interpersonal, interconnected, mutual interdependence. Hence family and carers' needs are recognized, as is the relevance of roles and life stages. The importance of seeing the network of relationships as a whole is crucial.
Inclusive model of health and well-being	Broader than diagnosis and treatment, with protection and safety for the vulnerable, this theme involves comfort, attachment, occupation, identity and inclusion, with attention to well-being and a biopsychosocial model of the person as a whole. This model includes an integrated holistic understanding of the individual's unique world with a recognition of his or her idiosyncratic and broader life-setting. It also includes attention to the prevention of disease, health promotion and the improvement of quality of life.
Expert lay knowledge	The legitimacy of individual's or the family's expert knowledge and experience is recognized. The possibility of consensus through negotiation, compromise, and active participation is encouraged. In addition, therefore, there is the possibility of service users contributing to service and professional development.
Shared responsibility	This suggests the sharing of power, responsibility, and control, with mutual agreement on plans and reciprocity, with involvement in decision-making, and an orientation towards the individual situated in context, but open to collaboration and partnership. Hence, a type of consumerism, with user involvement and awareness of rights.
Communication	This theme encourages communication with careful, sensitive, interactional dialogue, observational skills and authentic contact, including attentive listening, with the provision of accessible and unbiased information provided in ways that are affirming and useful.
Autonomy	This includes the person's ability to make his or her own decisions, with independence and recognition that individuals and families should be encouraged to live out their lives, make their own choices, in accordance with principles of self-determination, enhancing their control and independence in the process of receiving care.
Professional as a person	The emphasis is on valuing staff as well as service users and on the doctor's or professional's role as a person with emotions, who may need support to enable self-awareness and meaningful partnerships.

With kind permission from Springer Science + Business Media: Medicine, Healthcare and Philosophy, Types of Centredness in Healthcare: themes and concepts, **11**, 2008, 455–63, Hughes.

suggestion in the Nuffield Report and simply provide good quality care without worrying too much about what the care is called? (Perhaps like the State, which in Marxist theory was seen simply as a means to subjugate people, models should—to use the phrase concocted by Frederick Engels (1820–1895)—'wither away'![2]) Indeed, why do we bother with models at all?

A world without models

For the sake of transparency, there is a strategic move here that starts from the suggestion a little earlier that to be a human being, a being *qua human being* with the potential to draw Malcolm's sketch (whether or not one does *actually* draw such a sketch and whatever the actual *social* surround), is characteristically to have the potential to engage in such practices, where these are understood in a manner in keeping with the transcendental account of normativity, in which, therefore, there is (as a constitutive, immanent, and irreducible feature) meaning and significance. The strategy is to move from this understanding, via the discussion of clinical models, to the possibility of no models, in order to arrive at some further understanding of what it is to be a person in the world engaged in human encounters of the sort that people with acquired diffuse neurocognitive dysfunction have to face.

Models inevitably simplify reality. If they did more than this they would not be models, they would be the real thing. Models are ubiquitous in science, from representational models of phenomena and data[3]—the most obvious being the double helix model of deoxyribonucleic acid (DNA)—to theoretical models, such as the mathematical models of theoretical physics, from solid and quantum mechanics to string theory. Indeed, science as a whole, inasmuch as its observations lead to theories, relies on models, because theories can be thought of as models: they are statements about the world, which aim to capture some aspect or other of the world in order (usually) to make predictions with respect to the world.

There is a tension in the philosophy of science concerning whether (or the extent to which) scientific models are realist and are meant to capture nature as it really is, or the extent to which models are simply constructs that fit the world from a particular point of view at a particular time. This is not an area that I can discuss in any depth, but it is at least useful to see the importance of models in terms of their ability to frame the ideas and concerns of science. Thus, Ronald Giere, a philosopher of science, writes in the introduction to *Science Without Laws*:

> The fundamental concept in my particular understanding of scientific practice is that of a *model*. Models, for me, are the primary representational entities in science. Scientists, I claim, typically use models to represent aspects of the world. The class of scientific models includes physical scale models and diagrammatic representations, but the models of most interest are *theoretical* models. These are abstract objects, imaginary entities whose structure might or might not be *similar to* aspects of objects and processes in the real world. Scientists themselves are more likely to talk about the *fit* between their models and the world ... (Giere, 1999: 5)

There are two points in this that I wish to pick up, to do with representation and to do with the notion of fit.

We have come across the notion of representation, in connection with cognitive neuropsychology models in Chapters 5 and 6. We might wish to ask in what sense models are 'the primary representational entities in science'. A simple model of a molecule (with its simplifying assumptions, e.g. that atoms are like solid spheres which are held together by more or less rigid connecting bars!) is clearly a representational entity, but in what sense is a model defined by a complex mathematical formula a representational entity? There is a line of thought that takes us straight back to the representationalism of Fodor, which I discussed in connection with cognitive neuropsychology. For instance, Ducheyne (2008) argues that, 'Scientific models are a subset of mental representations'. Given the general points I have already made against representationalism (cf. pp. 162–68), I am unhappy to accept this conclusion. But the notion of metaphorical representation is more palatable, especially when combined with the thought that representations only make sense in the context of the public human world of meaning and narrative. Recall Gillett from Chapter 6:

> … representation, both to oneself and to others, depends on what is public and on the shared norms which persons follow to regulate and articulate activity. (Gillett, 1992: 118)

The representation as embedded in the world, however, takes us back to fundamental questions about how we see the world and what it is of the world that we see: do we see (a single) reality, or versions of it (as we saw in Chapter 1 being suggested by Goodman (1978))?

In turn, this takes us back to the second point to discuss from Giere, that of fit:

> The empirical question—the question of realism—is how well the resulting model fits the intended aspects of the real world. And here my central claim is that fit is always partial and imperfect. There is no such thing as a perfect model, complete in all details. That does not, however, prevent models from providing us with deep and useful insights into the workings of the natural world. (Giere, 1999: 6)

Gierre's preferred solution is to give weight to the importance of scientists making decisions about the versions they wish to adopt, where the rationality of the scientific judgement will often depend upon e.g. the utility of the model in specific circumstances and from a particular perspective.

> Science does not deliver to us universal truths underlying all natural phenomena; but it does provide models of reality possessing various degrees of scope and accuracy. (*ibid.*)

And, finally, this brings us back to the question about the use of models in thinking about dementia.

Notwithstanding uncertainties stemming from the debates about the use of models in science in general, I have already pointed out the various ways in which models help us in our thinking about acquired diffuse neurocognitive dysfunction and the ways in which they help people affected, directly and indirectly, by these sorts of condition. The disease (or biomedical), cognitive neuropsychology, social constructionist, person-centred, palliative care, and supportive care models all have something to contribute; as do the many models I have not discussed, such as relationship-centred and disability, citizenship, or recovery models, *et cetera*. Lumping all of these models together is, of course, not entirely appropriate, because (e.g.) the cognitive neuropsychology and the recovery models are intended to perform different functions. In one sense, then, there are no problems; it is just that different models will be used at different times for particular purposes. But this does point in the direction of a caution, which is that different models need to be used differently, according to the degree of fit. The effect of a drug on cognitive function is not best thought of in terms of the model of discursive psychology, whereas cognitive neuropsychology would be more apt. Trying to decide whether to admit someone from a nursing home to an acute medical ward because of a chest infection would require quite broad thought; so using a model that mostly focuses on the nature of the disease would be less apt than one that encourages thought about the person's previous beliefs and wishes, the views of the family, the legal framework, as well as the particular symptoms, the appropriateness of the social environment to meet the person's needs without an admission, and so on.

Let me make some bald statements about our actual use of models in clinical practice, thinking of acquired diffuse neurocognitive dysfunction in particular:

◆ We sometimes use specific models for a specific purpose;

◆ We often (and perhaps mostly) use models subconsciously, or in the background, in an unreflective way;

◆ We often (and perhaps mostly) use models eclectically, choosing from here and there depending on the circumstances.

Hence, I might very deliberately test cognitive function in order to demonstrate a particular deficit of processing because I need to make a statement about the person's capacity to make a certain sort of decision or, for example, about their ability to drive. Or again, mostly when I ask about a person's family history in the context of a routine assessment, it is not that I have in the front of my mind a model of genetic inheritance; but an understanding of the genetics of younger onset Alzheimer's disease is 'in my mind' somewhere (subconsciously or in the background). If I start to hear a story of a strong family history, the model of genetic inheritance comes into my mind in a conscious manner. But perhaps instead what I hear is that the family is large, that they live close by, and are willing and able to provide strong social support. The biomedical, genetic model does not need to be mobilized, but my thoughts are now in the groove of person-centred or supportive care. Still, I can be eclectic, because it might be that information about the person's difficult early life, successful marriage, but recent bereavement, may incline me to understand matters to some extent through the model of attachment theory (Bowlby, 1988).

This does not get me, however, as far as I need to go strategically. For the question I want to face is whether I need models at all. The answer will depend on my purposes. I have already acknowledged that for specific purposes certain models will serve me well. Sometimes these purposes will be scientific. But we should note that sometimes the type of science might be more like a *social* science. Clinical practice will often veer between the application of basic biological principles and the need to comprehend the social circumstances and facilitate a social solution.

This calls to mind the book *The Idea of a Social Science* by Peter Winch (1926–1997). This seminal work challenged the view that empiricism should be the basis of work in the social sciences. Social facts are not like physical facts and should be treated differently, indeed philosophically.

> For any worthwhile study of society must be philosophical in character and any worthwhile philosophy must be concerned with the nature of human society. (Winch, 1958: 3)

There is much in this work that would support the ideas of discursive psychology. Winch also provides, however, a powerful statement of the difference between causal and constitutive accounts of intentional mental states.

> 'Understanding' ... is grasping the *point* or *meaning* of what is being done or said. This is a notion far removed from the world of statistics and causal laws: it is closer to the realm of discourse and to the internal relations that link the parts of a realm of discourse. (Winch, *op. cit.*: 115)

So, if our task is to understand people with dementia, to understand what the world is like for them, to understand the situations they find themselves in, to understand their behaviour, then we need to understand their discourses. But this is to understand more than what is said at any one time. It is to understand a life perhaps. And the question here is whether we are enabled to do this by a model. And, if not, then it looks as if, *for these purposes and to this extent*, the approach of science will not be appropriate. I shall expand on this.

Understanding the person is the central endeavour. We can use models to understand certain aspects of the person. The amyloid cascade hypothesis, which was discussed in Chapter 5, presents a model to explain how Alzheimer's pathology develops. This will be useful in understanding some aspects of the person who has acquired diffuse neurocognitive dysfunction. But it does not give us a full view. Discursive psychology provides a broader view in one sense, but not necessarily a better view, except for specific tasks, when its model is more apt, more fitting. Thus, discursive psychology would be a better model than a narrow disease model to use in order to negotiate a tricky ethical issue. But the disease model would provide a better fit if the issue concerned the relationship between falls and a particular type of acquired diffuse neurocognitive dysfunction, such as Lewy body disease. All of these models, therefore, will have a place.

If the point, however, is 'to understand' in the sense that we wish to grasp the significance of things, what they mean, then we need to move, 'closer to the realm' of discourse and to the internal relations that link the parts of a realm of discourse' (*ibid.*). Ignoring the argument concerning whether or not this means that the person must be *actually* engaged in discourse or only *potentially* so, the point still places us in the realm of the normative, where to understand is to engage in practices in which meaning and normativity are embedded (constitutively, immanently, and irreducibly). To make the point differently, recall Wittgenstein writing early in *Philosophical Investigations*: 'And to imagine a language means to imagine a form of life' (PI §19). A little later he emphasizes that, 'the *speaking* of language is part of an activity, or of a form of life' (PI §23). Combining this with the quote from Winch, to enter the realm of discourse is to enter a 'form of life'. The activity that constitutes forms of life is, according to Wittgenstein, 'the given', which 'has to be accepted' (PI p. 226). Thus, to understand, in this sense, is to participate in the background, the form of life, which makes up human linguistic communities.

The question then is: what sort of model will enable one to participate in this way? The answer should be that there cannot be a model, because the only things that could count as models would necessarily fit only partially and imperfectly: 'There is no such thing as a perfect model, complete in all details' (Giere, 1999: 6). A model of the whole human being as he or she exists in the world would necessarily be a model of the whole human being (and the world)! In which case, it would either be inadequate as a model (because it would not capture the whole unless it were the whole), or (if the whole) it would not be a model. And the point is that, in the required sense, understanding needs to be holistic. To see the person, qua person (rather than to grasp some particular aspect of the person from his biology or her sociology), is to see the surround: it is to grasp the whole. But to do this is to operate without models.

The world without models is the world of real human encounters, where embodied subjects meet in the raw. But the world without models is also a world without science. It is where eyes meet and convey meaning, not by the sharing of a model of understanding, according to which there must be some sort of mutual interpretation, but on account of the form of life shared by human beings of this sort. To be of this sort is to be embedded in a world, authentically, where flesh and blood mingle with intentionality and normativity, where facts and values come together, where the inner and the outer interdigitate without difficulty. It is the everyday world (not the world of theory) where the background is taken-for-granted and meaning is embedded. It is also the world in which friendship and humour can show themselves through touch and through shared practices of care, not through the application of models. These aspects of our humanity are deeply embedded; they are the habitus and the embodied subjectivity of personhood. Thus we find Barbara Pointon writing of the 'essential Malcolm':

> It can be seen in his patience and serenity, in his abiding passion for music (he turns his head slightly towards the source of the sound, and a tear will roll down his face when a favourite piece is played) and in his eyes when kindly people talk or touch his hands. Even his mischievous, subversive sense of humour will out: while being fed, he will lift an eyebrow, look his favourite carer straight in the eye and thwart her by clamping his teeth on the spoon for no good reason. (Pointon, 2007: 118)

To understand his patience and serenity, his passion for music, or his sense of humour is not to be in possession of the correct model, it is rather to stand in the right relation, to have the correct perspective, which means to share a form of life, to share a pre-reflective background or surround (a habitus), possession of which is enough to ensure that meanings can be grasped and understood. This remains true even when it is difficult. A world without models is an atheoretical world, but it is not an easy world, because human encounters are not always straightforward. There can be strong tensions in this world, but they are not tensions that are always solvable by the application of a model. Often they will require instead the right stance, where this is conceived in ethical terms. Misunderstandings will be possible, but (again) these are not put right or avoided by the use of a model; superficial misunderstandings might be, but where the issue is the deep engagement of individuals, rather than mere instrumental exchanges, to misunderstand is simply to be in a different groove, a different background.

Where the misunderstandings are at the level of human-to-human contact, qua human, they are rectified or avoided by making attempts to improve human relations even under difficult circumstances; and this requires honesty, charity, bravery, compassion or love, and so on; in fact, just the sort of human dispositions or virtues that define what it is to flourish or do well as a good human being.

But the jump to the virtues is not the move I wish to make here. Instead, having commended the notion of the world without models, which is a world of human encounters as they are or could be if they were to be true reflections of life *as it is actually lived* by people, I want to suggest now that we should drill down to the rawness of the human (ethical) encounter, which must always be person to person. And I wish to consider what this amounts to as a phenomenon.

'To the things themselves!'[4]

Phenomenology is a lot of things and I neither propose at this point to try to summarize its precepts nor to lay bare its tensions (but see Fulford et al., 2006: 181–210). Its origins are chiefly found in the work of Edmund Husserl (1859–1938). He regarded phenomenology as a method, an approach which Heidegger endorsed:

> To have a science 'of' phenomena means to grasp its objects *in such a way* that everything about them which is up for discussion must be treated by exhibiting it directly and demonstrating it directly. (Heidegger, 1962: 59)

Heidegger's project in *Being and Time* (at least the part of the project that was completed) was to raise the question of the 'meaning of Being', by which he meant Being itself, not particular manifestations of it. Crudely, he was not interested in this or that thing, but in thingness itself. But he felt that the question of Being was raised most clearly by considering human beings, because they raised the question of the meaning of Being for themselves and in themselves. Concerning his concept *Dasein*, which literally means 'there-being', but is better understood as implying the human existent, Heidegger says:

> Dasein is an entity which does not just occur among other entities. Rather it is ontically distinguished by the fact that, in its very Being, that Being is an *issue* for it. But in that case, this is a constitutive state of Dasein's Being. ... It is peculiar to this entity that with and through its Being, this Being is disclosed to it. *Understanding of Being is itself a definite characteristic of Dasein's Being.* (Heidegger, *op. cit.*: 32)

In this sub-section, I wish to focus on what it is to be a human being of this sort, because this is what we share as people both with and without acquired diffuse neurocognitive dysfunction. In Chapter 3, I suggested that the mind was in some sense mystical; and I have also suggested, in Chapter 6, that getting to know someone intimately involves mystery. Similarly, in Chapter 4, I considered the mysterious way in which we can share in our understanding of music and recognize the Englishness of Elgar and the American nature of Copland. Quite generally, despite its everydayness, what constitutes the mind seems mysterious, as something that cannot be pinned down. At the end of Chapter 5, I suggested that *what* it is to remember is clouded in a degree of mystery: our words, our mental concepts, point to 'something', which is none the less out of reach.

> There are, indeed, things that cannot be put into words. They *make themselves manifest.* They are what is mystical. (TLP §6.522)

Here I want, albeit briefly, to elucidate the phenomenon, the shared nature of our being as human beings. This is precisely not to suggest that I am going to clarify this phenomenon by putting it plainly into words. That there is something mysterious precludes this possibility. But I wish to shed *some* light on these deeper inclinations.

At the start of *Being and Time*, Heidegger draws on the works of Aristotle and Thomas Aquinas. He says:

> Thomas is engaged in the task of deriving the '*transcendentia*'—those characters of Being which lie beyond every possible way in which an entity may be classified as coming under some generic kind of subject-matter (every *modus specialis entis*), and which belong necessarily to anything, whatever it may be. Thomas had to demonstrate that the *verum* is such a *transcendens*. He does this by invoking an entity which, in accordance with its very manner of Being, is properly suited to 'come together with' entities of any sort whatever. This distinctive entity, the *ens quod natum est convenire cum omni ente*, is the soul (*anima*). (Heidegger, 1962: 34)

If it were possible to live in a world in which we interacted *without* models, where there were no explanatory models or models of care for people with acquired diffuse neuro-cognitive dysfunction, what would be the basis of these person-to-person interactions? We can put this in a less conditional way: when we interact at the most basic level, as human beings meeting afresh with authentic friendship (*sans* models, *sans* preconceptions, *sans* ambitions, *sans* agendas, *sans* jealousies, *sans* everything that might be a form of selfishness, egocentricity, or narcissism), when we form that instinctive bond (which is a manifestation of love if not love itself), what is it that connects? I wish to say 'the soul'. In Chapter 3, I alluded to the mystery that surrounds the soul. It is the soul on which I now wish to shed some light.

In that basic interaction, which is certainly possible (even if worldly concerns often undermine the authenticity of the experience) especially between people who are in love (which is, perhaps, most immediately captured in poetry), I wish to say that the bond is at the level of the soul. We might be inclined to say such encounters are a meeting of minds—something metaphysical—which takes us in the direction of dualism. Or we might wish to argue that these instinctive interactions are a matter of bodily chemistry, of pheromones and surges in hormones and neurotransmitters, which would take us in the direction of physicalism. But there is a notion of the soul that takes the middle route. Whether Heidegger's use of ancient philosophers is accurate in its interpretation, it is certainly useful to look back at what they wrote, which turns out to be thoroughly modern in its implications.

Aristotle states in *De Anima*:

> … we should not ask whether the soul and body are one, any more than whether the wax and the impression are one, or in general whether the matter of each thing and that of which it is the matter are one. (Aristotle, 1968: 9 [412b6])

In other words, although we can talk of the wax and the impression in the wax as two different things, the wax is not separate from the impression and the impression is not other than the wax. For thinkers such as Aristotle (384–322 BC) and later St. Thomas Aquinas (c. 1225–1274), the soul is thought of as the animator, as that which gives life. Aquinas agrees with Aristotle that the soul and the body form a unity, which is staunchly anti-dualist, as is shown by his insistence that human beings are soul and body.

> ... it belongs to the very conception of 'human being' that there be soul, flesh and bone. (*Summa theologica* Ia. 75. 4; quoted in Davies, 1992: 210)

Aquinas is not a dualist, but nor does he think the soul is a body. As Brian Davies explains:

> ... though he denies that they are two distinct things [soul and body], he still feels obliged to distinguish between what is true of people and what is true of bodies. That is because he holds that the human soul cannot be something corporeal, though it must be something subsisting. (Davies, 1992: 211–12)

Aquinas holds that there must be a principle of life that marks the difference between living and non-living things; and this cannot be a body, otherwise any material thing whatsoever (e.g. my desk)—anything with a body—would be alive. But the soul is 'subsisting' and Davies explains this as follows:

> 'When Fred has knowledge, there is more to Fred than what can be seen, touched, weighed, and so on. As Aquinas puts it, there is intellect or intellectual life, and it is by virtue of this that Fred is the kind of thing he is (a rational animal). Aquinas calls this 'that by virtue of which Fred is the kind of thing he is' Fred's 'soul'. So he can say that Fred is bodily but also that Fred is (or has) both body and soul. The two cannot be torn apart in any way that would leave Fred intact. But they can be distinguished from each other, and the soul of Fred can therefore be thought of as something subsisting immaterially' (Davies *op. cit.*: 212–13).

The modernity of this view can be seen if we compare it with the notion of the body-subject derived from Merleau-Ponty (see Chapter 2, pp. 46–50), which suggests that our body has a subjective character and that our subjectivity is embodied. This is the embodied selfhood described by Kontos (2004). Or, as Merleau-Ponty says:

> The body is our general medium for having a world. (Merleau-Ponty, 1962: 169)

The implication is that our total mental life is intrinsically embodied; and yet we *have* a world: our subjective nature is a reality. Indeed, Eric Matthews suggests that the notion of the 'body-subject' places the body, 'on the subject-side of experience rather than the object-side' (Matthews, 1996: 92). But the body is still the 'general medium' for having subjective experience. Elsewhere, Matthews has summed this up as follows:

> On this view, in short, the subject of thought, feeling, intention, desire, hope etc. is neither a Cartesian 'mind', existing independently of anything material, nor a 'brain', in the sense of a piece of physical machinery, operating according to physicochemical laws, but a *person*, a human being with a body (including a brain) capable of formulating and expressing thoughts, feelings, intentions, etc. (Matthews, 2007: 98)

So we can point to a notion of the soul that sums up the kind of thing that a being is (Aquinas), which is intrinsically embodied, but none the less subjective (Merleau-Ponty) or immaterial (Aquinas). As Wittgenstein said:

> The human body is the best picture of the human soul. (PI p. 178)

But what is the phenomenon, the thing itself? We can gain a purchase on this by returning to the idea of the basic human interaction described above. Between 1932 and 1934 Wittgenstein wrote:

> The face is the soul of the body. (CV p. 23)

We should recall here the work of Emmanuel Lévinas (1906–1995), for whom the face had such significance, as described by Gillett:

> … the face of the other is the fundamental ethical stimulus because it signals a being who should call me to respond because of his or her very nature (hence ethics is grounded in ontology). (Gillett, 2008: 131)

It is, after all, through the face that we mainly (but certainly not entirely) judge emotions: hope and joy, sadness and anger, thoughtfulness and apathy are all seen in the face in ways that are infinitely subtle. Wittgenstein talks of 'reading' different emotions into a face (PI §537) and makes a direct comparison with music:

> The reinterpretation of a facial expression can be compared to the reinterpretation of a chord in music, when we hear it as a modulation first into this, then into that key. (PI §536)

Elsewhere, just after he has spoken of music as a means of communicating feelings, he writes of what it means to have the same facial expression (CV p. 38). Or again:

> A theme, no less than a face, wears an expression. (CV p. 52)

He goes on to say, 'The theme interacts with language' (*ibid.*).

This takes us back to the discussion in Chapter 4 concerning the understanding of music. A link is possible between the importance of the face as a means to understand the soul and the way in which music is understood. Music is like language in that both can be understood or misunderstood; and so too with human faces. There is the possibility of correct and incorrect interpretations, i.e. normativity is at work. I argued in Chapter 4 that the constitutive nature of normativity means that the mere possibility of engagement in patterned practices of the requisite type is enough in principle to support the claim that human life *as such* is characteristic of persons. Thus, Barbara's interpretation of Malcolm's love of music even in the severe stages of his illness is important, partly because it is a telling example of how interpretation depends on shared background knowledge, but also because it shows Malcolm engaging in human reactions (which amount to meaningful practices), as shown (in part) by his facial responses, which immediately situate him as a person in a particular surround (i.e. with a particular history, family, culture, habitus, set of values and social repertoires, and so on). The embedded nature of intentional mental states in these human practices—as shown by facial expressions—gestures in the direction of the situated, human-worldly context of persons.

The soul, as expressed by the face, is partly everyday and humdrum. In a sense, to see the soul *just is* characteristically how we see people, how we interpret and understand them: we see and understand them (in large measure through their faces) as *beings of this type*. Wittgenstein admits that we can think of people as automata (e.g. they would have fixed expressions and walk as if in a trance), but he then challenges himself, 'to keep hold of this idea in the midst of your ordinary intercourse with others, in the street, say!' (PI §420). His suggestion is that this cannot be maintained. Later he writes:

> 'I believe that he is not an automaton', just like that, so far makes no sense.
> My attitude towards him is an attitude towards a soul. I am not of the *opinion* that he has a soul (PI p. 178)

We know what it is to be a human person, largely through the human face. It is this—i.e. any particular authentic (or inauthentic) human exchange—that tells us something about the nature of our being qua human beings. And it is this, I am suggesting, that amounts to the human soul. In other words, we arrive at the level of the soul by looking at the phenomena of ordinary human life in detail, but we have to clear away the day-to-day concerns to arrive at what is essential in our human encounters. Perhaps this is captured in the letter Wittgenstein wrote to his former pupil and friend, Maurice O'Connor Drury (1907–1976), when Drury had experienced a bad time with a patient:

> 'Look at your patients more closely as human beings in trouble and enjoy more the opportunity you have to say 'good night' to so many people. This alone is a gift from heaven which many people would envy you. And this sort of thing ought to heal your frayed soul, I believe. ... I think in some sense you don't look at people's faces closely enough' (Rhees, 1981: 110)

So, in a sense, the soul is obvious as a phenomenon: 'that by virtue of which Fred is the kind of thing he is' (Davies *op. cit.*). But can we get a better conception of the soul or are we left at the level of human exchanges and the phenomena of everyday encounters? Can we move beyond the language that describes these encounters (which would be like asking if we can get to the thing we understand in music,—to its whatness)?

Well, even if the face of the Other, according to Lévinas, is the stimulus to a response that acknowledges the person's essentially ethical being, the Other also shows us 'strangeness'.

> Levinas argues that the face of the other is not encompassable within one's own view of the world and what goes on in it represents an unknown. (Gillett, 2008: 131)

But, according to Lévinas, this encounter with the Other as something unknown takes us to absolute Otherness, a sense of transcendence, beyond Being in a way that cannot be comprehended (Lévinas, 1981). According to Lévinas, awareness of this transcendent Otherness amounts to an encounter with God. For Lévinas, however, our sense of religion is rooted 'in our concern with fellow human beings' (Matthews, 1996: 162).

> Positively, we will say that since the Other looks at me, I am responsible for him, without even having *taken* on responsibilities in his regard; his responsibility *is incumbent on me*. (Lévinas, 1985: 96)

So, beyond the individual encounter with the face of the Other, the notion of transcendence (as used by Lévinas) still leads us to the centrality of our relationships with human beings, *merely because of the kind of beings that we are*. Our souls, that is to say, are manifest in the context of our being-with-others.

To get further than this, to the thing-in-itself, is to move beyond the phenomenon to Kant's concept of the noumenon, which we touched upon in Chapter 2 (see p. 31). The noumenon served the function of limiting the reach of sensibility. In Wittgenstein's philosophy, much the same point is made by talk of the limits of language. As Wittgenstein wrote early on: 'All philosophy is a "critique of language". . .' (TLP §4.0031), which obviously parallels (or parodies) Kant's *Critique of Pure Reason*. Later, Wittgenstein famously wrote: 'Philosophy is a battle against the bewitchment of our intelligence by means of language' (PI §109). He also wrote, in 1931, that as long as language remains the same, people will keep, 'stumbling over the same difficulties and find themselves staring at something which no explanation seems capable of clearing up' (CV p. 15). Hence, we shall always require philosophy. He continued:

> And what's more, this satisfies a longing for the transcendent, because in so far as people think they can see the 'limits of human understanding', they believe of course that they can see beyond these. (*ibid.*)

At which point, in our search for the soul, we need to see that we cannot penetrate the transcendent realm of *noumena*, even if such a realm is the result of rational analysis.

> The existence of things in themselves (*noumena*), including human beings, is necessitated by our rational and transcendental analysis of experience, but only knowable in so far as we have developed techniques for their characterization. Oneself as subject, the psychically informed centre of subjectivity, is inscrutable in just this way and knowable only as a psychological and embodied being. (Gillett, 2008: 82)

By satisfying ourselves with engagement in the world as it is, however, we can know what kind of things we are as human beings. This does, after all (especially in our encounters with others), give us rational access to something—albeit ineffable and inscrutable—that is immaterial in the sense used by Aquinas, but none the less a transcendent feature of our bodily lives as situated, agentive subjects. Our phenomenal lives in this sense are manifest as souls, not as separate from our bodies, but informing them (because having a soul is no more than to be a living being of this kind) as human beings interacting with the world. And, I have argued, being these kind of bodies and these kind of subjectivities—souls of this sort—means that the potential for people with acquired diffuse neurocognitive dysfunction to retain their standing as persons in the world persists through their sharing in the histories and bodily forms of human beings.

These reflections, on the nature of our being as embodied subjects, and the role of habitus, which can incorporate the background psychological and social histories of people, and combine with them in an embodied way to define the person's situated standing as a being-in-the-world of this kind with particular sorts of engagement with others in such a way as to show the soul, i.e. the form of being that we all share as human beings of this kind, are not merely theoretical. They find support in the experience of real people. For they are also seen in Barbara's reflections about her husband, Malcolm, even in the midst of her involvement with his care.

> Malcolm is surrounded by love. We reach out to communicate with him at a profound level—often through eye contact and gentle whispering and touch—and from him there flows a deep childlike trust, luminosity and reciprocating love—as though it were his very self, the self he was born with, that we are privileged to glimpse. ... Does it matter what we call it—spirit, soul, inner self, essence, identity—so long as we have experienced it?
>
> ... So the search for spirituality and the real Malcolm ends here—in the revelation of his essential self because of the loving care he receives and the trust that it engenders. (Pointon, 2007: 119)

The phenomenon emerges in the rawness of this intimate encounter, where, without models or theories, the self meets the self as beings (souls) of this kind in the world.

> To stand stripped of everything the world values and to see each other as we really are is a very precious and humbling experience, and one I would never have encountered were it not for the ravages of dementia (*ibid.*).

Dementia-in-the-world

Malcolm's sketch and his narrative, which is a shared narrative with Barbara, root us in the real world of human encounters. These everyday encounters, which are bodily and psychical, once seen as authentic (in some sense), as stripped of the ephemera of human busy-ness and egotism, occur at the level of the human soul. They define us as the kind of beings that we are. Before concluding this chapter, I want to refer back to Heidegger. In Chapter 2, I mentioned his notion of 'Being-with' (*Mitsein*) and the ways in which he regarded 'concern' (*Besorgen*) and 'solicitude' (*Fürsorge*) as of fundamental importance for Dasein (see pp. 45–48). For completeness, Heidegger also uses the concept of 'care' (*Sorge*). There is a gradation in terms of the level of engagement with Being and the world contained in these three technical terms. They are certainly not intended to be taken in their ordinary senses.

> Because Being-in-the-world is essentially care, Being-alongside the ready-to-hand could be taken ... as *concern*, and Being with the Dasein-with of Others as we encounter it within-the-world could be taken as *solicitude*. (Heidegger, 1962: 237)

The concept of 'care' emerges in response to Heidegger's treatment of anxiety, which is the human existent's (Dasein's) response to finding itself 'thrown' into the world.

The concomitant to this state of being-in-the-world, which intrinsically involves anxiety, is care: 'Dasein's Being reveals itself as *care*' (Heidegger, 1962: 227). The concept of 'concern' is more to do with what might be called the practical or instrumental dealings with the world. Heidegger refers to, 'circumspective dealings with the ready-to-hand within-the-world', which he then calls 'concern' (*op. cit.*: 157). But the most engaged of these concepts is 'solicitude':

> Concern is a character-of-Being which Being-with cannot have as its own, even though Being-with, like concern, is a *Being towards* entities encountered within-the-world. But those entities towards which Dasein as Being-with comports itself do not have the kind of Being which belongs to equipment ready-to-hand; they are themselves Dasein. These entities are not objects of concern, but rather of *solicitude*. (*ibid.*)

The reason for mentioning these technical distinctions from Heidegger is because I want now to introduce the notion of *dementia-in-the-world*.

Seeing the person with acquired diffuse neurocognitive dysfunction as having a soul, which defines the individual as a particular kind of being, as one potentially open to the possibility of engagement with normatively constrained practices that constitute intentional mental states, where this in turn entails (partly through the mind's externality) being-in-the-world as a narratively, historically, culturally, situated embodied agent, seeing the person in these ways puts emphasis on the notion of the world and what it might be to be-in-the-world. Heidegger devotes Chapter III of Part One of Division One of *Being and Time* to a discussion of 'The Worldhood of the World'. Without going into details, once again there is a gradation: from the world as the totality of entities that we come across and use in the world, to the nature of the Being of those entities, to the nature of the Being of the world in which human beings exist, to the 'a priori character of worldhood in general' (Heidegger, 1962: 93). I shall try briefly to capture some of the flavour of the discussion.

Heidegger notes that, '. . . the world is always the one that I share with Others', and he goes on to discuss what happens when Others are encountered (*op. cit.*: 155). His point (to paraphrase) is that such encounters are not disengaged events: it is not like seeing one among others and picking this person, nor is it a matter of talking with others using a model based on how we look at ourselves. Rather,

> They are encountered from out of the *world*, in which concernfully circumspective Dasein essentially dwells. Theoretically concocted 'explanations' of the Being-present-at-hand of Others urge themselves upon us all too easily; but over against such explanations we must hold fast to the phenomenal facts of the case which we have pointed out, namely, that Others are encountered *environmentally*. (*ibid.*)

We need to understand what Heidegger means by 'environmentally', but it is possible to note already that the message squares with the theme of this chapter: there is some sort of encounter with others that is outside models and beyond theories, which involves an engagement at the phenomenal level, person to person (soul to soul), in the context of concern and solicitude. To hammer the point home, this is the sort of engagement described by Barbara Pointon in connection with her husband, Malcolm, in the quotations at the end of the last section.

In the same passage, Heidegger refers to this 'elemental worldly kind of encountering, which belongs to Dasein and is closest to it'. He states:

> Dasein finds 'itself' proximally in *what* it does, uses, expects, avoids—in those things environmentally ready-to-hand with which it is proximally *concerned*. (*ibid.*)

This may be taken, according to my understanding, to mean that (potentially) the soul can be encountered in our ordinary, everyday encounters, in our comings and goings.

But what does he mean by the environment? Heidegger talks about discovering entities that one 'encounters environmentally', and then says:

> For the environment is a structure which even biology as a positive science can never find and can never define, but must presuppose and constantly employ. Yet, even as an *a priori* condition for the objects which biology takes for its theme, this structure itself can be explained philosophically only if it has been conceived beforehand as a structure of Dasein. (Heidegger, 1962: 84)

In other words, the environment is understood transcendentally, as a ground for the possibility of disciplines such as biology that study the world in one particular way, as physical entities. More importantly, however, the environment is part of what it is to be a human existent. This is to emphasize the characterization of Dasein precisely as Being-*in-the-world*. The world, the environment, is constitutive of the kind of beings that we are as human beings. In a particular (ontological) way, the world has significance for us. Later, Heidegger writes:

> And, significance, as worldhood, is tied up with the existential 'for-the-sake-of-which'. Since the worldhood of that world in which every Dasein essentially is already, is thus constituted, it accordingly lets us encounter what is environmentally ready-to-hand as something with which we are circumspectively concerned, and it does so in such a way that together with it we encounter the Dasein-with of Others. The structure of the world's worldhood is such that Others are not proximally present-at-hand as free-floating subjects along with other Things, but show themselves in the world in their special environmental Being ... (Heidegger, 1962: 160)

In short, we are not disengaged beings-in-the-world, but are characterized by our worldly engagements.

A person with dementia, therefore, is always a being-in-the-world. This follows from the Wittgensteinian transcendental account of normativity, where this establishes criteria of correctness for our use of language, for our understanding of music, and for the interpretation of faces, as being embedded (constitutively, immanently, and irreducibly) in worldly practices. So, to understand the person with dementia is always to understand something about the world. Moreover, dementia itself is a feature of the world, a phenomenon in its own right, which requires broad conceptualization. It is dementia-in-the-world, where this encompasses the understanding implied by the ascription of 'acquired diffuse neurocognitive dysfunction', where it suggests the need for solicitude, but where there can also be the 'luminosity and reciprocating love' described by Barbara Pointon (*vide supra*), as well as the possibility of meaningful engagement, communication difficulties, the possibility of humour, the need to attend to appropriate environments of care, and to enable a good death, to name but a few of the elements of the world of dementia. The view of dementia encouraged by the notion of dementia-in-the-world is a broadening one: it refuses to be reductive; it looks to the thing itself, acknowledging the impossibility of fully encompassing that which it is, but in the hope of shedding light on it; it embraces the world as a constitutive feature of dementia; it gives a perspective on the surround, on the notion of Being-with, on the need for solidarity[5] with those engaged in caring.

Acquired diffuse neurocognitive dysfunction involves a loss of cognitive function. The person with dementia is, to a lesser or greater extent, no longer able to enjoy the intentional mental states of understanding certain things, of remembering others, or of making calculations. To understand this phenomenon, however, we have to understand that the failure is not just of the brain, nor is it simply a functional failure of internal processing, nor is it just a failure in the field of social practices. It is a failure in the realm of normativity too, where normativity—as we have seen—is world-involving.

If I have acquired diffuse neurocognitive dysfunction I make mistakes: I refer to my daughter as my wife. This is a mistake in the rational realm where certain normative constraints operate. But the rational, normatively structured realm has to be understood, in accordance with the Wittgensteinian analysis, in terms of embedded practices in the world. This rational (normative) shaping of the world (which is potentially, but not essentially, public) gives sense to the notion of *failure* of (e.g.) episodic recall memory.

Furthermore, the description of the realm that I (as someone with acquired diffuse neurocognitive dysfunction) and others (at least potentially) inhabit must be rich in order to capture the full sense of normativity. The embedded practices in which normativity, as a constitutive, immanent, and irreducible feature, is transgressed in dementia will involve a history and cultural environment. This will itself depend upon individual histories of people, which will in turn depend upon numerous physical (both biological and geographical), psychological, social and spiritual factors. In other words, because normativity involves contextual embedding and because (as the Wittgensteinian analysis implies) intentional psychological states require an externalist account, the rational requirement for normativity entails the world. It is not that these factors are a necessary condition for normativity, it is simply that normativity brings into play (potentially) all that we mean by the world: its places, practices, traditions, cultures, history, physical features, and everything else. So, an understanding of acquired diffuse neurocognitive dysfunction entails an understanding of the world. This is itself a transcendental claim: in order to understand acquired diffuse neurocognitive dysfunction—as a prerequisite to such understanding—we must have an understanding of the world in all its features. In short, to understand dementia is to understand dementia-in-the-world.

Dementia-in-the-world brings awareness of the worldly embedding practices that make up the world of embodied agents-in-the-world. But it is the *human* world or, at least, the world from the human perspective. The shared background, context, culture, habitus, history and life, in which the practices that underpin the normativity of thought and language embed, is human. It is also true that we share the world with dolphins and primates, but the normative realm in which dementia is understood is specifically human. Although for other reasons we might wish to keep such anthropo-morphic sentiments in check,[6] it is important to note, with respect to the normativity of intentional psychological phenomena, that the issue is how such phenomena relate to the human realm, even if that realm is a part of (and only properly understood in the context of) the world we share with dolphins and primates. It might be that one day we have to acknowledge that other worldly creatures and extraterrestrials have a perspective on normativity. That would require an extension of our concepts and our thoughts, but there is no reason at present to deny that our understanding of dementia-in-the-world is, unavoidably, an understanding of the human world, by which I mean an understanding from the human perspective, which will feature in the discussion of Chapter 8.

Dementia-in-the-world is a concept that aims to make us aware of the full implica-tions of dementia. This is not *just* a matter of a technical fix. It is a matter that raises some of the most complex medical, psychological, social, ethical, and spiritual prob-lems that can arise anywhere in clinical and social care practice. In this sense, it is 'of the world'. Dealing with dementia involves dealing with a potentially broad array of different problems, which are decidedly in the world. Dementia-in-the-world, as a notion, also points in the direction of hope. If the problems associated with dementia can be alleviated, they will be alleviated by the world and by our (biological, psycho-logical, social, and spiritual) engagements with the world.

Conclusion

Much of this chapter has been concerned with the nature of human encounters and our understanding of such encounters in the light of the analysis of previous chapters. There are three aspects to consider. First, there is the background to the encounters, which is, after all, the world. But it is the world conceived broadly (and not through the narrowing lens of a model), as habitus for instance, and in such a way as to allow it to form a constitutive part of what it is to be a human being. It is against the particu-lar background of our knowledge of Malcolm Pointon's life narrative that we can attempt to understand the content of his sketch and of his other behaviours. In reality this means understanding behaviours and language used in the context of (against the background of) the world and our worldly engagements. By our nature, we cannot be disengaged inhabitants of the world. It is *our* world. Secondly, there is the phenome-nological aspect of these encounters, which turn out to reflect, once they are seen in the raw as ontological and ethical events, our Being at the level of the human soul. Once the face of the Other has been seen, what emerges is an appreciation of the kind of beings that we are as human beings-in-the-world. We cannot ultimately pin down (neither in language nor in reason) this phenomenon—the quiddity of the immaterial soul—except that in authentic everyday exchanges (such as those between Barbara and Malcolm even when he was in the advanced stages of the disease) we gain some sense of the transcendent reality of the soul as informing our lives as mutually engaged embodied subjects. Thirdly, there is the centrality of our relationships. These reflect our being as kinds of this sort—of flesh, blood, and soul—situated in the world. A human being *of this sort* occupies the world and shapes it in accordance with characteristic normatively constrained embedded worldly practices. And a person with dementia, such as Malcolm Pointon, will be a human person as an inevitable consequence of his or her situated and embodied life history.

Endnotes

[1] 'The Dreamtime (or Dreaming) is a term used to describe the period before living memory when Spirits emerged from beneath the earth and from the sky to create the land forms and all living things. The Dreamtime stories set down the laws for social and moral order and establish the cultural patterns and customs.' From: http://www.aboriginalartstore.com.au/aboriginal-art-culture/aboriginal-dreamtime.php [accessed 3 July, 2010].

[2] 'State interference in social relations becomes, in one domain after another, superfluous, and then dies down of itself. The government of persons is replaced by the administration of things, and by the conduct of processes of production. The state is not "abolished". It withers away.' From: Engels (1969): Part III, chapter 2: 332–3.

[3] For a fuller discussion of models in science than I can hope to give, see the comprehensive discussion by Roman Frigg and Stephan Hartmann (2006) on the extremely useful website (see Bibliography) of the *Stanford Encyclopedia of Philosophy*.

[4] This is Heidegger's shorthand for understanding 'phenomenology' (cf. Heidegger, 1962: 58).

[5] The notion of 'solidarity' emerges as a key part of the ethical framework suggested in *Dementia: Ethical Issues*. It is: '. . . the idea that we are all 'fellow-travellers' and that we have duties to support and help each other and in particular those who cannot readily support themselves. (Nuffield Council on Bioethics, 2009: p. 29, §2.43).

[6] See, for example, 'Is a dolphin a person?' in Midgley 1996: 107–17.

Part IV

Personhood and the world

Chapter 8

From dementia-in-the-world to the human-person-perspective

On the Move
Take yourself back to the first time
you saw them doing it. Hither and thither
and thither and thither.
It seems definitely not just
absentmindedly. It seems as if
people have something on their mind.
Going A to B to C to D to E ………
They seem to be so restless.
I think to myself they must get
awfully tired. There seems to be
an awful lot of movement.
It doesn't strike you at first.
But then everybody's doing it.
It is really rather shattering,
because you've been surprised
by others doing it, and then you find
that you are doing it yourself!
(*On the Move* from *Openings*;
John Killick & Carl Cordonnier, 2000)

Introduction

In the last chapter, I spoke of the possibility of a world without models, in which personal encounters might be at the level of the soul. Our interactions would then be of a fashion that acknowledged our mutual standing as beings *of this kind* in this human world. This is the asymptote for our explanatory models and models of care. The following quote is an expression of how the world might be for all of us (including those with acquired diffuse neurocognitive dysfunction) as we participate meaningfully in our shared world of concern and solicitude; (it might have been written by Tom Kitwood as he imagined residential and nursing homes putting into practice person-centred care):

> Supposing that we had [participated] in a human manner; each of us would in his [participation] have doubly affirmed himself and his fellow men. I would have: (1) objectified in my [participation] my individuality and its peculiarity and thus both in my activity enjoyed an individual expression of my life and also ... have had the individual pleasure of realizing that my personality was objective, visible to the senses and thus a power raised beyond all doubt. (2) In your enjoyment ... I would have had the direct enjoyment of realizing that I had both satisfied a human need by my [action] and also objectified the human essence and therefore fashioned for another human being the object that met his need. (3) I would have been for you the mediator between you and the species and thus been acknowledged and felt by you as a completion of your own essence and a necessary part of yourself and have thus realized that I am confirmed both in your thought and in your love. (4) In my expression of my life I would have fashioned your expression of your life, and thus in my own activity have realized my own essence, my human, my communal essence. (quoted in McLellan, 1975: 34–5)

If not Kitwood, then one might have thought this was a religious thinker, such as Martin Buber. In fact—apart from changing 'produced' to [participated], 'production' to [participation], and 'work' to [action]—this comes from the posthumously published *Economic and Philosophical Manuscripts* (EPM) of 1844 by Karl Marx (1818–1883). He wrote this to indicate how the world might be in the absence of *alienation*. Of course, Marx used the notion of 'alienated labour' in a technical sense, which mostly referred to the economic realities of capitalism as he saw it, but which he also used in connection with religion and the State. The notion of alienation, albeit interpreted freely, is one I shall come back to in this chapter. This is what Marx wrote elsewhere in the same work:

> Every alienation of man from himself and from Nature appears in the relation which he postulates between other men and himself and Nature. ... In the real world of practice, this self-alienation can only be expressed in the real, practical relation of man to his fellow men. (EPM, *Marx-Engels Gesamtausgabe* I/3: 91; quoted in Marx, 1961:177)

The concept of alienation seems to capture what it is like to have dementia. The lack of meaningful engagement for people with acquired diffuse neurocognitive dysfunction (in care homes for instance) means that they become estranged and alienated from those around them. Part of the work of this chapter is to look at how this is so and how it might be better. The notion of dementia-in-the-world, introduced in the last chapter, is intended to locate dementia in a broader field of concern, where people with acquired diffuse neurocognitive dysfunction are inherently more engaged with the worldly environment simply because of their standing as beings of this kind. If we are still playing the Marxist card, we might summarize the discussion of the last chapter by saying that the problem of models is precisely that they alienate us from our true selves. We start to see the person through the lens of the model and the person him or herself also starts to feel alienated from his or her true self because of the awareness of deficit. I shall say more about this in the first section of this chapter, where I draw on earlier comments from Chapter 3, on externalism of the mind, to make the link between dementia-in-the-world and the human-person-perspective.

In the second section, I want to expand the discussion of the human-person-perspective and make overt links with the SEA view of Chapter 2. I intend to focus on the issue of severe acquired diffuse neurocognitive dysfunction in order to understand the contribution the SEA view makes under these circumstances (this will allow further consideration of some of the views of Steve Sabat); and, to gain more understanding of the notion of the human-person-perspective, I shall also consider thought around the issue of behaviour that challenges in dementia. This discussion will lead to further reflections on the ideas of narrative and selfhood. The poem with which this chapter opens is the result of words transcribed and edited by John Killick, but spoken by a person with dementia. In the poem we catch a glimpse of the embodied subjectivity of someone with acquired diffuse neurocognitive dysfunction. It should be enough to convince us that 'challenging behaviour', pacing say, must be taken as a sign of something else: something yet to be interpreted, but reflective of the strength of persisting selfhood. As Kate Allan and John Killick say elsewhere:

> In our view a fundamental principle of supportive care should be to assume that no matter how disabled the person with dementia is, they continue to have strengths, and that those in a supporting role should seek to discover and work with these strengths to the greatest possible extent. This applies both broadly in working with the person, and specifically in relation to communication. (Allan & Killick, 2010: 220)

The idea of alienation resonates with Heidegger's idea that the human existent, Dasein, might lose itself in the 'they'. This is an explication of what it is, on Heidegger's view, to lead an inauthentic existence, that is, an existence that takes no account of the true nature of our Being, which is in part a 'Being-towards-death'. To absorb the idea of Being-towards-death, to anticipate this possibility in a way that makes the nature of human existence plain, is to open up the potential for a more authentic existence. But 'lostness in the "they" ' closes the possibility of authenticity down.

> So Dasein makes no choices, gets carried along by the nobody, and thus ensnares itself in inauthenticity. This process can be reversed only if Dasein specifically brings itself back to itself from its lostness in the 'they' (Heidegger, 1962: 312)

The idea of lostness in the 'they' is one that will also return, along with the idea of alienation, through the course of this chapter.

Thus, in the third section, I shall return to the problems of models and I shall raise anew the issue of diagnosis, which allows me to mention recent controversial views expressed by Peter Whitehouse with his colleague Daniel George. I shall also return to the tension discussed in Chapter 6, because it is still not clear how we should approach the individual: to what extent, if we are aiming for validity in our diagnoses, can we afford to make an individualized interpretation? It is through the type of individualized, personal encounter, which we saw in the last chapter between Barbara and Malcolm, that one can hope to arrive at phenomenological understanding, which, on my view, stands over against the type of understanding possible through models of any sort. Understanding the human existent will inevitably involve, on this view, care and solicitude.

In the final section of the chapter, before concluding, I want to emphasize the extent to which the human-person-perspective is uncircumscribable. It should impel us in the direction of a revolution in terms of our attitudes in which nothing that is part of broadly conceived human flourishing is out of the question. Hence, in this chapter I shall flesh out an account of the human-person-perspective:

◆ It is the perspective from and in which we understand dementia-in-the-world.

◆ It brings into view the normative nature of the world and makes use of the conception of persons as situated embodied agents.

◆ It can accommodate other models of acquired diffuse neurocognitive dysfunction, inasmuch as they are genuinely useful, but it is the lack of this perspective which makes them otherwise circumscribed.

◆ It is uncircumscribable, because what it is to be a person is open-ended.

The human-person-perspective and dementia-in-the-world

Dementia is dementia-in-the-world. It is a situated phenomenon. It has to be regarded in this light. To try to understand dementia without the background context of the world might succeed in explaining something, as e.g. the disease model clearly does, but it cannot give us the broad understanding that will allow the different views—those of the person with dementia and the family carer, as well as those of the neuroscientists—to come into full focus: the possibility of a surview is precluded. The broad understanding needs to accommodate the normative as well as the physical realms; it will provide a constitutive account as well as a causal one. For the point about dementia-in-the-world is precisely that a full understanding of acquired diffuse neurocognitive dysfunction inherently involves the world, with all that this entails when described in norm-rich detail.

The message from Chapter 1 was that our judgements about acquired diffuse neurocognitive dysfunction will reflect background understandings. Not only, therefore, does dementia-in-the-world imply that acquired diffuse neurocognitive dysfunction has to be regarded as an embedded phenomenon, but, in addition, we (as persons) are embedded in the selfsame world. For this reason, if for no other, we should show solidarity with all those involved. Hence, our understanding of the world, our grasp of the normatively structured concerns and worldly points of view, will impinge upon our understanding of dementia. If our view of the world is one in which we have a limited idea of what constitute cognitive phenomena, and cannot see that the normative structuring of such phenomena reaches right up to the world in which they are situated, if we operate with a limited 'cognitive paradigm', then our understanding of dementia will be limited too.

Dementia-in-the-world, therefore, highlights the importance of the worldly context from which and in which dementia must be understood if it is to be understood broadly. The idea of a metaphysical conceit, mentioned in Chapter 3, is again evident. Just as, in Marvell's poem (see p. 57), the Mind was conceived as transcendentally able to create, 'Far other Worlds, and other Seas', so too, dementia-in-the-world not only implies that we should think broadly about dementia, but it also implies that 'the world' is contained within dementia. Just as an understanding of Dasein involves understanding the way in which the world *is* for the human existent, not as something separate, but as something constitutive, so too for dementia-in-the-world. No real understanding of dementia—one that is not bounded by the perspective of a model—can ignore the constitutive role that the world plays. In part this is because of the link between the mind and dementia, whereby key features of acquired diffuse neurocognitive dysfunction must be understood as reflecting worldly embedded human practices, which show normativity as a constitutive, immanent, and irreducible feature. But this worldly context is the human context of persons. The perspective from which and in which dementia-in-the-world has to be understood becomes, accordingly, the human-person-perspective.

Dementia occurs, is lived with—by those who have the condition and by their carers—and is studied (e.g. by neuroscientists), in the context of human persons. Judgements about people with acquired diffuse neurocognitive dysfunction, such as Miss Breen, are made in comparison with other human persons: the normative constraints that allow us to judge that she is profoundly disoriented reflect human practices deeply embedded in the world. Furthermore, our understanding of Miss Breen will reflect our grasp of the significance of the concerns and values that surround her and which are rooted in the world. It is partly our shared grasp of these concerns and values, which shape the world, that allows us to understand Miss Breen. What we share, therefore, is the human-person-perspective, which is the perspective required to understand dementia-in-the-world. But, as we shall see, this perspective, precisely because it is 'in-the-world', cannot be bounded. Any tendency to say that our values are secure and the best will always be defeasible.

In Chapter 3, I made the point that the notion of the world being *constitutive* of the mind is central to externalism. If so, then this is still the case for people with acquired diffuse neurocognitive dysfunction. Their minds will be peopled by the external world. If this is a world from which they are alienated, either through their own disabilities, or through the behaviour of others, their mental lives become shallow. But it need not be so. All the more reason to enrich the environment for people with acquired diffuse neurocognitive dysfunction, if this is a way to enrich their (mental) lives. For, to enrich their (mental) lives is to confirm their standing as persons-in-the-world, which we should be inclined to do because of our standing alongside, our solidarity with them as beings-of-this-human-type-in-the-world. And this sharing of a background is to have a particular perspective on the surround that constitutes our world. There is, then, a direct pathway from our understanding of dementia-in-the-world, which draws on the externalist conception of mind, to the human-person-perspective.

The human-person-perspective and the situated embodied agent view

The situated embodied agent (SEA) view of the person helps us to understand dementia, because it helps to elucidate the human-person-perspective of dementia-in-the-world. This perspective involves all of the considerations that I outlined in considering the SEA view in Chapter 2. So, the person is situated in a richly textured context of culture, time and place; in a narrative history which has a past and future and which interconnects with the narratives of others; in a world shaped by certain normative concerns, which are themselves based upon deeply rooted practices and customs. And the situatedness is also a matter of embodiment, since to be a human person is to have a human body, which helps to provide the narrative continuity and connectedness that is a part of the wholeness of our lives. But our embodiment also contains the causal possibilities that explain and determine our lives (at least at a causal level). Meanwhile, as persons we are agents too: acting within the framework of our embodied and situated natures; reflecting both our experience of causal interactions with the world and our understanding of the world as structured in a systematic way by our thoughts (since the having of certain thoughts precludes others and means that our understanding of the world must be thus and so to accord with such normative constraints).

Our understanding of persons helps to flesh out our understanding of dementia because both notions are embedded in the world. I have worked towards that embeddedness by an analysis of intentional mental states, an understanding of which is crucial to our understanding of both acquired diffuse neurocognitive dysfunction and persons. Coming to understand the transcendental account of intentional psychological phenomena, according to which normativity is a constitutive, immanent, and irreducible feature of embedded practices that make up the world, has provided a means of assessing models of acquired diffuse neurocognitive dysfunction. It has also led us to the human-person-perspective as the way to understand acquired diffuse neurocognitive dysfunction more broadly.

The human-person-perspective allows an understanding of acquired diffuse neurocognitive dysfunction, which recognizes the normative nature of the world. For what it is to see acquired diffuse neurocognitive dysfunction from this perspective is to see it within a normatively structured context, in which we too are situated. The world of human persons is underpinned by, because thought and language are underpinned by, normatively structured and deeply embedded worldly practices, where normativity is constitutive, immanent, and irreducible. The Wittgensteinian analysis and the discussion of the human-person-perspective, therefore, are mutually supportive. Both require an appreciation of the contextual embedding that underlies the different concepts with which they deal. This is, after all, unsurprising. For the concept of a person makes links with the concept of intentional mental states. I do not think this link entails that to be a person requires there are *actually* intentional mental states (which might not be the case in severe learning disability, head injury, or acquired diffuse neurocognitive dysfunction), but the *potential* for such states is typical of these human persons. At a conceptual level, certain, typically human, normatively structured concerns must be implicit. Otherwise, it would not be possible to construct the notion of a human person from norm-free data. Persons are inevitably situated in a world of norms.

Narrative

It is often considered extremely important that persons are regarded as situated in narratives. I have already discussed, in Chapter 2, some of the ways in which philosophers have used the notion of narrative to support their accounts of personhood (see pp. 44–47). For instance, MacIntyre argues that, even if the person has forgotten or suffered a head injury so cannot give the requisite account, to be able to say that there is an intelligible narrative linking different descriptions of an individual just is to say that it is the same person.

> Thus personal identity is just that identity presupposed by the unity of the character which the unity of a narrative requires. Without such unity there would not be subjects of whom stories could be told. (MacIntyre, 1985: 218)

In this sense the notion of narrative gives unity to a life, even if the life has taken unexpected turns. MacIntyre also acknowledges that our lives are interdependent: 'The narrative of any one life is part of an interlocking set of narratives' (*ibid.*). The importance of the idea of narrative unity is, in part, that it argues against the suggestion that in dementia the person changes into a different person (which Hope (1994b) found counter-intuitive), or that (as suggested by Brock (1988) and quoted in Chapter 2) the individual ceases being a person altogether. But the unity of a life narrative gives the idea of coherence and shape to a life as well. Narrative shape and coherence provide the basis for judgements to be made about a life as a whole. In this vein, we find MacIntyre suggesting:

> The unity of a human life is the unity of a narrative quest. Quests sometimes fail, are frustrated, abandoned or dissipated into distractions; and human lives may in all these ways also fail. But the only criteria for success or failure in a human life as a whole are the criteria of success or failure in a narrated or to-be-narrated quest. (MacIntyre, *op. cit.*: 219)

The quest, according to MacIntyre, is for the good life as defined by the virtues. The importance of the virtues is not my concern here;[1] however, the idea that life as a whole has (ethical) meaning as a consequence of its narrative structure is compelling. It is also contested.

In her scholarly and compelling book, *The Long Life*, Helen Small raises questions about how suitable it is to use the notion of narrative in thinking about old age and conditions such as dementia. She notes the tendency for narrative to engender discussion of notions such as 'unity', 'progress', and 'completeness', but wonders whether these ideas are always relevant.

> … if there is severe loss of capacity, we may do better to reject the narrative view altogether. That is, we may find it kinder, and more in keeping with the person's ability to give shape to their own life, to place much less emphasis on narrative, preserving it only weakly, as a dotted line to indicate the fact of an ongoing life, but faded powers of self-direction. (Small, 2007: 104–5)

It might be that the type of formal coherence suggested by narrative is inappropriate in some of the circumstances that obtain in any life, but perhaps especially in the lives of people with acquired diffuse neurocognitive dysfunction. Small's use of literature helps to remind us that there can be meaning in lives that are less coherent, but none the less still open to quality on account of, 'images, scenes, moments, anecdotes, jokes' (Small, *op. cit.*: 106). From the human-person-perspective we can be very sympathetic to this view. The lives of people with acquired diffuse neurocognitive dysfunction might well be enlivened by moment-to-moment happenings irrespective of the overall shape or direction of their lives. Talk of narrative seems, from this viewpoint, to be superfluous.

And yet, Small does not really engage with the possibility of others holding the person's identity and maintaining his or her selfhood, which is one of the useful features of the narrative approach: our lives are co-authored, so even if I cannot recall my past, you can do this for me. Nor does Small place sufficient weight on the philosophical position of the body—the way it mediates our narratives—and the way in which this, in itself, can be viewed as providing a basis for the ascription of selfhood. We can describe our lives in various ways, with or without narrative playing a role, but this does not mean that it is illicit to use the notion for specific purposes.

Clive Baldwin has argued that the claim that the narrative approach is not relevant to people with acquired diffuse neurocognitive dysfunction is a matter of 'narrative dispossession', which probably results from,

> ... a definition of narrative that relies on verbalization, extended coherence, a limited sense of narrative agency, restricted opportunities to engage in narrative activity, and narrative illiteracy on the part of those around people with dementia. (Baldwin, 2010: 246)

Baldwin commends instead four aspects of care that might be helpful (Baldwin, 2010: 247ff.). First, 'Maintaining narrative agency', amounts to as little as talking with people, but includes the numerous ways in which we can encourage meaningful activity. Secondly, 'Establishing the emergent plot', recognizes that people can wish to maintain some control, e.g. through advance care planning, and others can engage with them to do this. Thirdly, 'A sensitivity to and an appreciation of narrative webs', which draws on our essential interdependency: the ways in which we engage with the Other (reflecting the work of Lévinas, discussed in the last chapter). Finally, 'The accumulation of narrative resources', refers to the possibility of maintaining a store of stories, which will help to maintain meaningful engagement with the person. It is sad to admit how frequently those of us who work in health and social care do not know the full histories of those we work with as patients or clients. The call for a narrative approach is no more, under these circumstances, than a plea that we should know the stories of the lives of those we seek to help, which should start from the time of assessment (Keady & Gilliard, 2002). So, my inclination, whilst accepting the force of the point encouraged by Small (2007), namely that there may be other ways to portray our lives as meaningful without narrative, is to hold onto the idea of narrative in connection with acquired diffuse neurocognitive dysfunction. For one thing, the human-person-perspective should not commit us to only one way of seeing the world: we need the broadest possible view, which can include narrative, but need not exclude other ways of understanding the person's way of being-in-the-world.

So, we are situated in our narratives, which give us a particular view of the world; and to understand others we must try to understand their narratives. In addition, it has been argued that,

> Narratives are essentially normatively structured, reason-based accounts of individual thought and action. They are the perspective from which a subject, as a person, comes into view. (Thornton, 2008)

We also need to be aware of the ways in which we co-author our lives through our mutual involvement in each other's stories. And these stories are the lives of beings like us: human beings-in-the-world. However we tell our stories (in words, in pictures, in music), they locate us in a whole way of life, with its own meanings, history, and normative constraints, which define us as the beings that we are.

> Blackfella law is really important: that's why we paint. They tell my life, my family story, they keep that story alive. My Dreaming is my painting. That story will not finish—my son will take him. (Ronnie Jackamarra Lawson, 1987).[2]

We can neither escape our situatedness, which is typically with others, nor the ethical imperatives that flow from our interdependence. The human-person-perspective must necessarily embrace these positions, which can be narratively construed or otherwise, but which form the surround to our encounters in the world.

Selfhood

This takes me back to the seminal work of Steve Sabat (2001). In Chapter 5, in connection with Sabat and Harré (1992), we came across the notions of self 1 and selves 2 (see p. 148). In Sabat (2001, 2002), the social construction of selfhood is given a broader framework.

- Self 1: '. . . is the self of personal identity which is experienced as the continuity of one's own singular point of view from which one perceives, and acts in, the world. . . . This aspect of selfhood is expressed discursively through the use of personal pronouns . . . "I," "Me," . . . "My," "Mine."' (Sabat, 2001: 17).
- Self 2: 'Such mental and physical attributes as we have at present, and have had over the course of a lifetime, along with our beliefs about those attributes, . . .' (ibid.).
- Self 3: '. . . are the ways in which one presents oneself in the world, the displays of one's personality and character' (ibid.: 18).

Even as these aspects of selfhood are described, it is apparent how they will be affected by acquired diffuse neurocognitive dysfunction.[3] Self 1 can persist late into the condition, because (e.g.) I can index my self with gestures. Self 2 can also persist, because my body persists (despite changes) and many of my mental attributes will still be identifiable late into the condition. Self 3, however, is particularly vulnerable, because, to maintain the personae that make up Self 3, I require the cooperation of others. To be the respected father, I need my children to respect me; and so on. Learning Miss Breen's narrative is, in part, for us to learn about the ways in which she has presented and would present herself to the world. We can support or undermine this presentation.

In the last chapter, I introduced Sabat's (2001, 2006a) notion of 'malignant positioning'. The ways in which the social environment can enrich or impoverish a self, which derives in part from Kitwood's (1997) 'malignant social psychology', are pervasive.

> Realistic, accurate positioning would require healthy others to take into account the effects not only of the disease itself, and the afflicted person's reactions to the effects of the disease, but also the effects of the social environment on the afflicted person's behavior. (Sabat, 2001: 111)

Positioning is evident even in the benign-seeming procedure of cognitive testing. As Sabat points out, psychometric testing which places the person below a statistically derived cut-off immediately positions the person with acquired diffuse neurocognitive dysfunction as inferior in some sense (Sabat, 2001: 166). Cognitive tests amount, therefore, to 'defectology': they show what the person cannot do, not what they can. Indeed, we know that formal cognitive testing can be upsetting both for the person afflicted with the condition and for the informal carer: having admitted that she and her husband had cried as a result of the testing, one spouse told me in an interview that she wondered why her husband could not have been more simply engaged in a conversation about politics to test his mental abilities (Hughes, Hope, Reader, and Rice, 2002). We also know that stigma can immediately follow diagnosis, which can also be described as harrowing. Indeed the whole assessment process requires careful thought (Keady & Gilliard, 2002). Corner and Bond (2006) describe a woman called Rose, in whose case (after diagnosis) there was,

> ... a marked decrease in participation in social activities because of the anxiety associated with telling friends and family and their anticipated negative reactions.

In commenting on this case, Sabat (2006b) pointed to two things:

> ... (1) the person with [Alzheimer's disease] is seen more and more in the light of the Self 2 attribute of the diagnosis and the defects present in the person's abilities and (2) this contributes to the social identity of the person becoming more and more limited to 'dysfunctional, burdensome, patient'.

Thus there is a real sense of alienation, which includes self-alienation, as the person regards him or herself as being deficient in some way, which helps to create an environment in which there is nothing to bolster the person's sense of self-esteem. It falls to others to do the positive work to create the right social encounters for the person with acquired diffuse neurocognitive dysfunction. Sabat describes this in a group setting:

> ... healthy others had to look into the totality of each person with Alzheimer's disease in the context of his or her own interests, needs, proclivities, values, and dispositions, as developed and maintained over the course of decades of healthy adult life, in order to gain clues about the social personae in which the afflicted found value. (Sabat, 2001: 159)

Here we see the role of narrative (the need to know the person's story); the need for a meaningful encounter in which there is a real engagement between the person and the Other (where the meeting is at the level of the soul), which is consonant with the human-person-perspective; the relevance of the SEA view as a way to help recognition of all aspects of the person's situatedness (the broad perspective), along with attention to his or her sense of persisting agency, whilst not losing sight of the person's embodiment.

Severe acquired diffuse neurocognitive dysfunction

But even if it is possible to accept that all of this makes sense for people with quite marked acquired diffuse neurocognitive dysfunction (Sabat's work was with people with moderate to severe dementia according to standard tests), a question still hovers concerning people with *severe* acquired diffuse neurocognitive dysfunction. The question is: in what sense can they be considered as persons? The Locke–Parfit view suggests that they might *not* qualify for consideration as persons. I suggest that the human-person-perspective supports the opposite view. It does so partly because it is premised upon the Wittgensteinian analysis of psychological mental states, which broadens our conception of what constitutes such states. An externalist construal of intentional mental states suggests that we do not have to rely solely on a person's verbal ability to describe inner psychological phenomena. What it is to be in a particular mental state can be shown externally. This does not just apply to intentional states, but might also apply, for instance, to being in pain. Even in severe acquired diffuse neurocognitive dysfunction, therefore, leaving aside signs of distress, there might be some evidence of comprehension, of recall, of intention, or of motivated action.

Moreover, even in the most severe cases of acquired diffuse neurocognitive dysfunction, from the human-person-perspective the situated nature of persons means that there is a sense in which personhood is sustained by our embeddedness. Thus, we are embedded in our histories or narratives, which are kept alive (at least to some extent) by those who care for us. Behaviour (the behaviour of someone with severe acquired diffuse neurocognitive dysfunction for instance) has to be characterized, not as isolated, but within a surround. Moreover, our lives are mutually involved; our narratives overlap. We are embedded, at root, in a realm of shared human concerns, which it is practically and rationally difficult to set aside. On these grounds, when Wiggins (1987) considers wilful killing, he states:

> … consider how much, how many habits of mind and feeling, you … have to put aside coolly to contemplate simply cutting off … another person. Obviously, all these things can be laid aside. But the point is not that they *cannot* be put aside, but the psychic and visceral cost—and the prima facie irrationality—of doing so.

We simply cannot help acknowledging our mutual embeddedness in a context of shared concerns, interrelated narratives, and normative constraints.

I wish to pursue this by considering how Heidegger's notion of 'solicitude' intersects with the notion of a situated being. The notion of solicitude, it will be recalled from the previous chapter, is to do with our encounters 'within-the-world' that allow us to Be-with the 'Dasein-with of Others' (Heidegger, 1962: 237). In alternative language, we might say that solicitude is to do with encounters at the level of the soul, where beings of this sort (i.e. embodied human beings with human souls) meet and interact precisely at the level of Being itself. Heidegger would call this level of interaction 'authentic'. Heidegger makes a link between the idea of the 'lostness in the "they"' and his notion of 'Resoluteness'. Resoluteness emerges as a concept in relation to Heidegger's understanding of conscience, something that calls us to an authentic way of Being-in-the-world. Resoluteness, then, is a manifestation of the human being's inclination to lead an authentic existence, in other words, to avoid being lost in the 'they'.

> To this lostness, one's own Dasein can appeal, and this appeal can be understood in the way of resoluteness. (Heidegger, 1962: 344)

Heidegger goes on to say that resoluteness is about our authentic existence and engagement with the world and, in particular, it connects to the notion of solicitude, where we engage with others as authentic human beings of this kind (i.e. souls). Thus,

> Resoluteness, as *authentic Being-one's-Self*, does not detach Dasein from its world, nor does it isolate it so that it becomes a free-floating 'I'. And how should it, when resoluteness ... is *authentically* nothing else than *Being-in-the-world*? Resoluteness brings the Self right into its current concernful Being-alongside what is ready-to-hand, and pushes it into solicitous Being with Others. (*ibid.*)

This is not just a matter of bumping into people and things in the world *en passant*, it is the deep engagement of authentic human encounters. Heidegger then moves on to introduce the notion of the '*Situation*'—'the "there" which is disclosed in resoluteness' (Heidegger, *op. cit.*: 346). By the 'Situation', Heidegger does not mean day-to-day circumstances, but the Being-in-the-world of authentic human beings who are *not* lost in the 'they'.

> For the "they", however, the Situation is essentially something that has been closed off. (*ibid.*)

For authentic human beings, on the other hand, the space indicated by the idea of the 'Situation' is one of meaning and significance. Once again, we might say, this is the space at which the human being (Dasein) authentically encounters the world, i.e. at the level of Being itself, or what I have called the level of the soul.

So much for Heidegger, who does, therefore, make a link between solicitude and being situated. To be situated, qua human being, is to be in that space where others necessarily evoke the response of solicitude, just because we are the sort of creatures that we are. And this takes me back to Wiggins and his point that we would have to give up, or set aside, so much in order to indulge in wilful killing; which in turn takes me back to the 'problem' of people with severe acquired diffuse neurocognitive dysfunction.

To care for someone with severe acquired diffuse neurocognitive dysfunction is to recognize a mutual situatedness. This will reflect a variety of factors, from shared culture and history, to the shared human form and agentive acts that can be comprehended in the context of human exchanges. Of course, it is open to anyone to deny that it makes sense to talk in terms of these factors in connection with Miss Breen when she reaches the terminal stages of her illness. But, in that case, an account must be given of situatedness that does *not* accommodate those with even severe acquired diffuse neurocognitive dysfunction. What this will involve is a restricted account of situatedness and, by implication, a restricted account of what it is to be a person, which is not open to the full elucidation of personhood from the human-person-perspective. Since intentional psychological phenomena are constitutive of persons, the externalist view implies that persons cannot be regarded solely in terms of their inner states and must be situated in the human world of which they are a part. Hence, a full elucidation of what it is to be a person, involving as it does (on my view) an externalist view of the person as a situated being, will also involve a notion of the mutual sharing of concerns which is characteristic of caring (or solicitude) between persons, even caring for persons with severe acquired diffuse neurocognitive dysfunction.

Engagement with Miss Breen, for instance, whether as brother or nurse, even if this involves little more than careful feeding or cleaning, exemplifies the values of care as understood in our culture (i.e. now using 'care' in its broader sense to include all that we ordinarily mean, which will also include an element of the solicitude to which Heidegger refers). But such actions, at the same time, help to construct care: 'It is in our actions and the way we treat one another that values come into being and are preserved in being' (Luntley, 1995: 218). Murphy (1984), for example, has suggested that through good clinical care dignity and the identity of a person may be preserved:

> Loss of dignity derives from the way we care for our sufferers from dementia, not from the illness itself ... More than at any other time of life the sufferer needs his personal identity preserved.

This, then, is an example of how, through care, which is a reflection of our engagement with the world in which we are situated, personhood can be preserved even in severe acquired diffuse neurocognitive dysfunction. This requires that the elucidation of 'care', which involves an acknowledgement of our situatedness, intersects with our notion of the person as a situated being.

The idea that care is constructed might seem more in keeping with the tenets of social constructionism and, accordingly, at odds with arguments I used earlier against that model. This is not the case, however, since social constructionism is *correct* to look to our public, shareable practices. The point against social constructionism is that those practices have to be regarded as embedded in the world in such a way as to secure normativity, so that their publicity is a secondary feature, rather than in itself the ground of the normativity. In the present case, our notions of care need public instantiation, by careful attention to Miss Breen, but they also reflect a deeper engagement between the values that underpin care and the manner in which the world is normatively structured by our embeddedness in it. The normativity of our thought and language is a feature of the world and helps to shape it.

Even at the stage where Miss Breen has severe acquired diffuse neurocognitive dysfunction, therefore, when she is unable to communicate in a meaningful way, and is totally dependent for all her needs on those around, we can argue that—qua situated embodied agent—she is still a person.

> For, to be an agent is to be an agent in the world. Our actions cannot simply and solely be regarded as the final outcome of a causal chain; they have some sort of meaning in the world. This is a reflection of our embeddedness in the human world.
>
> We reach this conclusion by ignoring the *causes* of actions and looking instead at what *constitutes* human action as the action of an agent. By doing this, however, we bring into play the embedding context of the world in which the person is situated as an embodied agent of this kind. (Aquilina & Hughes, 2006: 157)

Miss Breen must be seen as a *situated* agent, where *ipso facto* her actions have a certain meaning. She is also an *embodied* agent (Merleau-Ponty's idea of a body-subject again), whereby her bodily movements similarly in themselves have a particular significance.

> Treating our body as part of our subjectivity ... implies that not all aspects of our subjectivity—not all ways, for instance, in which we may be purposive—need necessarily be fully 'conscious' in the sense of being objects of explicit awareness. (Matthews, 1996: 92)

The link between the SEA view of the person and the human-person-perspective arises because both presume engagement with and a standing in the world that stems from being of this kind. This type of being engenders this type of solicitude, not as an added extra, but constitutively, immanently, and irreducibly. Once more, the characterization of normativity comes into play because beings of the kind—beings that are potentially minded—where intentionality is characteristic, are such as to engage in encounters of this type, which amount to normatively constrained practices in the world.

The human-person-perspective and models of dementia

Our models of dementia can be regarded as embedded within the broader human-person-perspective. Any particular model may contain errors, which will need to be corrected or jettisoned from the model, such as the *extreme* physicalist conception of the disease model, the representationalism of cognitive neuropsychology, or the over-emphasis on discourse in social constructionism. There is a general point, however, about what is genuinely (clinically and scientifically) useful in such models: I suggest that if there is such *genuine* usefulness, then it is likely that the model can be accommodated within the human-person-perspective. For why would this perspective wish to leave out something that is of genuine use? Our more causal models, which tend to supply specific explanations, tell us something of note, even if on their own they can only supply a circumscribed account. The human-person-perspective will take these *explanations* into account, but will be more concerned to achieve a broader *understanding* of what constitutes acquired diffuse neurocognitive dysfunction.

I want to illustrate this point by considering work in connection with behaviour that challenges. The biomedical model tends to refer to these behaviours collectively as the Behavioural and Psychological Symptoms of Dementia (BPSD), which typically have to be managed (Ballard, O'Brien, James, and Swann, 2001). The types of behaviour include wandering, aggression, agitation, screaming, repetitive questioning, sexual disinhibition, and so on. One initial point to make is that lumping all of these behaviours together is probably unhelpful in the first place, because each type of behaviour can probably be split into further sub-types. Thus, 'wandering' is not just one thing, but encompasses a variety of behaviours: seeking the reassurance of someone familiar by always going where they go is different from trying to find a door to get into the garden and different again from believing that one lives elsewhere (Hope et al., 1994c). It might also be, as suggested in the poem, *On the Move*, with which the chapter began, that pacing around is the only way to belong in an environment that seemingly has no other meaningful activities. But this leads to a second point, which is that rather than trying to treat or manage these conditions as if they are (simply) manifestations of dementia pathology, they need to be understood more broadly (Ballard et al., 2001). For some years, Graham Stokes has argued that,

> … behaviours that challenge are often attempts to communicate unmet need, and in most instances viewing these behaviours as symptoms of pathology is evidence of diagnostic overshadowing. (Stokes, 2010: 160)

Instead Stokes commends 'functional analysis', which involves a broad perspective to try to understand the meaning of the behaviour and the nature of the needs that are not being met, which are leading to the behaviour. In short, this is the human-person-perspective in action.

In a beautiful book, Stokes (2008) has recorded the stories of a number of people with dementia to hammer home the imperative of the broader view. In a particularly sad story, 'A man no longer known', he tells of Mr Bryan, a rather proud and reserved gentleman, who took to his garden to avoid the problems of his Alzheimer's disease (which were more to do with his social environment), but was eventually put in a long-term care home, where he was then denied access to the garden, with tragic consequences. As Stokes read the documents about him, he wondered when Mr Bryan's story would start:

> 'It talked of him "wandering outside" and the destruction he caused, the confrontations and arguments, the hazards and risk of accident and assault, and how his wife could no longer cope with the stress. But what about him?' (Stokes 2008: 56).

What was missing was a narrative account and one with a broad enough view—the human-person-perspective—to allow the right sort of help to be given to Mr Bryan and to his wife. Stokes reflects:

> People with dementia are different from each other. Move away from the cognitive disability, and what impresses us most is their uniqueness, not their similarity. So why do we degrade their behaviour to symptoms of a disease, rather than seeing it as evidence of efforts to survive in a world that resonates with fear, threat and mystery? Could it be that we no longer see them as people whose feelings need to be acknowledged and their opinions valued? Are we seduced by the simplicity and authority of the disease-model that not only fails to talk of people, but also absolves us of all responsibility? (Stokes, *op. cit.*: 54)

Once more, it is the human-person-perspective that is missing. For we do not wish to abandon the usefulness of the disease model, but we do not want its glare to overshadow how we approach and understand the person with acquired diffuse neurocognitive dysfunction.

But with this point still ringing, I wish to return to issues to do with diagnosis. I want to ask whether even the notion of 'dysfunction', which I have been using, might not itself be labelling and cause overshadowing: the person becomes perceived as mainly 'dysfunctional'. I shall also discuss afresh the broader context in which the problems of diagnosis look more like aesthetic judgements. In raising this question I shall then make some brief comments about the recent book by Peter Whitehouse with Daniel George, *The Myth of Alzheimer's* (Whitehouse & George, 2008). I shall end this section by discussing how it is possible to make individual, person-centred diagnoses.

Back to the diagnosis

Acquired diffuse neurocognitive dysfunction was intended, in Chapter 1, as a syndromal diagnosis, an umbrella term for nosological purposes covering a variety of more specific diseases. It might be useful as a way to explain to people what is happening to them, but it need not necessarily be the diagnosis that people are given. It is descriptive, but does not define pathology. It leaves unanswered questions about where to draw the limits around particular diseases, such as Alzheimer's disease. To be told your brain is 'dysfunctional' would not, of course, be reassuring and might be a source of labelling. How to eliminate stigma is a complex sociological problem. Whichever words are chosen, there is always the potential for stigma. Even the notion of ageing can be stigmatizing: a good deal of British humour is based on stigmatizing attitudes towards old age! My interest, however, is in the nature of the evaluative judgements that surround diagnoses of one or other form of dementia. In Chapter 1, I suggested that thinking through the concept of 'dementia' would be akin to making an aesthetic judgement. I implied this would be the case in at least three ways: first, there would have to be a degree of uncertainty about any diagnosis; secondly, there would inevitably be a degree of mystery around these conditions, because of the surround; and, thirdly, this would follow because the surround turns out to be the nature of human life in the human world.

If there is something controversial about these three suggestions it is probably, in some sense, because they seem to mount a challenge against (what might be perceived as) a more sensible, scientific, biomedical approach. My contention, contrariwise, is that these suggestions frame the only sensible way to approach a host of scientific problems. At the margins of any scientific endeavour there will always be uncertainty, because this is, after all, a driver for scientific research. Many scientific facts seem certain. The paradigm shift from Newton to Einstein should convince us that even certainties might change. But this point (that large paradigm shifts are possible) does not itself need to be over-egged. We simply need to note again the Second Principle of Values-Based Medicine (VBM), discussed in Chapter 1, namely the 'science-driven' principle (Fulford, 2004: 212). This suggests that values become more obvious and pervasive as science advances. These evaluative concerns have emerged and will continue to emerge as we learn more about how the brain and body work. There is, therefore, a perfectly ordinary way in which it is sensible to talk about the mysteriousness that surrounds scientific work in this area: at the margins of research things are uncertain and beyond the margins they are not known. The only challenge to this view would be the (rather extreme) opposing view that one day science might explain everything *completely* and there would be no uncertainty whatsoever. Such a view seems (to me at least) naïve. It is also a belief that cannot be falsified; it is only possible to present evidence (of previous misplaced certainty or of areas where one advance has raised many further questions) that would seem to make the belief unlikely. In any case, for the foreseeable future we have to live with uncertainty as a scientific reality, which is a way of saying we have to accept there is something mysterious.

The third point was that this mystery reflects the context (or surround), which is the human condition in the human world. Again, rather than this seeming to be a point that might be regarded as inimical to science, it is actually the inescapable reality that forms the background to scientific thought. It is the nature of our being as embodied creatures of this kind that accounts for the impulse to explain and to understand the world in which we are engaged. It is characteristic of human beings that they enquire: it is part of our way of being-in-the-world.

In a particular fashion, however, acquired diffuse neurocognitive dysfunction raises this sense of mystery, not just in a surface way—because there are all sorts of things still not known about the different types of disease—but also (in a deeper sense) because these conditions are a clear manifestation of our ageing. They raise deep questions about the purpose or meaning of life in that, more than many other diseases, they challenge our sense of self. The dual assault on personhood and narrative coherence posed by the conditions that fall under the syndromal diagnosis are an existential challenge. Even having met the challenge as best we can, we are left making sense of our standing as beings-in-the-world: there is an accommodation to be made, a sense of alienation to be overcome. The human-person-perspective, which gives us a way to make the accommodation, can only succeed if it can bring into view what is required to make sense of human existence with its vulnerabilities and dependencies. There has to be some sort of horizon against which other things have meaning. We may wish to refer only to the phenomenal world that we encounter, or we may wish to point beyond it (in some metaphorical sense) to the noumenal world. But, however we wish to proceed in justifying our world view, the existential question is raised by dementia in a more pointed way than by many other diseases. And this question does, finally, move beyond science. For it is a question that science cannot answer; rather science itself, including the science around acquired diffuse neurocognitive dysfunction, raises it. As Wittgenstein said:

> The facts all contribute only to setting the problem, not to its solution.
> It is not *how* things are in the world that is mystical, but *that* it exists. (TLP §§6.4321–6.44)

From my viewpoint, the mystical is the backdrop to scientific advance. It is the question that arises rationally from consideration of the surround perceived from the broad view, the human-person-perspective, of acquired diffuse neurocognitive dysfunction. Hence, the questions that arise in connection with decisions about where to draw lines around particular diagnoses *just are* questions about the *nature of our being as creatures of this kind in the world*, with all that this entails in terms of our engagement as situated embodied agents, as human beings seeking authentic existence as beings-in-the-world.

The ageing brain

Well, one way in which we are in the world is as ageing beings. Whitehouse and George have been keen to point us away from thinking about Alzheimer's disease to think instead about brain ageing. In summary form:

> *Defining brain aging as a disease and then trying to cure it is at its root unscientific and misguided. In short, Alzheimer's is a hundred-year-old myth that is over the hill. The entire scientific, technological, and political framework for aging needs to be reassessed to better serve*

> *patients and families in order to help people maximize their quality of life as they move along*
> *the path of cognitive aging.* (Whitehouse & George 2008: 6)

Whitehouse has been one of the foremost neuroscientists in the field of Alzheimer's research (Whitehouse, Price, Clark, Coyle, and DeLong, 1981). He now feels that the emphasis on the possibility of a cure for Alzheimer's disease is misplaced (partly because he does not regard 'it' as one thing). His book examines many of the possible reasons why there is such an emphasis. It reflects people's dread of the condition, for sure, but it also reflects institutional and political influences at work in university departments and in large pharmaceutical companies. Many people find Whitehouse's views egregious. It surely is not shocking, however, to suggest that prevention is better than cure, that quality of life is what counts, and that this should be considered broadly:

> Quality of life can be improved ... by staying mentally and physically active and address-
> ing the range of ecological factors that influence your cognitive health ... Having a sense
> of purpose in life and a sense of belonging to a family and community is also critical to
> individual well-being. If physicians spend all their time talking about drugs, there is little
> time to discuss other life options that may contribute to preserving and even enhancing
> quality of life. (Whitehouse & George, 2008: 147)

There is, however, a tension in the argument that because Alzheimer's is a manifestation of brain ageing, which seems indisputable, therefore it is not a disease. Here is how Whitehouse says he would put it to a patient:

> All people have brains that age over time, and all our brains age in different ways. ...
>   It's important that you know that ... you're not diseased, even though your memory
> loss may be more pronounced than others your age. (Whitehouse & George, 2008: 10)

This raises an obvious question about what *would* count as a 'disease', but it shows very clearly that there is an evaluative judgement being made. It is a judgement about the nature of ageing and how we should cope with it. As such, it is a judgement about the nature of our being-in-the-world. The previous quotation was specific in commending, 'a sense of purpose in life and a sense of belonging to a family and community' (*vide supra*). In fact, one way of framing Whitehouse's project is to say that he is raising a question about the context in which research on Alzheimer's, and Alzheimer's itself, is seen. The broader view raises a challenge concerning how we deal with Alzheimer's: not solely on the basis of a biomedical model because, as Whitehouse asserts, the issues are vaster. This is to see things from the human-person-perspective. It is not to deny the science, but to locate it against a broader canvas.

Giving a diagnosis

It does, however, raise again the type of tension with which I was concerned in Chapter 6. How can we provide an individualized account, which still allows the type of generalizability that is required in practice? How can we have valid diagnoses if everyone is different? How can we have narrative and yet correct interpretations, which preclude the possibility that just any story will do? The suggestion I have made before is that the broad view, the human-person-perspective, should allow both an individualized, narrative account and the more nomothetic, law-like account required for a valid diagnosis. But how will this work?

In practice, I do not think it raises particular concerns. It is already the case that we are used to dealing with classificatory systems that do not always quite match the reality of the patients we see. We search for the best fit. There are, of course, clear-cut cases. But often this is not so. This does not make the diagnostic systems unusable. The key thing is that the history, or narrative, should be personalized, individual, and full. This immediately means that the understanding of the person will be from his or her unique perspective, which is just the viewpoint that is required if the sort of background understanding advocated by Stokes (2008, 2010) or Sabat (2001) is going to be achieved. The process of diagnosis needs to include a formulation, which should amount to an interpretation of the history to the patient in such a way as to make him or her feel that they have been heard (McLean, 2006). And, at best, the interpretation should allow consensus. What is then required is a conversation that reflects the broad view, which may or may not focus on a particular diagnosis. If it does, this may need to be approached with appropriate circumspection, so that the person understands the level of certainty attached to the diagnosis. An explanation in appropriate language of what acquired diffuse neurocognitive dysfunction means might be a good place to start. But it will mean different things to different people in the context of their differing narrative histories.

The human-person-perspective, therefore, entails no more than making sure that the meaning of the diagnosis to the person concerned is understood. The account that is meaningful to the person is, after all, what counts. The particular code associated with the diagnosis is a secondary matter, which will be more or less important for specific reasons. The bigger issue is that the person is given help and hope concerning how to deal with their state. Once again, it is the broader surround that is the issue. The direction of movement initiated by this perspective, which reflects the concerns of Whitehouse and George (2008), is outwards to the embedding context, which is a situated one for the individual, where history, family, culture, moral and spiritual values, and so forth will be the real issues. The human-person-perspective brings in the normative concerns that characteristically accompany our thinking about human beings-in-the-world.

The uncircumscribable human-person-perspective

A similar line of argument was present in the work of the psychiatrist George L. Engel (1913–1999). His seminal paper (Engel, 1977) was cited in passing in Chapter 5. Engel's 'biopsychosocial model' aims to counter the 'crippling flaw' of the 'biomedical model', which 'does not include the patient and his attributes as a person, a human being' (Engel, 1980). 'Yet', as he says,

> … in the everyday work of the physician the prime object of study is a person … within the framework of an ongoing human relationship … (*ibid.*)

Engel uses a systems approach to locate the person in a hierarchy or continuum of natural systems that ultimately includes the biosphere. He explicitly discusses the interaction between different levels of the hierarchy and the movement between the different systems. Even this important account, however, of how models might be conceived in medicine, does not appear to me to go far enough.

Whilst Engel allows permeability between the boundaries of different systems or levels, the human-person-perspective suggests that the notion of boundaries is too concrete. The potential for a mistake here, I am suggesting, is at the first step: talk of 'models' itself brings to mind something definite and concrete. Talk of 'systems' again suggests something circumscribable. As my earlier discussion of the concept of a person suggested, this is a concept which should be uncircumscribable. There is always another field of concern, another way to describe the encounters between persons. It is not enough (although it is important) to expand outwards in the way Engel suggests towards the biosphere, for potential new fields of concern and ways of describing personal encounters should also add depth, precisely at the level of the person and not by moving to a new hierarchical level. Engel talks of experience and behaviour at the personal system level, but we also need to consider *at the same personal level*, ethics, aesthetics, spirituality, sexuality, race, culture and politics, *inter alia*. Speaking of these things as different systems, rather than as involved in the one perspective, allows the possibility of a mistake, as if the human person can be thought of as separate from, say, political concerns. The person as a system within a hierarchy of systems needs to be regarded instead as a being whose embedding in the world means that others and the environment are not separate systems with which the person can interact, but are constitutively involved (at least potentially) in the very notion of the human person. This conception of the human-person-perspective reflects the reality of dementia-in-the-world. The nature of our engagement with the world, in which we are embedded, means that the human-person-perspective cannot be circumscribed, nor partitioned.

And this means that, in connection with acquired diffuse neurocognitive dysfunction, we need a revolution on all fronts. Of course we still need basic biomedical research to continue, but my previous arguments suggest that this research needs to be viewed critically against a background of concerns that sets limits and provides focus. Meanwhile, the human-person-perspective sets no limits. This is the view that seeks to overcome the alienation caused by the diagnosis, which allows our models to 'wither away' to be replaced by authentic human encounters. Recall Marx, near the start of this chapter:

> Every alienation of man from himself and from Nature appears in the relation which he postulates between other men and himself and Nature.

> (EPM, *Marx-Engels Gesamtausgabe* I/3: 91; quoted in Marx, 1961: 177)

The inclusion by Engel of the biosphere in the biopsychosocial model is absolutely right. Our situatedness is not circumscribable. But the person with acquired diffuse neurocognitive dysfunction is often kept from enjoying the full fruits of the biosphere; like Mr Bryan (Stokes, 2008), many are prevented from even setting foot in the gardens of their care homes because of lack of staff as well as health and safety issues! They are left to 'wander' inside aimlessly.

> It doesn't strike you at first.
> But then everybody's doing it.
> It is really rather shattering,

because you've been surprised
by others doing it, and then you find
that you are doing it yourself! (*vide supra*).

People with acquired diffuse neurocognitive dysfunction are thus alienated from themselves and from the societies they have helped to create.

> This social life … is *life* itself, physical and cultural life, human morality, human activity, human enjoyment, real *human* existence. Human life is the *true social life* of man. As the irremediable exclusion from this life is much more complete, more unbearable, dreadful, and contradictory, than the exclusion from political life, so is the ending of this exclusion, and even a limited reaction, a *revolt* against it, more fundamental, as *man* is more fundamental than the *citizen, human life* more than political life. (*Marx-Engels Gesamtausgabe* I/3: 21; quoted in Marx, 1961: 242).[4]

The revolution, if it were to be guided by the human-person-perspective, would include a revolution in terms of research,[5] but would be much broader than that, to include every way in which it might be possible for people with acquired diffuse neurocognitive dysfunction to flourish as human beings in the world. In the ensuing paragraphs, before concluding this chapter, I shall gesture at the various ways in which this might be achieved. In no area shall I do more than scratch the surface of the good work that is being done. I shall undoubtedly omit areas that should be included. In each case, grasping the significance of the human-person-perspective is a way to bring people, those afflicted by these various conditions, along with their formal and informal carers, back from their lostness in the 'they', to a type of more authentic existence.

John Killick's work with people with acquired diffuse neurocognitive dysfunction, an example from which is the poem that starts this chapter, has spanned many years. Although poetry has led to several publications (e.g. Killick & Cordonnier, 2000) John's work embraces a variety of art forms. With Kate Allan he has established 'Dementia Positive'[6] to encourage communication, consultation and creativity with people with dementia. They undertook a pilot project in Australia a few years ago to see whether it was possible to encourage people with *severe* acquired diffuse neurocognitive dysfunction to communicate. Their encounter with one woman, Pat, was remarkable. She had not meaningfully engaged with anyone for a long time, not even her spouse. But John spoke with her, held her hand, synchronized his breathing with hers (a technique acquired from an approach to coma patients), and attempted eye contact. During the first two meetings there was no response; but then, during the third meeting,

> … gradually she raised her head, spoke, though I could not follow her words, and smiled. For a further ten minutes we were clearly in communication. I played her some music and she expressed interest and pleasure with her face, her gaze and through nonverbal sounds. She then went on to engage in a sustained sequence of speech-like sounds, only a few of which were recognizable to me but which were very definitely spoken in an Australian accent! (Allan & Killick, 2010: 223)

Pat then lapsed back into her non-communicative state. They comment:

> This brings us to what we believe is a capacity which acquires ever greater importance in interactions with persons with dementia, that of being *in the moment* with our attention

fully and open-mindedly focused on the person and our encounter with them. (Allan & Killick, *op. cit.*: 223–4)

I have highlighted the importance of the human encounter in the last chapter. It is the quality of the encounter that matters. The revolution required at the personal level is to make our human encounters matter in an authentic way.

One way to engage with people at a level that does not require words is through music. Barbara Pointon records (in the previous chapter) the powerful effects of music on her husband, Malcolm, even late into his disease. The story that people retain their musical abilities even into the severer stages of acquired diffuse neurocognitive dysfunction is a very common one. It inspired the title of the book by Graham Stokes: *And Still the Music Plays*. The particular story concerned a man called Colin with a diagnosis of Creuzfeldt-Jakob disease (CJD), whose distressing movements and grimaces in the severe stages were difficult to witness. His wife, Helen, wondered whether listening to the music he had always loved might help. The story, after music was introduced into his room, continues:

> The transformation, although by no means total, was both marvellous and a relief to see. For lengthy periods of time Colin was calm. Even on his most disturbed days his clumsy and ill-coordinated movements would in moments be less obvious and Helen was certain there was the occasional trace of a smile. (Stokes, 2008: 44)

The use of music as therapy for people with acquired diffuse neurocognitive dysfunction has become a recognized resource and means of recollecting and engaging with others (Aldridge, 2000). The difficulty is, however, that there is very little research of good quality to support music therapy. But this applies to almost all forms of non-pharmacological intervention for behaviours that challenge. For instance, in a systematic review of the effectiveness and acceptability of interventions to reduce 'wandering' in dementia, there was no robust evidence to support the use of any intervention, although there was weak evidence that exercise therapy might be helpful (Robinson et al., 2007). Only one randomized controlled trial (RCT) was found for music therapy (Groene, 1993), which did, however, seem to be an acceptable approach and raised no ethical concerns. An earlier Cochrane Review of music therapy had simply concluded: 'The methodological quality and the reporting of the included studies were too poor to draw any useful conclusions' (Vink, Birks, Bruinsma, and Scholten, 2004). All of which should elicit the response that lack of evidence is not evidence of lack of effect, it is just that adequate methodological studies have not been conducted.

There is no doubt that it is extremely difficult to conduct methodologically rigorous research of this kind with this population. For instance, measuring improvements may be difficult in the severer stages of acquired diffuse neurocognitive dysfunction, when the natural course of the disease is that things should worsen. In addition, there is the difficulty of communication. This might simply imply that researchers have to try harder!

Similar points can be made about dance therapies of various types, which have been tried in different settings: an example being a type of Latin American Ballroom Dance (Danzón) that has been tested in care homes, where (in a pilot study) the Danzón psychomotor intervention was found to enhance positive emotional states and general levels of satisfaction for both people with dementia and for the care staff involved

(Guzmán-García, Mukaetova-Ladinska, and James, in press). But the study (of 19 participants, 13 of whom had dementia) was not a RCT and used only one objective measure, which was a 'bespoke scale' of engagement; and was otherwise based on interviews.

Having suggested that it is simply a matter of trying harder, it may also be that the RCT is not the best method to capture improvements and benefits in this population. This is not the place to enter into a full-scale debate about research methodology, but there are some basic points to be made.

Group statistics, seeking to test the significance of a null hypothesis, will always have the potential to cover up the ways in which a particular intervention was excellent for one person and terrible for another. Given a specific instrument to measure change in, say, quality of life (but see the next chapter), it may be that it is highly likely that the group average score will go down over the course of a study of music or dance for people with acquired diffuse neurocognitive dysfunction; whereas quality of life might well have improved for a few. Even then, where quality of life as measured on this specific scale has deteriorated, the possibility that the individual benefited in some way from the music or from the dance (perhaps just by being an observer) is not precluded. The problem is one of measurement (Bond, 1999). Increasingly there is interest in other methodological approaches, such as the single case design, which is sometimes called the 'n=1' study (Kazdin, 1982; Morgan & Morgan, 2001). It may be that a mixed methods approach (i.e. using quantitative and qualitative techniques) to single cases, but employing multiple measurements before and after an intervention, where the scales used are specifically and individually tailored to the participants in the study, with detailed consideration—on the basis of both quantitative assessments and the results of interviews—of whether causal links can reasonably be established, would be the only way to establish benefit (Elliott, 2002).

Beyond the methodological arguments, however, the advantage of such an approach is that it allows a focus on individual human beings and, therefore, unique human encounters. In connection with music and dance there is a further point, which is that these art forms amount also to forms of communication (Coaten, 2002). Basic human encounters (of the body-subject)—especially at the level of the soul—are based on some form of communication, which is possible because the participants share an embodied form of life or way of being-in-the-world.

The obvious premise to approaches of this sort is that communication does not need to be oral or verbal, it may be non-verbal in various ways, from bodily to emotional or spiritual communication. Much reminiscence therapy is aimed at tapping into distant memories that 'may resonate with feeling' (Stokes, 2010: 164). So it makes perfect sense to use museums as a way to engage with people with acquired diffuse neurocognitive dysfunction, because it allows them to interact with others, with the artefacts in the museum, with the local community, and so forth. The Museum of Modern Art in New York (MoMA), for instance, has been running a programme for some while called *The MoMA Alzheimer's Project: Making Art Accessible to People with Dementia*.[7] Similar programmes have been run in other countries. The idea that some of the behavioural manifestations of acquired diffuse neurocognitive dysfunction might respond in a positive way to art has been encouraged by the formation of the

Artists for Alzheimer's programme (ARTZ).[8] These projects have been encouraged by John Zeisel, whose work has focused on the importance of the notion of the emotional self. His approach is summed up in his book, *I'm Still Here* (Zeisel, 2009). Zeisel stresses non-pharmacological treatments to promote the potential of the brain, despite dementia, and the creativity of the mind. Thus, trips to art museums, writing poetry, going to the theatre or cinema—these are all ways in which a person can stay active and engaged at a local level. Similarly, the emergence of Alzheimer's Cafés, first in the Netherlands and then in many other countries, has been a way to heighten a sense of participation in a supportive local environment.[9] There are thus a number of ways in which the sense of alienation can be countered at a local level.

Zeisel has also been instrumental in encouraging more thought to how environments themselves are designed to make them more appropriate for people with acquired diffuse neurocognitive dysfunction. The human-person-perspective should encourage a view that extends beyond the social environment to the designed and built environments. There has been increasing awareness that these environments can have an impact on how people with acquired diffuse neurocognitive dysfunction are able to live and be, which (on reflection) is not too surprising (Marshall & Hoskins, 2008)! Having available safe places to walk, different types of room to live and converse in, and gardens in which to enjoy feelings of freedom and beauty, must all potentially make a huge difference to a person's quality of life. Social and built environments which encourage meaningful occupation and human encounters of significance (which may be with others—e.g. through music-making or art therapy (Kahn-Denis, 2002)—or may be through quietly communing with nature) are another area where we require revolution.

What the world might look like after such a revolution, one which affects both the individual and community levels of engagement, is captured beautifully in the social documentary photography of Cathy Greenblat, whose images—e.g. in her book, *Alive with Alzheimer's* (Greenblat, 2004)—of people with acquired diffuse neurocognitive dysfunction from around the world attest to the possibilities that come from meaningful engagement (in music groups for instance) and significant encounters (between family members or professional carers and people with dementia).[10] These images are not carefully selected with the intention of only depicting the pleasant aspects of a life with Alzheimer's disease; they can also show anxiety, despair, and loneliness. They show dying. But the point is there are possibilities beyond the morbid. With the right political will—Marx might say *human* will—we can create environments in which people can live well with dementia. One seemingly simple idea has been proposed and put into practice by Peter Whitehouse and his wife Cathy: an intergenerational school, which older people, including those with dementia, can attend as volunteers to help with reading, say, and to participate in activities from computing to gardening. The children and the older people can both learn and benefit mutually (Whitehouse & George, 2008: 143–6). The effects are educative and therapeutic. Community and a sense of solidarity are achieved by older people pursuing voluntary occupations; which should, therefore, encourage the thought that people with acquired diffuse neurocognitive dysfunction might find some benefit in voluntary work more generally, in which they might, however, need to be supported (Stansell, 2002). The environments we wish to create will be social and physical environments in which the human-person-perspective holds sway (as in the intergenerational school, the Alzheimer's Café, music, art, or museum groups), where the importance of human encounters of significance is recognized.

If we are talking about environments, we must also consider the use of smart technology. There has been growing interest in the idea that, if acquired diffuse neurocognitive dysfunction is akin to a disability, people can be re-enabled by the use of assistive technology. It is well recognized, however, that in these conditions—where cognitive function is impaired and tends to worsen—there are complexities. Whether talking about individual items, such as an armband or notepad to enable the person (and carer) to know his or her position (Robinson, Brittain, Lindsay, Jackson, and Olivier, 2009), or about a whole 'smart home' (Orpwood, Gibbs, Adlam, Faulkner, and Meegahawatte, 2005), it is clearly important to have people with acquired diffuse neurocognitive dysfunction and their carers involved in the design. Early studies (such as those just cited) have tended to show the complexity of the design problem (because individual users have particular and sometimes changing needs), but in principle it should be possible to overcome design issues.

The bigger issues, however, are the *human* issues. In discussing the smart home, Orpwood et al. (2005) say the following:

> … the house should be able to act in a similar manner to a live-in carer, providing care for 24 h a day without becoming tired or frustrated. Of course, such technology could never replace human care and support, but it could augment such caring, and hopefully also provide some respite for personal carers. (p. 156)

This is an interesting statement. It expresses the laudable aspiration that it might be possible to help people, perhaps keep them independent, by using smart technologies, which sense what is happening and respond appropriately. But one might wish to probe the senses in which a 'house' can act like a 'carer'. The claim is not, of course, outlandish in many respects. But in the end, the house will not be able to care! It cannot, even in principle, because it cannot (even in principle) *Be-with* and, therefore, it is not open to the house to show solicitude towards the person who lives in the house. But the worry is that technological fixes *will* be used as ways to 'replace human care and support' (*vide supra*). This has also been a concern in connection with electronic tagging and tracking mechanisms (Hughes, Newby, Louw, Campbell, & Hutton, 2008), that they might be a way to reduce the number of staff in care homes. Such a worry might be misplaced—it might be that with less worry about people going missing, staff can spend more quality time with people. This helps to make the point that the issues around the use of assistive technology are actually to do with human responses. There is, at least, the possibility that, at the margins (where many moral abuses lurk), assistive technologies, such as electronic tagging, might be used in a manner that contravenes basic human liberties (Hughes & Louw, 2002a). This might be extraordinary, but the possibility has to be taken seriously when we are dealing with people who are essentially vulnerable. As Ruud ter Meulen and colleagues have wisely written (albeit in connection with enhancement technologies):

> Although these new possibilities are for some authors a reason to envisage a new utopia, and see the new application as essentially 'good', there are also serious ethical concerns.

> These concerns have to do with the impact of the new technologies on fundamental values like the freedom and autonomy of the individual, the nature of humanity and justice in society and health care. (ter Meulen, Nielsen, and Landeweerd, 2007: 803)

Assistive technologies may enhance the environment of care, but essentially care and solicitude are features of human interactions of the right sort. The revolution that is required is not a technological one, it needs to emanate from the human-person-perspective and lead to human encounters of significance.

Yet it is shocking that we should need to envisage a revolution to achieve such a basic *human* aim. There is every reason to pursue the ideals of the human-person-perspective, however, because they are fundamental to our standing as beings-in-the-world of this sort. The revolution is required by our inbuilt inclination, based on our situatedness, towards solicitude. This inclination is seen in the re-affirming encounters, which are thereby the opposite of alienating, that take place in support groups (Yale & Snyder, 2002; Snyder, 2006). Similarly, it is the inclination that is leading us to listen to the voices of people who actually endure these conditions (e.g. Davis, 1989; Wallace, 2010); and, with increasing frequency, we now see people with acquired diffuse neurocognitive dysfunction telling their stories and supporting one another through various websites and other means.[11] This in itself is a small revolution, which is based on and confirms the inclination to care. It is an inclination which points outwards to the world and places us, as human beings, in the broadest possible surround, of intergenerational concern, of Others, of personal ethics and the politics of ageing, of the environment and even the world.

> By placing ourselves on the continuum of brain aging and seeing it as a lifelong undertaking rather than an end-of-life 'disease', we will find solidarity with all the vulnerable members in our society—from our children to our elders. This solidarity can provide an ethical impetus to protect our fellow human beings from the complex environmental and social factors that contribute to brain aging, while expanding our compassion for those in the later stages of senescence. By doing so, we will create a greater sense of responsibility for future generations and for our planet—a collective wisdom that will nurture our growth as a species. (Whitehouse & George, 2008: 281)

Summary

In the sections above I have presented the human-person-perspective, which is the broad perspective intended to answer this central question: how are we to understand acquired diffuse neurocognitive dysfunction? I shall now summarize some of the arguments:

- ◆ Dementia-in-the-world suggests the rich context into which acquired diffuse neurocognitive dysfunction fits. Acquired diffuse neurocognitive dysfunction is understood within and from this context: the context in which, as situated embodied agents, we are all located. And it is this worldly context which provides the human-person-perspective within which we understand acquired diffuse neurocognitive dysfunction.

- ◆ The human-person-perspective allows an understanding which recognizes the normative nature of the world. Our understanding of persons, as situated embodied agents, helps to flesh out the human-person-perspective.

- It is a failure to recognize the constitutive, immanent, and irreducible normative features of intentional psychological states which accounts for the circumscribed nature of other models of acquired diffuse neurocognitive dysfunction; but this suggests the possibility that other models might be accommodated within this broader human-person-perspective too.

- The human-person-perspective is uncircumscribable, because what it is to be a human person is open-ended. That is, the concerns that shape our understanding of ourselves as persons cannot be pinned down once and for all. Instead, it is always possible for new fibres to be added to the thread which makes up our conception of ourselves as human beings.

- The human-person-perspective throws us in the direction of a revolution: at a national level, in terms of funding for services and for research of the right focus; at a local or regional level, which might mean broader thoughts about how to encourage meaningful activities; at a personal level in terms of our individual encounters and the need for sensitive communication and significant human exchanges.

Conclusions and implications

In this chapter, building on the Wittgensteinian analysis of Chapter 4, I have given substance to and supported the view of the person as a situated embodied agent from Chapter 2. I have suggested that this human-person-perspective is necessary for our understanding of dementia-in-the-world: it accommodates the models that shape our understanding already, but broadens the perspective to include the normativity that is a feature of our world. I have suggested that the standing of the person with acquired diffuse neurocognitive dysfunction makes him or her alienated. Carers, meanwhile, as well as people with dementia, are lost in the 'they', because it is so difficult to live an authentic life once it is blighted by this condition. But this sense of a life having been *blighted* itself arises from a sense of alienation, whereas life *could be* different and *could be viewed* differently. This would be possible if there were a revolution at the different levels that I have just sketched. We would then be able to live authentic lives. These would be lives in which we could show solidarity with people with acquired diffuse neurocognitive dysfunction and their carers. As the Nuffield Council report suggested,

> The concept of solidarity underpins the duty of individuals and of society to support those with dementia and their carers. It reinforces the responsibility of all of us to try to help research and to act to de-stigmatise dementia. Solidarity is relevant also to individual relationships: personal solidarity, in the form of love, loyalty and compassion, is the basis and motivation for giving care to one's partner, parent or friend. We suggest, therefore, that, under solidarity, society has a twofold obligation to provide resources and support to people with dementia and their carers: first as part of our obligations to help those who cannot readily support themselves; and secondly to enable carers to maintain their personal solidarity with the person for whom they are caring' (Nuffield Council on Bioethics, 2009: 30, §2.44)

And the basis of the duty of solidarity stems from the idea of the common good which arises from the way we are conceptually tied together as Beings-in-the-world-of-this-kind, whose nature is to Be-with, to demonstrate solicitude towards those Others who exist as situated embodied agents in a world we conceive broadly from the human-person-perspective.

Endnotes

1 But see Hursthouse, 1999; Hughes and Louw, 2005; Hughes and Baldwin, 2006: 88–93; Radden and Sadler, 2010; Hughes, forthcoming.

2 Ronnie Jackamarra Lawson was born around 1930. He is an aboriginal artist, whose native language is Warlpiri. This quote comes from the wall of The Indigenous Collection exhibited in the National Gallery of Victoria in Melbourne, Australia.

3 Sabat (2001) provides a detailed account of the ways in which the different manifestation of selfhood can be both maintained and undermined. It is based on Sabat's careful observation, recording, interpretation of, and engagement with, people with dementia. The surrounding commentary, in addition to the revealing, stimulating, humorous, and very moving verbatim dialogue, makes this an incisive critique of much that we take for granted in dementia care.

4 The full original reference is to: Karl Marx, (10 August 1844). *Kritische Randglosen zu dem Artikel: Der König von Preussen und die Sozial-reform. Von einem Preussen* in *Vorwärts*.

5 The Nuffield Council on Bioethics (2009) recommended a review of research funding given the inequity in terms of money spent on research on conditions such as cancer compared with funding for dementia research. This is reflected in the number of research publications in the field of dementia compared with other conditions. They also recommended that there should be more funding for qualitative research that might help us to understand the lived experience of dementia and ways to improve the quality of care.

6 See: http://www.dementiapositive.co.uk [accessed 17 July 2010].

7 See the websites from the Museum of Modern Art: http://www.moma.org/learn/programs/alzheimers and http://www.moma.org/meetme/index [both accessed 18 July 2010].

8 See: http://www.artistsforalzheimers.org [accessed 18 July 2010].

9 For information about the Alzheimer's Café UK see: http://www.alzheimercafe.co.uk/home.htm [accessed 18 July 2010].

10 See, for instance, Cathy Greenblat's series of pictures entitled *Love, Loss and Laughter: Seeing Alzheimer's Differently* at http://www.cathygreenblat.com/Portfolio.cfm?nK=1621&nL=1&nS=9#0 and *Alive With Alzheimer's* at http://www.cathygreenblat.com/Portfolio.cfm?nK=1641&nL=1&nS=9#0 [both accessed on 18 July 2010].

11 For instance, see the Talking Point website of the UK Alzheimer's Society: http://forum.alzheimers.org.uk/index.php [accessed 25 July 2010]; or the similar website for the Alzheimer's Association in the USA: http://alzheimers.infopop.cc/eve/forums/a/frm/f/375102261 [accessed 25 July 2010]; or the forum for people with dementia on the Canadian Alzheimer Society's website: http://www.alzheimer.ca/forum/index.php [accessed 25 July 2010].

Chapter 9

Dilemmas in dementia: a framework and philosophical approach

Introduction

In Chapter 1, I highlighted the real issues that arise in the context of care for people with dementia by sketching five dilemmas. I left these hanging. I introduced these dilemmas not because I wish to pursue a detailed ethical analysis of the sort that might be encouraged by a textbook of medical ethics (cf. Beauchamp & Childress, 2001). Rather, I wish to show the contribution made by the type of broader philosophical thought that I have been pursuing in these pages (cf. Dickenson & Fulford, 2000). It is inevitable, however, that these dilemmas, which are real-life, clinical, and ethical, must be dealt with using the principles and approaches that have developed over many years to deal with difficult decisions of this sort (cf. Hughes & Baldwin, 2006). Luckily, I do not need to present or justify a framework from scratch to approach these dilemmas. The report by the Nuffield Council on Bioethics (2009) sets out a framework that might be useful in approaching dilemmas in connection with dementia (see Box 9.1). The framework has six components and the Report makes plain that not all of the components will be of equal relevance in dealing with any particular dilemma.

In this Chapter, I shall, first, outline the Nuffield Council's framework; but I shall discuss this using the themes that have emerged during the course of thinking through dementia. In the second section, I shall consider each of the dilemmas from Chapter 1. I shall use the framework in a fairly free way to approach the dilemmas, but again I shall be drawing on the broader philosophical discussion in order to demonstrate the context in which the dilemmas must be approached. Needless to say, the context (or surround) is one in which facts and values are intermingled. What we have to do is negotiate and navigate our way through a world that is inherently normative.

The framework: philosophical underpinnings

The first component of the ethical framework is that there should be a 'case-based' approach to ethical decisions. This is also called casuistry, which is an approach with a long history (Jonsen & Toulmin, 1988). Casuistry suggests an inductive process according to which decisions are made on the basis of immersion in the particularities of the case, rather than an appeal (as in deductivism) to already established principles. Having looked at the realities of the particular case, a process of interpretation follows in the light of relevant values and with reference to the decisions made in relevant and similar

Box 9.1: Dementia: an ethical framework

(from: Nuffield Council on Bioethics (2009). *Dementia: Ethical Issues*. Table 2.1)

Component 1: A 'case-based' approach to ethical decisions: Ethical decisions can be approached in a three-stage process: identifying the relevant facts; interpreting and applying appropriate ethical values to those facts; and comparing the situation with other similar situations to find ethically relevant similarities or differences.

Component 2: A belief about the nature of dementia: Dementia arises as a result of a brain disorder, and is harmful to the individual.

Component 3: A belief about quality of life with dementia: With good care and support, people with dementia can expect to have a good quality of life throughout the course of their illness.

Component 4: The importance of promoting the interests both of the person with dementia and of those who care for them: People with dementia have interests, both in their autonomy and their well-being. Promoting autonomy involves enabling and fostering relationships that are important to the person, and supporting them in maintaining their sense of self and expressing their values. Autonomy is not simply to be equated with the ability to make rational decisions. A person's well-being includes both their moment-to-moment experiences of contentment or pleasure, and more objective factors such as their level of cognitive functioning. The separate interests of carers must be recognized and promoted.

Component 5: The requirement to act in accordance with solidarity: The need to recognize the citizenship of people with dementia, and to acknowledge our mutual interdependence and responsibility to support people with dementia, both within families and in society as a whole.

Component 6: Recognizing personhood, identity and value: The person with dementia remains the same, equally valued, person throughout the course of their illness, regardless of the extent of the changes in their cognitive and other functions.

cases (Murray, 1994). The conclusions made in any particular case according to this approach are still regarded as presumptive in the sense that they can be revised in the light of new facts or experience. In short, the casuistical process mirrors that of case law, which builds on precedent and paradigm cases in order to determine current cases. The approach can easily be used in connection with many types of ethical decision in connection with acquired diffuse neurocognitive dysfunction (Louw & Hughes, 2005).

The relevance of the case-based approach is in one sense obvious enough. It encourages an individual approach to individual cases, where the unique person is considered in his or her own context. But this sends us in the direction of something deeper. Casuistry demands an immersion in the particular facts of a particular case. In so doing, however, it forces us to consider the individual being in his or her individual world, where not only will there be particular facts, but these will be interwoven with individual values. And the being of the person, as a situated embodied agent, will necessarily interact with the narrative lives of others. This is Heidegger's notion of Being-with. Any approach to ethics that does not grasp the reality of this complicated nexus that makes up the surround of any dilemma will simply be inadequate. It is not that casuistry is the only ethical approach able to take these broader considerations into account (for instance, virtue ethics would do much the same thing), but the case-based approach helps to focus attention on the real complexities of real cases in an open-ended way. By this I mean that the case-based approach will encourage a broad view. Any new piece of information or different perspective will be potentially relevant. It is an approach that allows the human-person-perspective. The normative concerns that surround any piece of information (any fact) are simply there as part of the furniture of the world.

The second component is a belief about the nature of dementia. The point about this component is that it recognizes that acquired diffuse neurocognitive dysfunction is harmful under all sorts of circumstances to the individual. Hence, this component takes seriously the notion of embodiment. Agency in the dilemmas that arise will always be embodied agency. Moreover, because of the narrative structure of our lives and the way in which our potentially harmed bodies interact within our ongoing narratives, this component of the framework sets up the possibility of our *inter-dependencies*. People with acquired diffuse neurocognitive dysfunction are more or less dependent on others. This is in the nature of the condition. However, the harm that is done to any individual in a world of beings characterized by solicitude will have an impact on those around. This component, therefore, in itself, commends a broad view in order to understand the potential harm that might result for society.

Although acquired diffuse neurocognitive dysfunction is harmful, the third component adds the corrective thought that, nevertheless, it is possible to maintain a good quality of life if the person is cared for well. Dementia-in-the-world carries with it the implication that we should not simply look at harm, but should look at the potentially rich surroundings that can contribute in a way that might enhance the person's quality of life. This is not to deny component two, but is to see it in the broader human-person-perspective. Part of the value of this perspective is that it opens up the possibility of avoiding stigma and alienation. We must attend not only to the physical pathology, but also to the psychosocial and spiritual environment. Once again, this component reflects our being-with-others-in-the-world. In addition, particularly thinking about people with acquired diffuse neurocognitive dysfunction, where it might be thought (mistakenly) that the person was a 'shell', this component suggests otherwise. In doing so it draws on two potential sources. First, there is the notion of the externality of mind. As we have seen, this tells us that mindedness is not just in the head. My memories are, in part, maintained by others. What it is to have a memory, what constitutes memory, is something that is (at least potentially) shareable in the public domain. Therefore, whether I am actually a 'shell' will depend on whether or not I am treated like a 'shell'. I can be malignantly positioned: my Self 3 can be undermined by a malignant psychosocial environment.

The second source supports the first. The evidence is that good communication helps to demonstrate the ways in which the person is much more than a 'shell'. There is also the evidence of 'lucid intervals' (Normann, Asplund, and Norberg, 1998). These are episodes in which a person with quite severe dementia suddenly says something that is absolutely relevant to the circumstances, or which clearly carries meaning. It is also possible to point to gestures, where we can invoke the notions of the body-subject or embodied agency to argue in favour of persisting subjectivity. The various ways, therefore, in which the person remains as a situated embodied agent should encourage the thought that quality of life not only *can* be maintained, but *should* be maintained into the later stages of the condition.

Component four is to do with promoting the interests of the person with acquired diffuse neurocognitive dysfunction and his or her carers. It emphasizes both autonomy and well-being. One thing that should be obvious is that promoting interests can potentially cause conflicts. For instance, respecting a person's autonomy, that is allowing them to do what they wish, might threaten their well-being. In addition, the autonomous wishes of a patient might conflict with the wishes of the family carers. Thus, we see once again the potency of our situatedness.

Another theme that could be picked up in this connection is that of the uncircumscribable nature of personhood. This has a bearing on ideas around well-being, as it does concerning quality of life. It means that those making decisions need to think as broadly as possible in order to recognize the many fields in which people are situated. This full-field view (Fulford, 1989) is the human-person-perspective. There are obvious links to be made to the Heideggerian notion of Being-with. This can be seen by considering two other notions that are discussed in the literature.

The first is that of *relational* autonomy (Mackenzie & Stoljar, 2000). The second notion is that of *inter*-dependence, which I have already mentioned. The point is that none of us lives independently. Our autonomous decisions will almost always affect other people. My ability to make my own life choices is more often than not predicated on my presumption that certain other things will happen, which in itself implies that I am not fully autonomous, but actually dependent. The notion of dependence is often regarded as a bad thing in that it emphasizes the differential power relationship between people. But, as George Agich (2003) has so eloquently argued in connection with long-term care, dependence and autonomy can be regarded as opposite sides of the same coin. In other words, my ability to exercise my autonomy often reflects my dependency. As Agich suggests,

> ... the concept of autonomy properly understood requires that individuals be seen in essential inter-relationship with others and the world. (Agich, 2003: 174)

The exercise of my autonomous wish to be in the garden may well only be possible in the context of my dependency, because I depend on others to help me to the garden. But this dependency does not negate my autonomy, it allows me to fulfil my autonomous wishes. Autonomy will most often have to be thought of in the context of relationships. All of this can also be regarded as a feature of our situated nature as beings of this sort in a context of Being-with, which is characterized by solicitude.

The final two components of the framework refer to ideas that have been considered throughout this book, namely those of solidarity and personhood. No more needs to be said at this point, except to pick out the notion of *citizenship*. This is most naturally connected to the idea of solidarity. If we are bound together in societies, then it is a natural move to consider how we are located in the *polis*. As such, people with acquired diffuse neurocognitive dysfunction should also be regarded as citizens. Seeing people in this light does convey benefit in the sense that it stresses the potential for people with dementia to remain engaged in society: they should not be marginalized (Bartlett & O'Connor, 2007). The move to citizenship can also be regarded as a way to push forward the claim that personhood entails broader commitments. People with acquired diffuse neurocognitive dysfunction can none the less remain engaged in civic duties as citizens. However, although seeing things through the lens of citizenship might be a way of encouraging participation and allows (as the Nuffield Council on Bioethics (2009) has suggested) a link to be made to the whole notion of disability rights (Shakespeare, 2006). This is undoubtedly an avenue worth pursuing. It has to be remembered, however, that Karl Marx himself stated: '. . . *man* is more fundamental than the *citizen, human life* more than political life' (quoted p.243). Thus, I might argue that the notions of personhood and solidarity are more foundational than the idea that the person with acquired diffuse neurocognitive dysfunction is a citizen in the *polis*. But, if we are interested in pushing forward the political agenda (Redley, Hughes, and Holland, 2010), then the notion of citizenship is clearly of central importance, even if it is underpinned by the notions of solidarity and personhood.

Back to the dilemmas

Mr Siders

The dilemma for Mr Siders was whether he should present himself to the doctor for referral to the memory clinic for assessment and investigation. He was being told by various friends, for instance from the bridge club, that his memory was causing problems. But Mr Siders had anxieties about this because he was worried he might lose his driving licence, which would have been a disaster. He was also a little annoyed that people were telling him there was something wrong with him when he felt perfectly fine.

If we look at the particular details of this case, it has to be said that Mr Siders was not causing problems for anyone else. It was sometimes embarrassing when he forgot someone's name and frustrating if he went to the shops and then forgot what he was meant to be buying, but Mr Siders had a sense of humour about such events. It was only because someone else from the bridge club had taken his wife to the memory clinic that the discussion about him seeking such help had arisen. Dementia is definitely a harm, which is the second component of the Nuffield Council's framework, but it was not doing any harm to Mr Siders. There was the thought, put to him by his friend, that if he were diagnosed early, it might be that treatment would be forthcoming, which would be worthwhile in the longer term. At that point, however, he felt more inclined to exercise his own autonomous decision-making capabilities and not seek help. Against this, it could be said that his well-being would be served better by early assessment. In addition, it has to be recognized that if there were worries about his driving it would be better for these to be picked up and properly assessed as soon as possible. However, Mr Siders knew for sure that he had not been involved in any accidents, nor had anyone passed any critical comments about his driving at any stage.

On balance, therefore, particularly taking into account his own feelings on the matter, it does not seem right for pressure to be put on Mr Siders to seek assessment unless he particularly wishes to do so. This might change if, for instance, the difficulties caused by any forgetfulness were becoming more marked; and it would certainly be the case that he should seek assessment if his driving were to start to cause concern.

None the less, there is a line of thought that would suggest that early diagnosis is beneficial come what may. This takes us into arguments concerning mild cognitive impairment (MCI) (O'Brien, 2008). This is regarded as a pre-dementia state. The *conceptual* difficulty arises because some people with MCI will not progress to full-blown dementia. At present, the conversion rate from MCI to dementia is about 10% per year (Bruscoli & Lovestone, 2004); but there are reports of a conversion rate of 80% over six years (quoted in O'Brien *op. cit.*). In part this depends on where and how the subjects of studies were recruited and how strictly particular diagnostic criteria have been applied: there is a distinction between amnestic and non-amnestic MCI for instance (O'Brien, *op. cit.*). The *conceptual* problem arises because it is tempting to ask what kind of thing is MCI? It is not a diagnosis of an illness, because even in the most rigorously selected and diagnosed 'patients', 20% are still well (in the sense that they do not have dementia) six years later. MCI is clearly a construct, but is it useful? It might be (Petersen, 2006), but we know that receiving a diagnosis of MCI is not entirely benign. It can have negative effects because of the stigma (including self-stigma), sense of alienation, and anxiety caused simply by being told that you have a condition that might or might not progress to one that you perhaps fear (more or less rationally) more than any other (Corner & Bond, 2006; Sabat, 2006b). It just is the case that there is 'an essential ambiguity' about the status of MCI, about whether or not it is pathological (Thornton, 2006). We have to recognize that there is a variety of institutional and cultural factors that influence the clinical use of the 'diagnosis' of MCI (Moreira et al., 2008). Although the concept of MCI has now gained considerable currency (Petersen, 2006), it remains a contested notion (Graham & Ritchie, 2006a, 2006b). I have already discussed the views of Peter Whitehouse, who would contend that MCI, just as Alzheimer's disease, should be seen as a manifestation of normal ageing and not as a disease (Gaines & Whitehouse, 2006; Whitehouse, 2006).

There are different motivating forces at work pushing us either in the direction of early diagnosis in order to encourage early advice and treatment, or in the direction of encouraging people to accept difference without regarding this as pathological (Hughes, 2006c). The worry is that a 'diagnosis' such as MCI given in old age will tend to suggest impairment rather than mere difference.

The attention being paid to the mild cognitive problems being experienced by Mr Siders is, perhaps, a function of our hyper-cognitive society (Post, 1995, 2006). What is missing is the human-person-perspective. From this point of view it would seem reasonable to argue that Mr Siders should attend the memory clinic if he wishes, but should be under no pressure to do so. The important thing is that he is living his life well and enjoying companionship without any sense of stigma and alienation. If stigma and alienation are creeping in on the grounds of very minimal evidence of dysfunction, rather than this being a sign that Mr Siders should seek diagnosis, it may signify instead a deeper malaise affecting society.

Mrs Brownwell

The dilemma for the doctor looking after Mrs Brownwell is that her daughter wishes to know what is going on but the doctor knows that Mrs Brownwell will not wish to have anyone else meddling in her affairs. It is, therefore, to do with confidentiality.

Once again, the case-based approach of the Nuffield Council on Bioethics (2009) would suggest that we need to enquire carefully concerning the amount of harm that may or may not be caused by Mrs Brownwell's problems. In discussing this issue, the Nuffield Council working party took the view that capacity and best interests would have to be assessed very carefully. If Mrs Brownwell has capacity to make decisions about who should be involved in her care, which necessitates that she has good insight into the nature of any difficulties that she might be having and whether or not these are having an effect on anyone else, then her wishes must be abided by. If she lacks this capacity, because, for instance, she is unaware of how many times she telephones her daughter, then the doctor may reasonably make a decision that it would be in Mrs Brownwell's best interests for her daughter to be involved more fully in decisions about her care. However, even under these circumstances, this would not give Mrs Brownwell's daughter the right to know absolutely everything about her mother, but only those things that are necessary. Recognizing the personhood of Mrs Brownwell and not wishing to undermine her standing as an independent Self would suggest that Mrs Brownwell's views should be given a good deal of weight, even though she lacks capacity. The issue is to do with respecting her autonomy, but it is also to do with ensuring her well-being. Her daughter may contribute to her well-being and, of course, we need to be aware of aspects of relational autonomy that should push us in the direction of sharing relevant information in order to help Mrs Brownwell. The notion of solidarity should encourage us, in any case, to be supportive of both Mrs Brownwell and her daughter. In the end, however, much of this will depend on the nature of the doctor's communication both with Mrs Brownwell and with her daughter. The facts of the case may mean that the evaluative judgements are all on the side of maintaining Mrs Brownwell's confidences. If not, then the doctor will have to strive very hard to negotiate with Mrs Brownwell so that she accepts there should be more openness about what is happening. One practical tactic would be for the doctor to encourage Mrs Brownwell's daughter to attend an appointment with her mother. The real onus here should, perhaps, be on encouraging good, honest, straightforward communication between mother and daughter. The doctor's underlying duty is towards Mrs Brownwell, as the patient, but the arguments which stem from our understanding of persons as situated, and from the needs of solidarity, would suggest that the doctor has some obligation to encourage the sort of authentic encounter that will allow appropriate honesty. Elsewhere we have written:

> The more sophisticated philosophical picture ... involves people who are embedded in a shared human-worldly context ... The relationship between the doctor and the patient is—at its best—a matter of mutual engagement within this context. Confidentiality is a token of the trust that should exist as an element of this mutual engagement, but not necessarily as an overriding principle. This trust, therefore, exists within a shared context

in which others are likely to become involved as a matter of routine and for the good of the patient. (Hughes & Louw, 2002b)

Thus, whilst the direction of the decision making will be governed by laws and professional guidelines, the underlying issue is to do with our standing as human beings of this kind with these sorts of relationship, where certain manifestations of concern, in the context of certain kinds of relationship, must be taken seriously and cannot simply be set aside. In the absence of malign intent, the daughter's solicitude must be taken seriously and the doctor's judgement must be guided accordingly, even if Mrs Brownwell's right to confidentiality must be respected.

Dorothy Galpin

Dorothy Galpin's case raises a dilemma for her social worker. The question is whether, despite evidence of cognitive impairment, she should be allowed to go home as she wishes. Once again the facts of the matter will have to be considered very carefully. However, we should see straight away that the relevant facts are not completely easy to discern because values are tightly intermingled with the facts. The facts are value-laden. Dorothy Galpin may well say that she wishes to go home because she has lived there for so many years and she is familiar with it, and this fact in itself expresses a number of significant values. Another fact is that she performed poorly when assessed by the occupational therapist in the ward kitchen, but (over against that fact) what weight should be given to Mrs Galpin's insistence that she return to live in the home in which she lived for so many years with her now deceased husband? In particular, on what grounds can we presume that the problems in the ward kitchen would occur in Mrs Galpin's familiar environment in her home kitchen? The legal situation, at least under the *Mental Capacity Act 2005*, which covers England and Wales, is quite straightforward. Mrs Galpin lacks capacity to make this decision, or so it has been determined, and a decision has to be made in her best interests. Most of the multi-disciplinary team seem to feel that Mrs Galpin should go into long-term care, but the social worker is the decision-maker in this particular case and the social worker's view is that Mrs Galpin might be supportable with a significant homecare package. Other members of the multi-disciplinary team are pointing to the risks of harm because they feel Mrs Galpin is unsafe. These risks and concerns certainly have to be taken seriously. It is also important to think of Mrs Galpin's general quality of life. We know that people with acquired diffuse neurocognitive dysfunction can enjoy a good quality of life if the psychosocial environment is appropriate. It might be that Mrs Galpin, once at home, will feel very lonely and may feel happier when surrounded by others. But this cannot be presumed. There will have to be some weighing up of how best to promote her interests. We know that to respect her autonomous wishes we would have to allow her home, but there is the question of her well-being. However, her well-being may also be impaired in long-term care if she cannot accept this. Either way, the claims of solidarity would suggest that we must do all we can to support Mrs Galpin and, if we are to think of her personhood from a phenomenological point of view, with attention not just to her cognitive function, but also to her emotional state, we should seek the option that will take all of these factors into consideration. In other words, we need a broad view, the human-person-perspective. This will also be a view of Mrs Galpin's life story: the narrative view is important here. Mrs Galpin is suggesting how she wishes the narrative of her life to be continued and, perhaps, how it should end. It might, then, be a travesty to put her into care if this is something she will hate for her remaining days. The human-person-perspective should encourage us to make judgements based on a broad view. We should be able to see Mrs Galpin as a citizen who has rights and whose liberty should not be restricted. Or, if it must be restricted, the restriction of liberty should be as minimal as possible. These points might almost seem mundane, except that on a daily basis in developed countries all over the world, people with acquired diffuse neurocognitive dysfunction have decisions made for them concerning where they should live with very little attention paid to their wishes and with little hope that they can alter the decisions that are made. This would be less of a problem if the quality of long-term care were uniformly good, but this is (sadly) not the case. Hence, older people all over the world are having their liberty restricted (and possibly deprived) with very little concern for their human rights, their rights as citizens, or their rights as people. It will, of course, sometimes be entirely right to ensure a person's safety by arranging for long-term care in some form of institutional facility. None the less, our standing as situated embodied agents in the world, where the values of autonomy and well-being are part of the fabric of our being as creatures whose lives have significance, should entail: (a) that every possible effort is made to enable us to pursue our life stories in the way we wish; and (b) that, if we require care, this should be of the highest possible standard. The standard should itself be dictated by the needs of personhood, where the self should not be undermined, but where aspirations to improve the quality of life should be encouraged. In addition, as well as valuing the person, the person's position as a valuer (Jaworska, 1999) should be recognized as a matter of solidarity based (again) on our standing as situated beings who co-author each other's lives in the context of solicitude arising from our being-with as a constitutive feature of our worldly existence.

Mr Gupta

Mr Gupta's family feels that his quality of life is not good, whereas the nursing assistants in the home where he now lives are ambivalent about this. They see more evidence of well-being in their day-to-day encounters with Mr Gupta. But they are very concerned that feeding Mr Gupta now tends to lead to aspiration and pneumonia. The dilemma for the nursing assistants is that they feel, as they feed him, that they might be shortening his life since he definitely has difficulty swallowing. But they are uncertain whether they wish to see Mr Gupta being fed artificially either by a nasogastric tube or by a percutaneous endoscopic gastrostomy (PEG) tube. Both possibilities seem too invasive to them.

In all of these cases, there would be further facts to be elicited in order to help make decisions. For instance, we do not know whether Mr Gupta had ever expressed any views in the past about this sort of situation, either in connection with his own illness or in connection with someone else's. In addition, we do not know whether there are any strong religious views that might influence the decisions that have to be made. These are the facts that need to be clarified as we immerse ourselves in the particularities of Mr Gupta's case. There is no doubt that he is now suffering very distinct harm from his acquired diffuse neurocognitive dysfunction. He was probably suffering harm when he was agitated and somewhat aggressive, but that behaviour settled and it has to be said that his quality of life appeared reasonable until he started to have problems with swallowing and then chest infections. One thought, concerning his quality of life, is that if only the feeding difficulties could be circumvented, his quality of life would once again be good. Understanding what his interests are is now difficult in any direct sense, but we do know that his family has always been involved and their expressions concerning his interests, in particular what he would say himself, must be taken very seriously. A narrow understanding of his well-being would suggest that artificial nutrition would be of benefit. The notion of solidarity in this case would seem to suggest that a priority is to make sure that everyone feels as comfortable as possible with whatever the decision may be, which means that people need to be involved, whether they are nursing assistants or family. Doctors and other health and social care workers involved in Mr Gupta's case need to communicate effectively. The importance of recognizing Mr Gupta's personhood means paying attention to his subjective well-being, whilst also recognizing that his subjectivity is embodied, so that bodily care of the most appropriate sort will be a way to maintain his continuing standing as a person of value. The question is, however, what might constitute the most 'appropriate' type of bodily care: does this mean feeding him by hand despite the fact that he might then choke, or does it mean using artificial means?

There is some important empirical work upon which we can draw in order to make decisions about Mr Gupta. Finucane, Christmas, and Travis (1999) helped to confirm that tube feeding offered no significant advantages over oral feeding for people with advanced dementia. This might have seemed counter-intuitive, on the grounds that it might be thought that having bypassed the larynx there should be no way for food to get into the lungs. Unfortunately, aspiration still occurs in people with severe acquired diffuse neurocognitive dysfunction. It might also have been thought that ensuring proper calorie intake would be a way of ensuring that the person did not lose weight, but again this is not the case because people in the severer stages of the disease suffer weight loss as a consequence of the disease process even despite good intake. On these and other grounds, Gillick (2000) persuasively argued that there would be no moral imperative to use artificial feeding and nutrition for someone in the advanced stages of dementia. But there are further considerations. For instance, many people wish to stress the importance of the human contact that occurs during feeding of people with severe acquired diffuse neurocognitive dysfunction. Many describe this as quality time in a situation where staff can find it difficult to provide one-to-one attention to residents in care homes. This personal contact would be lost during artificial feeding. It is often the time when basic forms of communication can be established. This was described in Barbara Pointon's account of Malcolm's sense of humour, which could emerge when he was being fed (see Chapter 7). What we might perceive here is the existence of the background habitus, where deeply ingrained social responses still linger, where the body-subject can be sensed through embodied intentions. (I discussed these matters in Chapter 7 too.) Wim Dekkers has used the philosophy of

Merleau-Ponty to argue in favour of the notion of 'bodily autonomy'. Dekkers writes as follows:

> The lived body is the expression of one's existence and is concretely lived by oneself. It is through one's lived body that one manifests oneself to the world. ... The lived body possesses its own knowledge of the world, which implies the existence of a 'tacit knowledge' that functions without conscious control. (Dekkers, 2010: 257)

Dekkers goes on to apply this sort of thought directly to acquired diffuse neurocognitive dysfunction:

> Cognitive capabilities of persons with severe dementia gradually disappear until the moment they are no longer capable of exercising their autonomy by making explicit decisions. This does not mean, however, that their bodily knowledge, which has been developed in the course of their lives, necessarily also disappears. Tacit bodily knowledge is based on the sedimentation of life narratives. Although automatisms get gradually lost, persons with severe dementia still have routine actions stored in their body. Behavioural patterns of persons with severe dementia may be interpreted as a remainder of what once has been 'real', that is, rational autonomy. They have nothing else at their disposal than these bodily movements. Although the body in severe dementia increasingly shows dysfunctions, it still remains a lived body and a body in which previous forms of autonomy have been inscribed. (Dekkers, op. cit.: 258)

Dekkers argues, therefore, that when the person pushes away attempts at artificial feeding, when they pull out naso-gastric tubes, or indicate irritation with PEG tubes, these gestures should not be regarded as lacking in meaning. Indeed, as representations of bodily autonomy, they are full of significance. The natural inclination to pull out tubes should not be regarded as having no significance whatsoever. Hence, this would in itself be an argument against the use of artificial nutrition and hydration for somebody like Mr Gupta.

The other issue that is raised by Mr Gupta is to do with our thinking about quality of life. In general, we think we know what this means, and therefore we feel that we can make judgements about the quality of life of others. But this is fraught with difficulties. There is a particular difficulty associated with the idea that quality of life can be measured in people with acquired diffuse neurocognitive dysfunction (Bond, 1999; Hughes, 2003). Quality of life has to be thought about individually for individual people (Bond & Corner, 2004). This stems precisely from the point that personhood cannot be circumscribed. In which case, nor is it possible to pin down all of those factors that should be taken into account when quality of life is being judged (Hughes, 2003). To make such a judgement we require detailed information about the person's narrative, to include their previous wishes and beliefs, as well as to pay attention to their current likes and dislikes. The externality of mind suggests that one way to understand the person's inner subjectivity is precisely to consider their outward engagement with the world. This is to make Wim Dekkers' point about bodily autonomy in a different way. The worry in discussing quality of life is that, at any point, we are in danger of making a judgement about the person *qua person*, that perhaps their type of life is one unworthy of being lived (Jennings, 2000). But beings of this kind engaged in the world as we are should not think in this way because it is characteristic of our situation in the world that we should show concern and solicitude towards others of our nature. To think of others as unworthy is to demean our own standing as beings of this kind.

Dr Montagna

The dilemma for Susan, Dr Montagna's daughter, was whether or not she should allow her father to be admitted to hospital when he developed a fever. She had always wished to look after him at home. Once more, the detailed facts of the case are clearly important. For instance, we would wish to know whether Dr Montagna is still able to take tablets by mouth. Is he still drinking? But if we presume that he is no longer able to take oral medication, nor fluids, then the feeling that he needs to be admitted to hospital tends to grow stronger. The nature of Dr Montagna's condition is such that any infection has an increased chance of leading to his death because of his frailty. The question is then whether there should be a ceiling to the care that is offered to him. The first judgement is whether or not he should go into hospital, but if he does go into hospital there will then be questions concerning how far people should go in terms of treatment. We might presume that there is little doubt that the quality of Dr Montagna's life has been good because of the care that Susan has been able to give him. But she does not have adequate knowledge or expertise to treat him when he is physically unwell. To keep him at home might, therefore, increase the chances that he would die. But this is a difficult judgement to make. If it could be determined that he was going to die in any case, then it might be argued that his quality of life would be better if he could be cared for at home in familiar surroundings. A recent study in London by Liz Sampson and colleagues showed that mortality was independently associated with the severity of cognitive impairment (Sampson, Blanchard, Jones, Tookman, and King, 2009). Acquired distributed brain dysfunction increases the risks after hospital admission and there is a question, therefore, concerning whether hospital admission achieves anything other than inconvenience and distress; this seems especially pertinent if it is the case that people with more severe acquired diffuse neurocognitive dysfunction die within a short time of being admitted. There are also empirical points to consider in connection with specific treatments. For instance, rather than pneumonia being a pleasant way to die—the old man's friend—Jenny van der Steen and her colleagues have shown that there can be more discomfort associated with pneumonia in the context of dementia than might have been anticipated (van der Steen et al., 2002, 2009). They have also shown that evaluative decisions play a significant role in the type of treatment that people receive and whether or not treatment is withheld. Treatment, for instance, was more often withheld for pneumonias in the Netherlands than in the United States (van der Steen et al., 2004). It is becoming clear that quite complicated judgements have to be made concerning the use of antibiotics in infections in the context of severe acquired diffuse neurocognitive dysfunction. Antibiotics can be used to prolong life, but they can also be used simply as a palliative measure, because, for instance, they help with breathing. All of this might be considered to weigh in favour of Dr Montagna being admitted to hospital.

Against this we have to weigh up the possibility that he might acquire further infections in the hospital and that over-investigation and over-treatment in the hospital might in themselves cause him discomfort. Because of his close relationship with Susan, her views should be of significance. She is likely to be a good judge of her father's well-being and, in any case, the notion of solidarity should suggest that the decisions made should be supportive in the sense that they should take careful note of her opinions. Dr Montagna's personhood is, in part, at least held and maintained by his relationship with his daughter: their narratives are entwined.

We can see, therefore, that there are difficult clinical judgements to be made on the basis of somewhat conflicting and uncertain empirical evidence. So it might be more reasonable to make a clinical decision with a good deal of attention being paid to the values expressed by Susan given her closeness to her father. The conceptual analysis concerning personhood encourages and underpins this view. Dr Montagna is situated in such a way that his best interests must square with those of Susan. Her instincts seem likely to be extremely close to his wishes, given how well she knows him and given the quality and amount of care that she has given him. Under these circumstances, we might wish to say that her view should carry the day over and above any more factual evidence, but she needs adequate support. It would seem entirely apt for this decision to be made after a very careful conversation with Susan concerning her thoughts and wishes and her judgement about what her father would have wanted himself. Not only is there the likelihood that narrative coherence will be achieved by paying attention to Susan's views, but the issue is also to do with the ethics of care, where the nature of the relationship between Susan and her father is critical since it is most likely to reflect *genuine* care, or what Heidegger refers to as solicitude. The nature of the authentic encounters between Susan and Dr Montagna mean that she is most likely to have some understanding of his wishes and emotional needs as reflected by his embodied subjectivity, as well as by anything else he may have said earlier in their relationship. This is to say that she will be closer to her father's phenomenology because of her greater understanding of his mentality. This understanding is based on years of relationship, as well as on the more intimate encounters that are a feature of genuine holistic care both at a physical and spiritual level. More than anyone else, Susan has encountered her father at the level of the soul, so it would seem most appropriate for her views to be taken into consideration and given great weight at this moment of existential crisis. For the same reason, because of the need for solidarity and solicitude, she will now require considerable support. Because of the nature of her *Being-with*, the dilemma for Susan does not just concern her father; it concerns her own sense of authenticity and narrative coherence. But these are items in the normative world and must be taken seriously in the human-person-perspective.

Conclusion

What we have found in discussing these cases is that judgements are made against a particular background or surround. Not only is there a great variety of facts to be taken into consideration, and not only do the facts alter in each case, but there are also numerous evaluative judgements to be made, which are partly connected with the facts, but which also reflect broader considerations in the background of *particular* cases.

The inner subjectivity of persons is embodied. Just as intentionality is played out in the world in terms of practices, where normativity is a constitutive, immanent, and irreducible feature of those practices, so too our sense of right and wrong in particular cases is often determined by judgements about behaviours and histories, as recorded in discourse, which can be taken to reflect the person's sense of what is significant, meaningful, or important to them in their lives. The necessary interpretation that must occur will not always be easy and sometimes judgements will have to be made on the basis of partial understanding. None the less, in each case it is the broad view that is required: the human-person-perspective. So, we must act on the basis of seeing the world from a perspective that makes sense of our decisions. Once the surround is seen clearly—once we have a surview—the right decision is likely to be made.

What we see in these stories is that dementia is always dementia-in-the-world. Decisions must always, therefore, take into account everything that makes up the person's world. If this can be done then it is more likely that the right decisions will be made. But often, in situations of uncertainty, which will frequently obtain where there is acquired diffuse neurocognitive dysfunction, the important thing will be the nature of the communications that have occurred. In the end, good decisions will be made when those involved have had the courage to look with some intensity at the face of the Other; when encounters, however brief, are at the level of the soul. At this point, reflecting the mutual engagement of beings of this kind, there may be some sense of the ground for the possibility of knowing what might be right or wrong under the particular circumstances. But this ground is likely to be beyond our ability to enunciate, because at this level judgements are aesthetic. We are in the area of Keats' 'negative capability',

> ... when man is capable of being in uncertainties, Mysteries, doubts, without any irritable reaching after fact & reason ... (Keats, 1990: 370)

Our moral dilemmas, therefore, are solved by judgements that are akin to aesthetic judgements, where the key ingredient is that we should see things aright, and we shall do this if we can adopt the human-person-perspective. Aesthetic judgements involve reason. But they also involve a sense of normativity, which is based on our ways of being-in-the-world. In the end, we do not make these judgements on the basis of pure reason, but on the basis of our mutual participation in a form of life that sees things in *this* way and not *that*.

Chapter 10

Conversion and revolution

Introduction

Thinking through dementia is a matter of seeing our surroundings, of gaining a surview. Our view is always from somewhere and, like an aesthetic judgement, brings with it a host of intellectual, but also emotional, cultural, spiritual, and other preconceptions and background understandings. Our view incorporates a particular perspective, but this is by no means solely a rational one: it reflects our whole way of being-in-the-world, which is also volitional and intuitive. Thinking through dementia, therefore, involves unpacking this form of life, this kind of being. We are beings of this kind. Considering the implications of this statement, which is what thinking through dementia entails, is a vast undertaking. There are three aspects I shall consider here: mindedness, the world, and personhood; and these lead to a fourth: a sense of mystery.

First, then, we are minded. The key issue that arises in this context is to consider how our mental states make contact with the world. This is the problem of intentionality. As I have suggested, externalism helps to solve the problem: the mind just is populated by the world. We cannot conceive anything without conceiving the world. When we remember, we remember the world. Moreover, the normativity of intentional mental states makes direct contact with the world too. The transcendental account shows the way in which our intentional mental states are normative. That is, there are criteria of correctness that allow us to comment on the veridical nature of our thoughts and memories, that allow us to say whether or not a face has been *truly* recognized, but these criteria are pre-conditions for there being such things as thoughts and memories. They are built into our basic understanding of what it is to think, intend, or remember. The grounds for the possibility that a memory is true are not to be found elsewhere, they are found in the practices of remembering as constitutive, immanent, and irreducible. Our mental states reflect practices and a transcendental feature of such practices is that they are normative. Thus, at the heart of our mindedness is a quintessential worldly embedding.

Hence, secondly, we have to turn to the world, not as a separate thing, but because it is constitutive of our make-up. We are the kind of things that we are, our souls are such, on account of the world. It informs our being. This is true in a literal, albeit causal, sense. For it is the worldly carbon atom that Primo Levi (1919–1987) identified—at work in his brain—as responsible for his writing (Levi, 1975). But it is true in another sense, because 'the world' is constituted by values and norms too. They are *our* values, which may be modified and altered over time, but they are as much a part of the furniture of the world as the rest of the atoms in the Periodic Table. Our mode of being-in-the-world is enough to ensure that the world is populated in a manner that cannot be norm-free. Thinking in our world *just is as it is*, it cannot be otherwise. We are embedded in our worldly practices. This raises a related environmental issue. Our standing in the world is, inherently, a standing in relationship with the things of nature. Our engagement with the natural world is not optional, it is inevitable and, more than this, it too constitutes our being, so we ignore it at our peril (Midgley, 2001). Our deep embedding in practices is a deep embedding in the world itself.

But the things of the world, about which we must care, are not, however, beings like us. We are, instead, persons with the capacity to enjoy Being-with. The third aspect, therefore, is that of personhood. As I have suggested, being a person is to be a situated embodied agent. We are situated in a multifaceted surround. Our subjectivity is embodied, which is to restate the notion of the externality of mind. This, in turn, ensures that our agency is partly manifest through the enduring possibility of our gestures and behaviours being interpreted by others with whom we share cultures, histories, habitus, and the like. Our situatedness in the environment as persons is, amongst many other things, to be open to the ethical imperatives that flow from Being-with: the demands of solicitude. But, as we have seen, our situatedness and the nature of the world are such that our personhood cannot be circumscribed. Our world-view is always, potentially (however limited an individual perspective might be), of a broader surround.

Our mindedness, the world, and our personhood give rise to the fourth aspect I wish to highlight in connection with our being-in-the-world, which is the sense of mystery to which I have several times returned. There is a mystery associated with our mindedness, especially when, for instance, we think of consciousness and our inability to pin it down, despite attempts by scientists to provide causal accounts of its physical underpinnings (Shear, 1997). Once again, it is the constitutive understanding of consciousness that eludes us. Recall that the world itself, *that* it exists, is—according to Wittgenstein (TLP §6.44)—mystical. And being a person, in particular given the nature of our personal encounters –when we see the soul in the face of the Other—and given the way in which meaning can be interpreted without words—the way in which we can share a mutual understanding of music—this too is in an ultimate sense mysterious. In Chapter 7, I discussed how the mysterious aspects of our thinking through dementia are both mundane and quotidian—in the eyes of the Other, in our everyday encounters—whilst at the same time they point beyond our phenomenal grasp to something noumenal that cannot be captured in language or thought.

But perhaps this is not so. For perhaps it is precisely in poetry, art, architecture, sculpture, and music (and probably a host of other manifestations of the human spirit) that we do manage to gain some sort of perspective on the transcendent. This more mystical appreciation of nature and the world is less to do with reason and rationality and more to do with intuition. It is the stuff of the Romantics, but it brings us back to our topic.

It turns out that thinking through dementia, since this entails thinking about the kind of beings that we are, leads us beyond any circumscribed biomedical or cognitive neuropsychological models, beyond the discursiveness of social constructionism, to a broader view akin to making an aesthetic judgement, where what counts is not always definable (entirely) in rational terms, but is rooted in our human responses, incorporating all of our instincts, intuitions, emotions, drives, cultural narratives, historical contexts, our moral, and artistic sensibilities.

So we need the broadest possible perspective because thinking through dementia reveals that dementia is nowhere near straightforward. Even the biopsychosocial lens does not provide the right perspective. For dementia is about our place in the world. It is about us as minded, worldly persons, yet bounded by something spiritual or mystical. Dementia, to be considered appropriately, must be thought of as dementia-in-the-world. And to obtain the perspicuous surview that this notion demands, we cannot be constrained by any particular model. We need to approach dementia with the broadest possible lens. This is provided by the human-person-perspective, because this is a view without bounds.

This is the view that brings in, at least potentially, every aspect of human life, from our discursive practices to our silent encounters with the eyes of the Other. This is the view that demands we think broadly about what might be in someone's best interests, about what might constitute quality of life, about the possibilities for enhancing care and showing solicitude. The human-person-perspective is no soft option; it is a challenge to us not to accept what we see immediately, but to look beyond to what might be uncomfortable territory, to a world in which rights are fully respected and basic care is delivered without recourse to confining protocols. It is a perspective—reflecting the possibilities for human beings like us—that shows us how bad things are. It is not an easy perspective to consider. It shows us how life should be, but how shoddy it is now (by and large) for people with acquired diffuse neurocognitive dysfunction unless they experience the authentic encounters that are characteristic of solicitude.

Implications

The implications of the human-person-perspective, of dementia-in-the-world, and of the situated embodied agent view of the person have all been touched upon already. But I wish to point a little further in the direction of the philosophical and ethical implications and then in the direction of the clinical implications of this thinking through dementia.

For philosophy

From the philosophical point of view I shall say just two things. First, I hope I have shown how philosophical work can have practical relevance. Our understanding of the mind, for instance, is not without consequence for how we treat someone such as Miss Breen, as I indicated in Chapter 3. Secondly, a key feature of the philosophy of psychiatry is that there is the possibility of two-way traffic between practice and philosophy (Fulford, 1991). Yesterday I reviewed some of the patients (or residents) on our continuing care ward, people with severe acquired diffuse neurocognitive dysfunction. These particular people are totally dependent for all of their bodily needs on the dedicated nursing staff. They do not talk. They are immobile and doubly incontinent. I was struck afresh by the disparity between what I witness in this unit and the discussions I read in some of the ethics and philosophy literature. These are the 'shells' who have lost all personhood, whose lives seem to lack all quality or even worth. But the man I reviewed last week watched me intently yesterday as I went to review someone on the other side of the room, then turned his attention to someone new as they entered. The report is that he enjoys the television when it is on. The person I was reviewing meanwhile responded to my presence, looked somewhat anxious, but can occasionally show humour, and still manifests characteristics of his previous personality. The family carer I spoke to, who has not exchanged a word with his spouse for many years, nevertheless showed his complete commitment to his wife and his concern for her well-being. These were very ordinary encounters. There is no doubt about the sadness of the plight of these people. But there is also no room to deny them personhood, no doubt that they engage with their worlds in an individual way, no doubt that they are minded, however damaged they might also be. We feel their subjectivity through their behaviours; we perceive their humanity through their bodily gestures; and we witness the solicitude, the Being-with, of the family carers and the nursing staff. This is not sentimentality. It is, however, raw data for philosophers. I talked in Chapter 7 of flesh and blood mingling with intentionality and normativity, of facts and values coming together, and of the interdigitation of inner and outer (see p. 208). This is what I witness on our continuing care ward. Philosophy is rightly concerned with these matters at a conceptual level and philosophers would wish to interrogate some of the claims that I have just made. But we are dealing here with real people and, whatever the conclusions of our philosophizing, there has to be a sense in which these conclusions square with the practices and phenomenology of care.

Perhaps the crucial aspect here is talk of phenomenology. Purely rational arguments about the nature of the mind will tend to miss something unless they can make contact with phenomenological experience. In Chapter 5, I quoted Sisson writing about Edward Thomas (see p. 120), when he talked about the importance of 'human relationships'. I have laid store by the authentic human encounter, which does not require words, which Barbara Pointon describes in her relationship with her husband Malcolm, even when he was severely affected by Alzheimer's disease (see Chapter 7). To miss out this dimension of human experience in explications of mind, personhood, meaning, and the like, may be legitimate in particular circumstances; but any such discussion can never then lay claim to anything more than partial authority. Moreover, conditions such as acquired diffuse neurocognitive dysfunction test our notions of authenticity and, as such, are worthy of further philosophical thought. In any case, the idea that practice has something to offer philosophy (as well as the other way around) need not be argued further here (see Fulford, Morris, Sadler, and Stanghellini, 2003; Widdershoven, McMillan, Hope, and van der Scheer, 2008).

For ethics

In Chapter 9, I hope I have made a point about the implication of this work for ethics too. There I tried to show how the framework of the Nuffield Council on Bioethics (2009) was underpinned by the sort of philosophical considerations discussed in this book. That point was easily won because the Nuffield Council's framework itself used concepts that have been important in these pages, such as personhood. Similarly, the notion of solidarity has deep conceptual roots. The importance of broader philosophical thought as an antidote to the application of principles of medical ethics as a matter of rote learning needs to be emphasized. *Psychiatric* ethics is, in any case, another antidote to this tendency because it inevitably involves concepts that raise philosophical complexities (such as mind, person, freedom, coercion, normality, perception, consciousness, and so on) and because real cases in psychiatric practice tend to put stress on our more straightforward principles (as we saw in the discussion of 'autonomy' as 'relational autonomy' in connection with the Nuffield Council's framework) (see also Dickenson & Fulford, 2000). There is a further point, which is that psychiatric ethics involves more conceptual difficulties because of its 'more complex values structure' (Fulford et al., 2006: 479), which might account for the lack of attention paid to mental health issues in bioethics more generally. Issues around diagnosis emerge more readily in connection with psychiatric practice than they do in other areas of medicine because the evaluative judgements required to make psychiatric diagnoses are more apparent (Sadler, 2004). It might have been thought that dementia was more straightforward precisely because it looks like an 'organic' brain disorder, similar to other physical illness diagnoses and unlike those of mental illness; but the discussion of Chapter 1 (and elsewhere in this book) has shown how this is not the case (see also Thornton, 2007: 44–6). These complexities are particular to dementia because of the difficulties in discriminating normal from abnormal ageing. The construct of mild cognitive impairment (MCI) epitomizes these conceptual struggles (see the discussion on p. 256 above) and, hence, MCI warranted a special issue of the journal *Philosophy, Psychiatry, & Psychology* (Volume 13 (1), March 2006).

The major implication for ethics, however, is probably a political one. Stemming from the sort of concerns to which I have already referred, the underpinning ethical issue is to do with the standing of older people in the *polis* generally, but especially when they have acquired diffuse neurocognitive dysfunction. The tendency for older people to be marginalized or discriminated against, the tendency for their standing as selves to be undermined (i.e. Sabat's (2006a) 'malignant positioning'), the possibility of alienation from themselves, these are all political matters. The cry of solidarity and the demand for citizenship should be our response to the undermining of the human rights of large parts of our societies worldwide simply because they are ageing and, in particular, because of dementia.

For clinical practice

I hope my thoughts about the clinical implications of thinking through dementia will already be apparent from my comments earlier in this chapter as well as elsewhere in the book. In brief, the human-person-perspective means that we should think about our patients in the broadest possible light. If this sounds like motherhood and apple pie, then so be it; but we should not be comfortable. For a start, it means that almost no one in this field is doing well enough: not the average home carer, nor the average nurse or doctor, nor the Government Minister for Health. It also means that those who pursue a biomedical cure for dementia should accept, as Whitehouse and George (2008) in effect suggest, that they are chasing rainbows. We are extremely unlikely to 'cure' the ageing brain. But meanwhile it means that those who rile against the use of medications of various sorts should acknowledge the good that can be done by the judicious use of a variety of different drugs. And if it is highly unlikely that we can cure ageing and probably impossible that we shall find *a* cure for dementia (because it is not one thing, but about one hundred things), none the less, we might ameliorate (as we have done) age-related diseases and we might find cures for particular types of acquired diffuse neurocognitive dysfunction. Those who espouse the use of psychosocial interventions, where it can always be said that the problem is there has been less attention to these approaches because of the dominance of the biomedical model, must also admit that there will be no one approach to any particular behaviour that will succeed. Indeed, we shall find that individuals have to be approached individually, that a variety of approaches will work, but many will fail, and that these approaches will include the use of medications.

It is worth clarifying that this is not a stance, therefore, against a neuroscientific approach to acquired diffuse neurocognitive dysfunction. But the human-person-perspective suggests that we must temper our claims and focus our efforts. Indeed, this is the implication for the whole of the research community: we need good quality researchers pursuing both quantitative and qualitative research of real value. This was the message of the Nuffield Council on Bioethics (2009). The human-person-perspective demands a sense of balance between factions: more dialogue and cooperation between bioscientists and psychosocial researchers.

For clinicians and social care workers, the right perspective is one that embraces all possible approaches. There should be no reason not to try alternative, complementary therapies as well as more conventional ones and assistive technologies where these are genuinely useful. We should certainly insist that we know our patients or clients better: that more attempts are made to understand their needs, which (if unmet) may be driving their behaviour. To this extent we should be favouring psychosocial approaches to care. We should not be tolerating poor physical environments. But, perhaps more importantly, we should be fostering care environments in which the social milieu is enhancing, in which patients or clients, as well as their informal (usually family) and formal carers feel supported. This is to put into effect the precept of solidarity and it is to respect the personhood of all concerned.

Conclusion

But the human-person-perspective on dementia-in-the-world digs deeper. It suggests an important *metanoia*: a change of mind, a conversion, a change of one's life. For what is at stake is the way in which we think of our *own* lives. It is the way we view ageing and decline. It is to do with the way we view each other. The human-person-perspective is importantly about how I encounter the Other, about whether I look in his or her eyes and about what happens as a result. It is about the *authentic* nature of my being-in-the-world and my engagement with others. It is about communication at the level of the soul, that is, where we can communicate our humanity. It is about having the correct (physical, psychological, social, and spiritual) environments in which to let this occur. It is about *being in the moment* with the person. It is about genuine care and making manifest the possibility of solicitude.

From the personal to the governmental levels, therefore, as suggested in Chapter 8, the human-person-perspective calls for revolution. To quote Sisson again on Edward Thomas: 'All passion for the truth is revolutionary . . .' (quoted by Wright in Thomas, 1981: 25). The human-person-perspective is not one view once and for all: it will seek all the possibilities for truth that surround the human being in the world.

For the human-person-perspective is about our place in our world. It is, then, as Whitehouse has suggested, about relationships between generations and with the world. It is about solidarity as beings-in-the-world. It is about compassion and solicitude. It is about,

> ... a greater sense of responsibility for future generations and for our planet. (Whitehouse & George, 2008: 281)

The human-person-perspective is about how we stand in relation to others and to creation. We should be artists and scientists, philosophers, and artisans; for we must both think and do. Our connections with the world are made up of our thoughts and our actions, and how we make those connections is constrained by the norms that shape our lives. These norms are lived out in our practices, which are embedded in the world and defined constitutively by the criteria that make the way we live and the things we say right or wrong. These immanent and irreducible features of our lives are what the human-person-perspective is ultimately about. It is about a type of being that is inherently constrained by its normative features, but in the face of dementia-in-the-world our *Being-with* alters the space of our solicitude. We must not just have the right perspective, we must act on it. Our approach to dementia-in-the-world is akin to an aesthetic judgement, because we must be willing to contemplate broadly, emotionally, and intuitively, as well as rationally. But we cannot simply stand by and contemplate. Confronted by acquired diffuse neurocognitive dysfunction, we have to act; and the ultimate justification for doing one thing rather than another will not be some further justification, it will be immanent in the nature of the actions that make up our practices. What we end with is, '. . . an ungrounded way of acting' (OC §110). But it is a way of acting that is in the world, where it must cohere with our broader patterns of practice (Hughes, 2006d). In the end, for better or for worse, what we do shapes our surround.

Bibliography

Agich, G.J. (2003). *Dependence and Autonomy in Old Age: An Ethical Framework for Long-Term Care*. Cambridge: Cambridge University Press.

Aldridge, D. (ed.) (2000). *Music Therapy in Dementia Care*. London and Philadelphia: Jessica Kingsley.

Allan, K. and Killick, J. (2010). Communicating with people with dementia. In: *Supportive Care for the Person with Dementia* (eds. J.C. Hughes, M. Lloyd-Williams, and G.A. Sachs), pp. 217–25. Oxford: Oxford University Press.

Alzheimer, A. (1907). Über eine eigenartige Erkrankung der Hirnrinde. *Allgemeine Zeitschrift für Psychiatrie und Psychisch-Gerichtliche Medizin*, **64**, 146–8. Translated in R.H. Wilkins and I.A. Brody (1969). Alzheimer's disease. *Archives of Neurology*, **21**, 109–10.

Alzheimer's Disease International (ADI) (2009). *World Alzheimer Report (2009): Executive Summary*. London: Alzheimer's Disease International.

Ames, D., Burns, A., and O'Brien, J. (eds.) (forthcoming). *Dementia* (4th edition). London: Arnold Health Sciences.

Anderson, E. (2008). Cognitive change in old age. In: *Oxford Textbook of Old Age Psychiatry* (eds. R. Jacoby, C. Oppenheimer, T. Dening, and A. Thomas), pp. 33–50. Oxford: Oxford University Press.

Anscombe, G.E.M. (1975). The first person. In: *Mind and Language* (ed. S. Guttenplan), pp. 45–65. Oxford: Clarendon Press.

Anscombe, G.E.M. (1976). The question of linguistic idealism. *Acta Philosphica Fennica*, **28**, 188–215. Reprinted in The Collected Philosophical Papers of G.E.M. Anscombe, Volume One: From Parmenides to Wittgenstein, pp. 112–33. Oxford: Blackwell (1981).

Anscombe, G.E.M. (1991). Wittgenstein. Whose philosopher? In: *Wittgenstein Centenary Essays* (ed. A. Phillips Griffiths), pp. 1–10. Cambridge: Cambridge University Press.

Aquilina, C. and Hughes, J.C. (2006). The return of the living dead: agency lost and found? In: *Dementia: Mind, Meaning, and the Person* (eds. J.C. Hughes, S.J. Louw, and S.R. Sabat), pp. 143–61. Oxford: Oxford University Press.

Aristotle (1968). *De Anima*, Books II and III (trans. D.W. Hamlyn). Oxford: Clarendon Press.

Armstrong, D.M. (1968). *A Materialist Theory of the Mind*. London: Routledge & Kegan Paul.

Arrington, R.L. (1991). Making contact in language: the harmony between thought and reality. In: *Wittgenstein's Philosophical Investigations: Text and Context* (eds. R.L. Arrington and H.-J. Glock), pp. 175–202. London: Routledge.

Baker, G.P. and Hacker, P.M.S. (1984). *Scepticism, Rules and Language*. Oxford: Basil Blackwell.

Baldwin, C. (2010). Narrative, supportive care, and dementia: a preliminary exploration. In: *Supportive Care for the Person with Dementia* (eds. J.C. Hughes, M. Lloyd-Williams, and G.A. Sachs), pp. 245–52. Oxford: Oxford University Press.

Baldwin, C. and Capstick, A. (2007). *Tom Kitwood on Dementia: A Reader and Critical Commentary*. Maidenhead, Berkshire: McGraw Hill, Open University Press.

Ballard, C. and Aarsland, D. (2010). Pharmacological management of neuropsychiatric symptoms in people with dementia. In: *Supportive Care for the Person with Dementia* (eds. J. C. Hughes, M. Lloyd-Williams, and G. A. Sachs), pp. 105–15. Oxford: Oxford University Press.

Ballard, C.G., O'Brien, J., James, I., and Swann, A. (2001). *Dementia: Management of Behavioural and Psychological Symptoms.* Oxford: Oxford University Press.

Bamford, C., Lamont, S., Eccles, M., Robinson, L., May, C., and Bond, J. (2004). Disclosing a diagnosis of dementia: a systematic review. *International Journal of Geriatric Psychiatry,* **19,** 151–69.

Bamford, C., Arksey, H., Poole, M., Kirkley, C., Hughes, J., Corner, L. et al. (2009). *Person- and carer-centred respite care for people with dementia: developing methods of evaluating the effectiveness of different models.* Report for the National Institute for Health Research Service Delivery and Organisation Programme. Available at: http://www.sdo.nihr.ac.uk/ files/project/113-final-report.pdf [accessed 4 July 2010].

Banfield, S. (1997). *Gerald Finzi: An English Composer.* London and Boston: Faber and Faber.

Barber, R., Gholkar, A., Scheltens, P., Ballard, C., McKeith, I.G., Morris, C.M., et. al. (1999). Apolipoprotein E epsilon 4 allele, temporal lobe atrophy, and white matter lesions in late-life dementias. *Archives of Neurology,* **56,** 961–5.

Bartlett, R. and O'Connor, D. (2007). From personhood to citizenship: broadening the lens for dementia practice and research. *Journal of Aging Studies,* **21,** 107–18.

Beauchamp, T.L. and Childress, J.F. (2001). *Principles of Biomedical Ethics* (5th edition). Oxford: Oxford University Press.

Berlin, I. (1999). *The Roots of Romanticism* (ed. H. Hardy). London: Pimlico.

Berrios, G.E. (1987). Dementia during the seventeenth and eighteenth centuries: a conceptual history. *Psychological Medicine,* **17,** 829–37.

Blackburn, S. (1984). The individual strikes back. *Synthese,* **58,** 281–301.

Bloor, D. (1973). Wittgenstein and Mannheim on the Sociology of Mathematics. *Studies in History and Philosophy of Science,* **4,** 173–91.

Bloor, D. (1996). The question of linguistic idealism revisited. In: *The Cambridge Companion to Wittgenstein* (eds. H. Sluga and D. G. Stern), pp. 354–82. Cambridge: Cambridge University Press.

Bloor, D. (1997). *Wittgenstein, Rules and Institutions.* London: Routledge.

Boghossian, P.A. (1989). The rule-following considerations. *Mind,* **98,** 507–49.

Bolton, D. (1997). Encoding of meaning: deconstructing the meaning/causality distinction. *Philosophy, Psychiatry, & Psychology,* **4,** 255–67.

Bolton, D. and Hill, J. (1996). *Mind, Meaning, and Mental Disorder: The Nature of Causal Explanation in Psychology and Psychiatry.* Oxford: Oxford University Press.

Bond, J. (1999). Quality of life for people with dementia: approaches to the challenge of measurement. *Ageing and Society,* **19,** 561–79.

Bond, J. and Corner, L. (2004). *Quality of Life and Older People.* Buckingham: Open University Press.

Boorse, C. (1975). On the distinction between disease and illness. *Philosophy and Public Affairs,* **5,** 49–68.

Bowlby, J. (1988). *A Secure Base: Clinical Applications of Attachment Theory.* London: Routledge.

Boyd, C.M. (1954). Gerald Finzi and the solo song. *Tempo,* **33** (Autumn), 15–18.

Braak, H. and Braak, E. (1991). Neuropathological stageing of Alzheimer-related changes. *Acta Neuropathologica*, **82**, 239–59.

Brock, D.W. (1988). Justice and the severely demented elderly. *Journal of Medicine and Philosophy*, **13**, 73–99.

Brooker, D. (2004). What is Person Centred Care for people with dementia? *Reviews in Clinical Gerontology*, **13**, 215–22.

Brooker, D. (2008). Person centred care. In: *Oxford Textbook of Old Age Psychiatry* (eds. R. Jacoby, C. Oppenheimer, T. Dening, and A. Thomas), pp. 229–40. Oxford: Oxford University Press.

Bruscoli, M. and Lovestone, S. (2004). Is MCI really just early dementia? A systematic review of conversion studies. *International Psychogeriatrics*, **16**, 129–40.

Buber, M. (2004). *I and Thou* (2nd edition) (trans. R.G. Smith, 2004). London: Continuum. (Ich und Du first published in 1923; translation first published in 1937).

Budd, M. (1989). *Wittgenstein's Philosophy of Psychology*. London: Routledge.

Burns, A., O'Brien, J., and Ames, D. (eds.) (2005). *Dementia* (3rd edition). London: Arnold Health Sciences.

Burton, E.J., Barber, R., Mukaetova-Ladinska, E.B., Robson, J., Perry, R.H., Jaros, E., et. al. (2009). Medial temporal lobe atrophy on MRI differentiates Alzheimer's disease from dementia with Lewy bodies and vascular cognitive impairment: a prospective study with pathological verification of diagnosis. *Brain*, **132**, 195–203.

Buscema, M., Grossi, E., Snowdon, D., Antuono, P., Intraligi, M., Maurelli, G. et al. (2004). Artificial neural networks and artificial organisms can predict Alzheimer pathology in individual patients only on the basis of cognitive and functional status. *Neuroinformatics*, **2**, 399–416.

Churchland, P.M. (1984). *Matter and Consciousness: A Contemporary Introduction to the Philosophy of Mind*. Cambs., Mass.: Bradford Book, MIT Press.

Churchland, P.M. and Churchland, P.S. (1992). Intertheoretic reduction: a neuroscientist's field guide. In: *Neurophilosophy and Alzheimer's Disease*, (eds. Y. Christen and P. Churchland), pp. 18–29. Berlin: Springer-Verlag. (First published in *Seminars in the Neurosciences*, 1990, **2**, 249–56.)

Coaten, R. (2002). Movement matters: revealing the hidden humanity within dementia through movement, dance and the imagination. *Dementia: The International Journal of Social Research and Practice*, **1**, 386–92.

Corder, B., Saunders, A.M., Strittmatter, W.J., Schmechel, D.E., Gaskell, P.C., Small, G.W., et. al. (1993). Gene dose of apolipoprotein E type 4 allele and the risk of Alzheimer's disease in late onset families. *Science*, **261**, 921–3.

Corner, L. and Bond, J. (2006). The impact of the label of mild cognitive impairment on the individual's sense of self. *Philosophy, Psychiatry, & Psychology*, **13**, 3–12.

Coulter, J. (1979). *The Social Construction of Mind. Studies in Ethnomethodology and Linguistic Philosophy*. London and Basingstoke: Macmillan Press.

Damasio, A.R., Damasio, H., and van Hoesen, G.W. (1982). Prosopagnosia: anatomic basis and behavioral mechanisms. *Neurology*, **32**, 331–41.

Damasio, H. and Damasio, A.R. (1992). Memory, language and decision-making: contributions from the lesion method in humans. In: *Neurophilosophy and Alzheimer's Disease* (eds. Y. Christen and P. Churchland), pp. 108–22. Berlin: Springer-Verlag.

Davidson, D. (1980). *Essays on Actions and Events*. Oxford: Clarendon Press.

Davies, B. (1992). *The Thought of Thomas Aquinas*. Oxford: Clarendon Press.

Davies, B. and Harré, R. (1990). Positioning: the discursive production of selves. *Journal for the Theory of Social Behaviour*, **20**, 43–63.

Davis, R. (1989). *My Journey into Alzheimer's Disease: Helpful Insights for Family and Friends.* Wheaton, Illinois: Tyndale House.

Dekkers, W. (2010). Persons with severe dementia and the notion of bodily autonomy. In: *Supportive Care for the Person with Dementia* (eds. J.C. Hughes, M. Lloyd-Williams, and G.A. Sachs), pp. 253–61. Oxford: Oxford University Press.

Dennett, D.C. (1969). *Content and Consciousness.* London and Henley: Routledge & Kegan Paul.

Dennett, D.C. (1978). *Brainstorms. Philosophical Essays on Mind and Psychology.* Montgomery, VT: Bradford Books. (References here are to (1997) Penguin edition, Harmondsworth.)

Dennett, D.C. (1987). *The Intentional Stance.* Cambridge, MA: MIT Press.

Dennett, D.C. (1991). *Consciousness Explained.* Harmondsworth: Allen Lane; The Penguin Press.

De Renzi, E., Perani, D., Carlesimo, G.A., Silveri, M.C., and Fazio, F. (1994). Prosopagnosia can be associated with damage confined to the right hemisphere–an MRI and PET study and a review of the literature. *Neuropsychologia*, **32**, 893–902.

Descartes, R. (1954). *Descartes: Philosophical Writings* (trans. E. Anscombe and P.T. Geach). Sunbury-on-Thames: Nelson's University Paperbacks, The Open University.

Dickenson, D. and Fulford, K.W.M. (2000). *In Two Minds: A Casebook of Psychiatric Ethics.* Oxford: Oxford University Press.

Downs, M., Clare, L., and Mackenzie, J. (2006). Understandings of dementia: explanatory models and their implications for the person with dementia and therapeutic effort. In: *Dementia: Mind, Meaning, and the Person* (eds. J.C. Hughes, S.J. Louw, and S.R. Sabat), pp. 235–58. Oxford: Oxford University Press.

Ducheyne, S. (2008). Towards an ontology of scientific models. *Metaphysica: International Journal of Ontology and Metaphysics*, **9**, 119–27.

Duffy, C. (2005). *Shelley and the Revolutionary Sublime.* Cambridge: Cambridge University Press.

Dummett, M. (1958–59). Truth. *Proceedings of the Aristotelian Society*, **59**, 141–62. (Also in: *Philosophical Logic* (ed. P.F. Strawson), pp. 49–68. Oxford: Oxford University Press.)

Eccles, J.C. (1986). Do mental events cause neural events analogously to the probability fields of quantum mechanics? *Proceedings of the Royal Society of London*, **227**, 411–28.

Eccles, J.C. (1990). A unitary hypothesis of mind-brain interaction in the cerebral cortex. *Proceedings of the Royal Society of London*, **240**, 433–51.

Editorial (January 1965). *Music and Letters*, **XLVI** (1), 1–3.

Eldridge, R. (1986). The normal and the normative: Wittgenstein's legacy, Kripke, and Cavell. *Philosophy and Phenomenological Research*, **46**, 555–75.

Elliott, R. (2002). Hermeneutic single-case efficacy design. *Psychotherapy Research*, **12**, 1–21.

Ellis, A.W. and Young, A.W. (1988). *Human Cognitive Neuropsychology.* Hove, UK: Erlbaum.

Engel, G.L. (1977). The need for a new medical model: a challenge for biomedicine. *Science*, **196**, 129–36.

Engel, G.L. (1980). The clinical application of the biopsychosocial model. *American Journal of Psychiatry*, **137**, 535–44.

Engels, F. (1969). *Anti-Dühring. Herr Eugen Dühring's Revolution in Science.* Moscow: Progress Publishers. Originally published in 1877. Full text (slightly different translation by

Emile Burns from 1894 edition). Available at: http://www.marxists.org/archive/marx/works/1877/anti-duhring/index.htm [accessed 11 July 2010].

Esiri, M. (1997). Neuropathology. In: *Psychiatry in the Elderly* (2nd edition) (eds. R. Jacoby and C. Oppenheimer), pp. 79–103. Oxford: Oxford University Press.

Esiri, M.M., Matthews, F., Brayne, C., and Ince, P.G. (2001). Pathological correlates of late-onset dementia in a multicentre, community-based population in England and Wales. *Lancet*, **357**, 169–75.

Evans, G. (1982). *The Varieties of Reference* (ed. J. McDowell). Oxford: Clarendon Press.

Finucane, T.E., Christmas, C., and Travis, K. (1999). Tube feeding in patients with advanced dementia. *Journal of the American Medical Association*, **282**, 1365–70.

Fodor, J.A. (1976). *The Language of Thought*. Hassocks: The Harvester Press. (First published 1975; Scranton, PA.: Crowell.)

Fodor, J.A. (1985). Fodor's guide to mental representation: the intelligent auntie's vade-mecum. *Mind*, **94**, 76–100.

Fodor, J.A. (1987). *Psychosemantics: The Problem of Meaning in the Philosophy of Mind*. Cambridge, Mass.: MIT Press.

Folstein, M.F., Folstein, S.E., and McHugh, P.R. (1975). 'Mini-mental state'. A practical method for grading the cognitive state of patients for the clinician. *Journal of Psychiatric Research*, **12**, 189–98.

Frigg, R. and Hartmann, S. (2006). Models in Science. *Stanford Encyclopedia of Philosophy*. Available at: http://plato.stanford.edu/entries/models-science [accessed 6 July 2010].

Fulford, K.W.M. (1989). *Moral Theory and Medical Practice*. Cambridge: Cambridge University Press.

Fulford, K.W.M. (1991). The potential of medicine as a resource for philosophy. *Theoretical Medicine*, **12**, 81–5.

Fulford, K.W.M. (Bill), (2004). Facts/Values. Ten principles of values-based medicine. In: *The Philosophy of Psychiatry: A Companion* (ed. J. Radden), pp. 205–34. Oxford: Oxford University Press.

Fulford, K.W.M. (Bill), Morris, K., Sadler, J., and Stanghellini, G. (eds.) (2003). *Nature and Narrative: An Introduction to the New Philosophy of Psychiatry*. Oxford: Oxford University Press.

Fulford, K.W.M. (Bill), Thornton, T., and Graham, G. (eds.) (2006). *Oxford Textbook of Philosophy and Psychiatry*. Oxford: Oxford University Press.

Gadamer, H-G. (1960). *Wahrheit und Methode*. Tübingen. (Translated as Truth and Method, revised edition (1989), trans. J. Weinsheimer and D.G. Marshall. London: Continuum.)

Gadenne, V. (1989). Does introducing the social require eliminating the mental? A commentary on Rom Harré: 'Metaphysics and methodology: some prescriptions for social psychological research'. *European Journal of Social Psychology*, **19**, 455–61.

Gaines, A.D. and Whitehouse, P.J. (2006). Building a mystery: Alzheimer's disease, mild cognitive impairment, and beyond. *Philosophy, Psychiatry, & Psychology*, **13**, 61–74.

Gardner, H. (ed.) (1972). *The New Oxford Book of English Verse 1250-1950*. Oxford: Oxford University Press.

Gearin-Tosh, M. (2002). *Living Proof: A Medical Mutiny*. London: Simon & Schuster.

Gergen, K.J. (1985). The social constructionist movement in modern psychology. *American Psychologist*, **40**, 266–75.

Gergen, K.J. (1991). *The Saturated Self*. New York: Basic Books.

Giere, R.N. (1999). *Science Without Laws*. Chicago: University of Chicago Press.

Gillett, G. (1989). Representation and cognitive science. *Inquiry*, **32**, 261–76.

Gillett, G. (1992). *Representation, Meaning, and Thought*. Oxford: Clarendon Press.

Gillett, G. (2008). *Subjectivity and Being Somebody: Human Identity and Neuroethics*. Exeter UK: Imprint Academic.

Gillick, M.R. (2000). Rethinking the use of feeding tubes in patients with advanced dementia. *New England Journal of Medicine*, **342**, 206–10.

Goldfarb, W. (1985). Kripke on Wittgenstein on rules. *Journal of Philosophy*, **82**, 471–88.

Goodman, N. (1978). *Ways of Worldmaking*. Indianapolis: Hackett Publishing Company.

Graham, J.E. and Ritchie, K. (2006a). Mild cognitive impairment: ethical considerations for nosological flexibility in human kinds. *Philosophy, Psychiatry, & Psychology*, **13**, 31–43.

Graham, J.E. and Ritchie, K. (2006b). Reifying relevance in mild cognitive impairment: an appeal for care and caution. *Philosophy, Psychiatry, & Psychology*, **13**, 57–60.

Greenblat, C.S. (2004). *Alive with Alzheimer's*. Chicago: University of Chicago Press.

Groene, R.W. (1993). Effectiveness of music therapy-1:1 intervention with individuals having senile dementia of the Alzheimer's type. *Journal of Music Therapy*, **30**, 138–57.

Grossi, E., Buscema, M.P., Snowdon, D., and Antuono, P. (2007). Neuropathological findings processed by artificial neural networks (ANNs) can perfectly distinguish Alzheimer's patients from controls in the Nun Study. *BMC Neurology*, **7**, 15 [doi:10.1186/1471-2377-7-15].

Guzmán-García, A., Mukaetova-Ladinska, E., and James, I. (in press). Introducing a Latin Ballroom dance class to people with dementia living in care homes, benefits and concerns: a Pilot Study, *Dementia: The International Journal of Social Research and Practice*.

Hachinski, V. (2008). Shifts in thinking about dementia. *Journal of the American Medical Association*, **300**, 2172–3.

Hacker, P.M.S. (1972). *Insight and Illusion. Wittgenstein on Philosophy and the Metaphysics of Experience*. Oxford: Oxford University Press.

Hacker, P.M.S. (1987). Languages, minds and brains. In: *Mindwaves: Thoughts on Intelligence, Identity and Consciousness*, (eds. C. Blakemore and S. Greenfield), pp. 485–505. Oxford: Blackwell.

Hacker, P.M.S. (1993). *Wittgenstein: Meaning and Mind, Volume 3 of an Analytical Commentary on the Philosophical Investigations, Part I: Essays*. Oxford: Blackwell.

Hacker, P.M.S. (1996). *Wittgenstein's Place in Twentieth-Century Analytic Philosophy*. Oxford: Blackwell.

Hacking, I. (1982). Wittgenstein the psychologist. *New York Review of Books*, **29**, 42–4.

Harré, R. (1983). *Personal Being. A Theory of Individual Psychology*. Oxford: Blackwell.

Harré, R. (1989a). Language and the science of psychology. *Journal of Social Behavior and Personality*, **4**, 165–88.

Harré, R. (1989b). Metaphysics and methodology: some prescriptions for social psychology research. *European Journal of Social Psychology*, **19**, 439–53.

Harré, R. (1992). What is real in psychology? A plea for persons. *Theory and Psychology*, **2**, 153–8.

Harré, R. (1993). *Social Being*. (2nd edition. First published 1979.) Oxford: Blackwell.

Harré, R. (1994). Emotion and memory: the second cognitive revolution. In: *Philosophy, Psychology and Psychiatry,* (ed. A. Phillips Griffiths), pp. 25–40. Cambridge: Cambridge University Press.

Harré, R. and Gillett, G. (1994). *The Discursive Mind.* Sage, Thousand Oaks, London and New Delhi.

Hanson, N.R. (1958). *Patterns of Discovery: An Inquiry into the Conceptual Foundations of Science.* Cambridge: Cambridge University Press.

Haynes, J.-D. and Rees, G. (2006). Decoding mental states from brain activity in humans. *Nature Reviews Neuroscience,* 7, 523–34.

Heidegger, M. (1962). *Being and Time* (trans. J. Macquarrie and E. Robinson), Malden MA, Oxford, and Carlton (Australia): Blackwell. Sein und Zeit was first published in 1927.

Hodges, J.R., Salmon, D.P., and Butters, N. (1992). Semantic memory impairment in Alzheimer's disease: failure of access or degraded knowledge? *Neuropsychologia,* 30, 301–14.

Hodges, J.R., Salmon, D.P., and Butters, N. (1993). Recognition and naming of famous faces in Alzheimer's disease: a cognitive analysis. *Neuropsychologia,* 31, 775–88.

Hoerder-Suabedissen, A. and Molnár, Z. (2008). Principles of cerebral cortical development. In: *Oxford Textbook of Old Age Psychiatry* (eds. R. Jacoby, C. Oppenheimer, T. Dening, and A. Thomas), pp. 129–43. Oxford: Oxford University Press.

Holmes, C. (2008). The genetics and molecular biology of dementia. In: *Oxford Textbook of Old Age Psychiatry* (eds. R. Jacoby, C. Oppenheimer, T. Dening, and A. Thomas), pp. 103–17. Oxford: Oxford University Press.

Hope, T. (1994a). Commentary on 'The Alzheimer's disease sufferer as a semiotic subject'. *Philosophy, Psychiatry, & Psychology,* 1, 161–2.

Hope, T. (1994b). Personal identity and psychiatric illness. In: *Philosophy, Psychology and Psychiatry* (ed. A. Phillips Griffiths), pp. 131–43. Cambridge: Cambridge University Press.

Hope, T., Keene, J., Fairburn, C.G., Jacoby, R., and McShane, R. (1999). Natural history of behavioural changes and psychiatric symptoms in Alzheimer's disease: a longitudinal study. *British Journal of Psychiatry,* 174, 39–44.

Hope, T., Tilling, K.M., Gedling, K., Keene, J.M., Cooper, S.D., and Fairburn, C.G. (1994c). The structure of wandering in dementia. *International Journal of Geriatric Psychiatry,* 9, 149–55.

Hopkins, J. (1975). Wittgenstein and physicalism. *Proceedings of the Aristotelian Society,* 75, 121–46.

House of Commons (16 December 2008). *Hansard,* c677W. Also available at: www.publications.parliament.uk/pa/cm200809/cmhansrd/cm081216/text/81216w0033.htm#08121714000065 [Accessed on 4th December 2010].

Hudson, W.D. (ed.) (1969). *The Is-Ought Question: A Collection of Papers on the Central Problem in Moral Philosophy.* London and Basingstoke: Macmillan Press.

Hughes, J.C. (2001). Views of the person with dementia. *Journal of Medical Ethics,* 27, 86–91.

Hughes, J.C. (2003). Quality of life in dementia: an ethical and philosophical perspective. *Expert Review of Pharmacoeconomics and Outcomes Research,* 3, 525–34.

Hughes, J.C. (2006a). Beyond hypercognitivism: a philosophical basis for good quality palliative care in dementia. *Les Cahiers de la Fondation Médéric Alzheimer,* 2 (June), 17–23.

Hughes, J.C. (ed.) (2006b). *Palliative Care in Severe Dementia.* London: Quay Books.

Hughes, J.C. (2006c). The heat of mild cognitive impairment. *Philosophy, Psychiatry, & Psychology,* 13, 1–2.

Hughes, J.C. (2006d). Patterns of practice: a useful notion in medical ethics? *Journal of Ethics in Mental Health,* 1, 1–5. Available at: www.jemh.ca [Accessed on 4th December 2010]

Hughes, J.C. (2008). Being minded in dementia: persons and human beings. In: *Excellence in Dementia Care: Research into Practice* (eds. M. Downs and B. Bowers), pp. 119–32. Maidenhead, Berkshire: McGraw Hill, Open University Press.

Hughes, J.C. (forthcoming). Justice, guidelines, and virtues. In: Lesser, H. (ed.) *Justice and the Elderly*. Amsterdam and New York: Rodopi.

Hughes, J.C. and Baldwin, C. (2006). *Ethical Issues in Dementia Care: Making Difficult Decisions*. London and Philadelphia: Jessica Kingsley.

Hughes, J.C., Bamford, C., and May, C. (2008). Types of centredness in health care: themes and concepts. *Medicine, Health Care and Philosophy*, **11**, 455–63.

Hughes, J.C., Graham, N., Patterson, K., and Hodges, J.R. (1997). Dysgraphia in mild dementia of Alzheimer's type. *Neuropsychologia*, **35**, 533–45.

Hughes, J.C., Hedley, K., and Harris, D. (2006). The practice and philosophy of palliative care in dementia. In: *Palliative Care in Severe Dementia* (ed. J.C. Hughes), pp. 1–11. London: Quay Books.

Hughes, J.C., Hope, T., Reader, S., and Rice, D. (2002). Dementia and ethics: the views of informal carers. *Journal of the Royal Society of Medicine*, **95**, 242–6.

Hughes, J.C., Jolley, D., Jordan, A., and Sampson, E. L. (2007). Palliative care in dementia: issues and evidence. *Advances in Psychiatric Treatment*, **13**, 251–60.

Hughes, J.C., Lloyd-Williams, M., and Sachs, G.A. (eds.) (2010). *Supportive Care for the Person with Dementia*. Oxford: Oxford University Press.

Hughes, J.C. and Louw, S.J. (2002a). Electronic tagging of people with dementia who wander. *British Medical Journal*, **325**, 847–8.

Hughes, J.C. and Louw, S.J. (2002b). Confidentiality and cognitive impairment: professional and philosophical ethics. *Age and Ageing*, **31**, 147–50.

Hughes, J.C. and Louw, S.J. (2005). End of life decisions. In: *Dementia* (3rd edition) (eds. A. Burns, J. O'Brien, and D. Ames), pp. 239–43. London: Arnold Health Sciences.

Hughes, J.C., Louw, S.J., and Sabat, S.R. (2006a). Seeing whole. In: *Dementia: Mind, Meaning, and the Person* (eds. J.C. Hughes, S.J. Louw, and S.R. Sabat), pp. 1–39. Oxford: Oxford University Press.

Hughes, J.C., Newby, J., Louw, S.J., Campbell, G., and Hutton, J.L. (2008). Ethical issues and tagging in dementia: a survey. *Journal of Ethics in Mental Health*, **3**, 1–6. Available at: www.jemh.ca [Accessed on 4th December 2010].

Hume, D. (1962). *A Treatise of Human Nature* (ed. D.G.C. Macnabb). Glasgow: Fontana/Collins. (First published in 1739.)

Hume, D. (1975). *Enquiries Concerning Human Understanding and Concerning the Principles of Morals*, (ed. L. A. Selby-Bigge, from posthumous edition of 1777: Third edition with revision by P. H. Nidditch). Oxford: Clarendon Press.

Hursthouse, R. (1999). *On Virtue Ethics*. Oxford: Oxford University Press.

Jacoby, R., Oppenheimer, C., Dening, T., and Thomas, A. (eds.) (2008). *Oxford Textbook of Old Age Psychiatry*. Oxford: Oxford University Press.

Jaspers, K. (1923). *Allgemeine Psychopathologie*. Springer Verlag, Berlin. (English translation by J. Hoenig and M.W. Hamilton (1963). *General Psychopathology*. Manchester: Manchester University Press.)

Jaworska, A. (1999). Respecting the margins of agency: Alzheimer's patients and the capacity to value. *Philosophy and Public Affairs*, **28**, 105–38.

Jennings, B. (2000). A life greater than the sum of its sensations: ethics, dementia, and the quality of life. In: *Assessing Quality of Life in Alzheimer's Disease* (eds. S.M. Albert and R.G. Logsdon), pp. 165–78. New York: Springer Publishing Company.

Joachim, C.L., Morris, J.H., and Selkoe, D.J. (1988). Clinically diagnosed Alzheimer's disease: autopsy results in 150 cases. *Annals of Neurology*, **24**, 50–6.

Jobst, K.A., Hindley, N.J., King, E., and Smith, A.D. (1994). The diagnosis of Alzheimer's disease: a question of image? *Journal of Clinical Psychiatry*, **55** (11, supplement), 22–31.

Jolley, D. (2010). An introduction to the dementias: a clinical view. In: *Supportive Care for the Person with Dementia* (eds. J.C. Hughes, M. Lloyd-Williams, and G.A. Sachs), pp. 11–19. Oxford: Oxford University Press.

Jonsen, A.R. and Toulmin, S. (1988). *The Abuse of Casuistry: A History of Moral Reasoning.* Berkeley: University of California Press.

Kahn-Denis, K. (2002). The person with dementia and artwork: art therapy. In: *The Person with Alzheimer's Disease: Pathways to Understanding the Experience* (ed. P.B. Harris), pp. 246–69. Baltimore and London: The Johns Hopkins University Press.

Kandel, E.R. (1998). A new intellectual framework for psychiatry. *American Journal of Psychiatry*, **155**, 457–69.

Kandel, E.R. (2005). *Psychiatry, Psychoanalysis, and the New Biology of Mind.* Washington DC and London, England: American Psychiatric Publishing, Inc.

Kant, I. (1993). *Grounding for the Metaphysics of Morals* (3rd edition) (J.W. Ellington, trans.). Indianapolis/Cambridge: Hackett Publishing Company. (First published 1785.)

Kant, I. (2007). *Critique of Pure Reason* (M. Weigelt, trans. and ed.; based on translation by M. Müller). London: Penguin Books. (First published in Germany 1781 and 1787.)

Kazdin, A.E. (1982). *Single-Case Research Designs: Methods for Clinical and Applied Settings.* New York: Oxford University Press.

Keady, J. and Gilliard, J. (2002). Testing times: the experience of neuropsychological assessment for people with suspected Alzheimer's disease. In: *The Person with Alzheimer's Disease: Pathways to Understanding the Experience* (ed. P.B. Harris), pp. 3–28. Baltimore and London: The Johns Hopkins University Press.

Keats, J. (1990). *The Major Works.* (E. Cook, ed.). Oxford: Oxford University Press.

Kennedy, M. (1970). *Elgar Orchestral Music.* London: British Broadcasting Corporation.

Kenny, A. (1968). *Descartes: A Study of his Philosophy.* New York: Random House.

Kenny, A. (1984). *The Legacy of Wittgenstein.* Oxford: Basil Blackwell.

Kenny, A. (1989). *The Metaphysics of Mind.* Oxford: Clarendon Press.

Killick, J. and Cordonnier, C. (2000). *Openings: Dementia Poems & Photographs.* London: *Journal of Dementia Care* and Hawker Publications.

Kim, J. (1985). Psychophysical laws. In: *Actions and Events. Perspectives on the Philosophy of Donald Davidson* (eds. E. Le Pore and B. P. McLaughlin), pp. 369–86. Oxford, Basil Blackwell.

Kipps, C.M. and Hodges, J.R. (2008). Clinical cognitive assessment. In: *Oxford Textbook of Old Age Psychiatry* (eds. R. Jacoby, C. Oppenheimer, T. Dening, and A. Thomas), pp. 155–63. Oxford: Oxford University Press.

Kitwood, T. (1970). *The Christian understanding of man. First published in What is Human?* London: Inter-Varsity Press. Republished in: Tom Kitwood on Dementia: A Reader and

Critical Commentary (eds. C. Baldwin and A. Capstick), pp. 188–208. Maidenhead, Berkshire: McGraw Hill, Open University Press; 2007.

Kitwood, T. (1989). Brain, mind and dementia: with particular reference to Alzheimer's disease. *Ageing and Society*, **9**, 1–15.

Kitwood, T. (1990). The dialectics of dementia: with particular reference to Alzheimer's disease. *Ageing and Society*, **19**, 177–96.

Kitwood, T. (1993). Towards a theory of dementia care: the interpersonal process. *Ageing and Society*, **13**, 51–67.

Kitwood, T. (1997). *Dementia Reconsidered: The Person Comes First.* Buckingham: Open University Press.

Kitwood, T. and Bredin, K. (1992a). Towards a theory of dementia care: personhood and well-being. *Ageing and Society*, **12**, 269–87.

Kitwood, T. and Bredin, K. (1992b). A new approach to the evaluation of dementia care. *Journal of Advances in Health and Nursing Care*, **1**, 41–60.

Knapp, M. and Prince, M. (2007). *Dementia UK*. London: Alzheimer's Society.

Kontos, P.C. (2004). Ethnographic reflections on selfhood, embodiment and Alzheimer's disease. *Ageing and Society*, **24**, 829–49.

Kontos, P.C. (2006). Embodied selfhood. An ethnographic exploration of Alzheimer's disease. In: *Thinking About Dementia: Culture, Loss, and the Anthropology of Senility* (eds. A. Leibing and L. Cohen), pp. 195–217. Piscataway, New Jersey: Rutgers University Press.

Kripke, S. (1982). *Wittgenstein on Rules and Private Language: An Elementary Exposition.* Oxford: Basil Backwell.

Kurz, A.F. and Lautenschlager, N.T. (2010). The concept of dementia: retain, reframe, rename or replace? *International Psychogeriatrics*, **22**, 37–42.

Larsson, T., Sjogren, T., and Jacobsen, G. (1963). Senile dementia: a clinical, sociomedical and genetic study. *Acta Psychiatrica Scandinavica*, **39** (supplement 167), 1–259.

Lesser, A.H. (2006). Dementia and personal identity. In: *Dementia: Mind, Meaning, and the Person* (eds. J.C. Hughes, S.J. Louw, and S.R. Sabat), pp. 55–61. Oxford: Oxford University Press.

Levi, P. (1975). *The Periodic Table* (translated by R. Rosenthal). London: Penguin Books.

Lévinas, E. (1981). *Otherwise than Being or Beyond Essence* (trans. A. Lingis). The Hague: Martinus Nijhoff. Originally published as: Autrement qu'être ou au-delà de l'essence. The Hague: Martinus Nijhoff (1974).

Lévinas, E. (1985). *Ethics and Infinity* (trans. R.A. Cohen). Pittsburgh: Duquesne University Press. Originally published as: Éthique et Infini. Paris: Librarie Arthème Fayard and Radio France (1982).

Lewis, H.D. (1982). *The Elusive Self.* London: Macmillan.

Locke, J. (1964). *An Essay Concerning Human Understanding* (edited and abridged by A.D. Woozley). Glasgow: William Collins/Fount Paperbacks. (First published in 1690.)

Louw, S.J. and Hughes, J.C. (2005). Moral reasoning – the unrealized place of casuistry in medical ethics. *International Psychogeriatrics*, **17**, 149–54.

Lowe, E.J. (2000). *An Introduction to the Philosophy of Mind.* Cambridge: Cambridge University Press.

Lowe, E.J. (2006). Can the self disintegrate? Personal identity, psychopathology, and disunities of consciousness. In: *Dementia: Mind, Meaning, and the Person* (eds. J.C. Hughes, S.J. Louw, and S.R. Sabat), pp. 89–103. Oxford: Oxford University Press.

Luntley, M. (1991). The transcendental grounds of meaning and the place of silence. In: *Meaning Scepticism* (ed. K. Puhl), pp. 170–88. Berlin: De Gruyter.

Luntley, M. (1995). *Reason, Truth and Self: The Postmodern Reconditioned*. London: Routledge.

Luntley, M. (1999). *Contemporary Philosophy of Thought: Truth, World, Content*. Oxford UK and Malden USA: Blackwell Publishers.

Luntley, M. (2002). Patterns, particularism and seeing the similarity. *Philosophical Papers*, **31**, 271–91.

Luntley, M. (2003a). *Wittgenstein: Meaning and Judgement*. Malden USA: Blackwell Publishing.

Luntley, M. (2003b). Non-conceptual content and the sound of music. *Mind & Language*, **18**, 402–26.

Luntley, M. (2006). Keeping track, autobiography, and the conditions for self-erosion. In: *Dementia: Mind, Meaning, and the Person* (eds. J.C. Hughes, S.J. Louw, and S.R. Sabat), pp. 105–21. Oxford: Oxford University Press.

Lyman, K.A. (1989). Bringing the social back in: a critique of the biomedicalization of dementia. *The Gerontologist*, **29**, 597–605.

MacIntyre, A. (1985). *After Virtue: A Study in Moral Theory* (2nd edition). London: Duckworth.

Mackenzie, C. and Stoljar, N. (eds.) (2000). *Relational Autonomy: Feminist Essays on Autonomy, Agency, and the Social Self*. New York: Oxford University Press.

Macquarrie, J. (1968). *Martin Heidegger*. London: Lutterworth Press.

Malcolm, N. (1986). *Nothing Is Hidden*. Oxford: Blackwell.

Malcolm, N. (1989). Wittgenstein on language and rules. *Philosophy*, **64**, 5–28.

Marshall, M. and Hoskins, G. (2008). Good design for dementia means a better building for everyone. In: *Oxford Textbook of Old Age Psychiatry* (eds. R. Jacoby, C. Oppenheimer, T. Dening, and A. Thomas), pp. 371–88. Oxford: Oxford University Press.

Marx, K. (1961). *Selected Writings in Sociology and Social Philosophy* (2nd edition) (eds. T.B. Bottomore and M. Rubel; trans. T.B. Bottomore). Harmondsworth: Penguin Books.

Matthews, E. (1996). *Twentieth-Century French Philosophy*. Oxford: Oxford University Press.

Matthews, E. (2002). *The Philosophy of Merleau-Ponty*. Chesham: Acumen.

Matthews, E. (2005). *Mind: Key Concepts in Philosophy*. London and New York: Continuum.

Matthews, E. (2006). Dementia and the identity of the person. In: *Dementia: Mind, Meaning, and the Person* (eds. J.C. Hughes, S.J. Louw, and S.R. Sabat), pp. 163–77. Oxford: Oxford University Press.

Matthews, E. (2007). *Body-Subjects and Disordered Minds: Treating the Whole Person in Psychiatry*. Oxford: Oxford University Press.

McCulloch, G. (2003). *The Life of the Mind. An Essay on Phenomenological Externalism*. London and New York: Routledge.

McDonough, R. (1989). Towards a non-mechanistic theory of meaning. *Mind*, **98**, 1–21.

McDonough, R. (1991). Wittgenstein's critique of mechanistic atomism. *Philosophical Investigations*, **14**, 231–51.

McDowell, J. (1984). Wittgenstein on following a rule. *Synthese*, **58**, 325–63.

McDowell, J. (1991). Intentionality and interiority in Wittgenstein. In: *Meaning Scepticism* (ed. K. Puhl), pp. 148–69. Berlin: De Gruyter.

McDowell, J. (1994). The content of perceptual experience. *The Philosophical Quarterly*, **44**, 190–205.

McGinn, C. (1984). *Wittgenstein on Meaning.* Oxford: Blackwell.

McGinn, C. (1989). *Mental Content.* Oxford: Blackwell.

McKenna, P.J. (1991). Memory, knowledge and delusions. *British Journal of Psychiatry,* **159** (suppl. 14), 36–41.

McLean, A.H. (2006). Coherence without facticity in dementia. The case of Mrs. Fine. In: *Thinking About Dementia: Culture, Loss, and the Anthropology of Senility* (eds. A. Leibing and L. Cohen), pp. 157–79. New Jersey: Rutgers University Press.

McLellan, D. (1975). *Marx.* Glasgow: Fontana/Collins.

McMillan, J. (2006). Identity, self and dementia. In: *Dementia: Mind, Meaning, and the Person* (eds. J.C. Hughes, S.J. Louw, and S.R. Sabat), pp. 63–70. Oxford: Oxford University Press.

Mead, G.H. (1934). *Mind, Self, and Society from the Standpoint of a Social Behaviorist* (ed. C.W. Morris, 1962), Chicago and London: University of Chicago Press.

Mendez, M.F., Martin, R.J., Smyth, K.A., and Whitehouse, P.J. (1992). Disturbances of person identification in Alzheimer's disease. A retrospective study. *Journal of Nervous and Mental Diseases,* **180,** 94–6.

Merleau-Ponty, M. (1962). *Phenomenology of Perception* (trans. C. Smith). London: Routledge. First published as Phénomènologie de la Perception by Gallimard, Paris (1945).

Midgley, M. (1996). *Utopias, Dolphins and Computers: Problems of Philosophical Plumbing.* London and New York: Routledge.

Midgley, M. (2001). *Science and Poetry.* London and New York: Routledge.

Moreira, T., Hughes, J.C., Kirkwood, T., May, C., McKeith I., and Bond, J. (2008). What explains variations in the clinical use of mild cognitive impairment (MCI) as a diagnostic category? *International Psychogeriatrics,* **20,** 697–709.

Morgan, D.L. and Morgan, R.K. (2001). Single-participant research design. *American Psychologist,* **56,** 119–27.

Morris, R.G. (1997). Cognition and ageing. In: *Psychiatry in the Elderly* (2nd edition) (eds. R. Jacoby and C. Oppenheimer), pp. 37–62. Oxford: Oxford University Press.

Morton, A. (1990). Why there is no concept of a person. In: *The Person and the Human Mind: Issues in Ancient and Modern Philosophy* (ed. C. Gill), pp. 39–59. Oxford: Clarendon Press.

Mulhall, S. (1990). *On Being in the World.* London: Routledge.

Murphy, E. (1984). Ethical dilemmas of brain failure in the elderly. *British Medical Journal,* **288,** 61–2.

Murray, T.H. (1994). Medical ethics, moral philosophy and moral tradition. In: *Medicine and Moral Reasoning* (eds. K.W.M. Fulford, G. Gillett, and J.M. Soskice), pp. 91–105. Cambridge: Cambridge University Press.

Myrdal, G. (1958). *Value in Social Theory: A Selection of Essays on Methodology* (P. Streeten, ed.). London: Routledge & Keegan Paul.

Nagy, Z. and Hubbard, P. (2008). Neuropathology. In: *Oxford Textbook of Old Age Psychiatry* (eds. R. Jacoby, C. Oppenheimer, T. Dening, and A. Thomas), pp. 67–83. Oxford: Oxford University Press.

National Institute for Health and Clinical Excellence and Social Care Institute for Excellence (NICE-SCIE) (2007). *A NICE-SCIE Guideline on Supporting People with Dementia and their Carers in Health and Social Care. National Clinical Practice Guideline Number 42.* Leicester and London: The British Psychological Society and Gaskill (The Royal College of Psychiatrists).

Newson, A.J. (2007). Personhood and moral status. In: *Principles of Health Care Ethics* (2nd edition) (eds. R. E. Ashcroft, A. Dawson, H. Draper, and J. R. McMillan), pp. 277–83. Chichester: John Wiley & Sons.

Norberg, A. (1994). Ethics in the care of the elderly with dementia. In: *Principles of Health Care Ethics* (1st edition) (eds. R. Gillon and A. Lloyd), pp. 721–31. Chichester: John Wiley & Sons.

Normann, H.K., Asplund, K., and Norberg, A. (1998). Episodes of lucidity in people with severe dementia as narrated by formal carers. *Journal of Advanced Nursing*, **28**, 1295–300.

Nuffield Council on Bioethics (2009). *Dementia: Ethical Issues*. London: Nuffield Council on Bioethics.

O'Brien, J. (2008). Mild cognitive impairment. In: *Oxford Textbook of Old Age Psychiatry* (eds. R. Jacoby, C. Oppenheimer, T. Dening, and A. Thomas), pp. 407–15. Oxford: Oxford University Press.

O'Brien, J. and Barber, B. (2000). Neuroimaging in dementia and depression. *Advances in Psychiatric Treatment*, **6**, 109–19.

Orpwood, R., Gibbs, C., Adlam, T., Faulkner, R., and D. Meegahawatte. (2005). The design of smart homes for people with dementia – user-interface aspects. *Universal Access in the Information Society*, **4**, 156–64.

Parfit, D. (1984). *Reasons and Persons*. Oxford: Oxford University Press.

Parfit, D. (1987). Divided minds and the nature of persons. In: *MindWaves: Thoughts on Intelligence, Identity and Consciousness* (eds. C. Blakemore and S. Greenfield), pp. 19–26. Blackwell, Oxford.

Park, S.B.G. and Young, A.H. (1994). Connectionism and psychiatry: a brief review. *Philosophy, Psychiatry, & Psychology*, **1**, 51–8.

Patterson, K. (1986). Lexical but nonsemantic spelling? *Cognitive Neuropsychology*, **3**, 341–67.

Pears, D. (1988). *The False Prison. A Study of the Development of Wittgenstein's Philosophy. Volume II*. Oxford: Clarendon Press.

Pericak-Vance, M.A., Bebout, J.L., Gaskell, P.C. Jr., Yamaoka, L.H., Hung, W.-Y., Alberts, M.J., et. al. (1991). Linkage studies in familial Alzheimer's disease: evidence for chromosome 19 linkage. *American Journal of Human Genetics*, **48**, 1034–50.

Perry, E.K., Tomlinson, B.E., Blessed, G., Bergmann, K., Gibson, P.H., and Perry, R.H. (1978). Correlation of cholinergic abnormalities with senile plaques and mental test scores in senile dementia. *British Medical Journal*, **2**, 1457–9.

Petersen, R.C. (2006). Mild cognitive impairment is relevant. *Philosophy, Psychiatry, & Psychology*, **13**, 45–9.

Pettit, P. (1990a). The reality of rule-following. *Mind*, **99**, 1–21.

Pettit, P. (1990b). Affirming the reality of rule-following. *Mind*, **99**, 433–9.

Plato, (1987). *The Republic* (trans. D. Lee). London: Penguin Books (first published around 375 BCE; first published in this translation 1955; second edition 1974; revisions 1987).

Pointon, B. (2007). Who am I?–The search for spirituality in dementia. A family carer's perspective. In: *Spirituality, Values and Mental Health: Jewels for the Journey* (eds. M.E. Coyte, P. Gilbert, and V. Nicholls), pp. 114–20. London and Philadelphia: Jessica Kingsley.

Pointon, B. (2010). The view of the family carer. In: *Supportive Care for the Person with Dementia* (eds. J.C. Hughes, M. Lloyd-Williams, and G.A. Sachs), pp. 27–32. Oxford: Oxford University Press.

Popper, K.R. and Eccles, J.C. (1977). *The Self and its Brain*. Berlin: Springer International.

Post, S.G. (1995). *The Moral Challenge of Alzheimer Disease* (1st edition) Baltimore: Johns Hopkins University Press.

Post, S.G. (2006). *Respectare*: moral respect for the lives of the deeply forgetful. In: *Dementia: Mind, Meaning, and the Person* (eds. J.C. Hughes, S.J. Louw, and S.R. Sabat), pp. 223–43. Oxford: Oxford University Press.

Putnam, H. (1981). *Reason, Truth and History*. Cambridge: Cambridge University Press.

Radden, J. and Fordyce, J.M. (2006). Into the darkness: losing identity with dementia. In: *Dementia: Mind, Meaning, and the Person* (eds. J.C. Hughes, S.J. Louw, and S.R. Sabat), pp. 71–88. Oxford: Oxford University Press.

Radden, J. and Sadler, J. (2010). *The Virtuous Psychiatrist: Character Ethics in Psychiatric Practice*. Oxford: Oxford University Press.

Rapoport, S.I. (1992). Alzheimer's disease: disruption of mind-brain relations. In: *Neurophilosophy and Alzheimer's Disease* (eds. Y. Christen and P. Churchland), pp. 86–107. Berlin: Springer-Verlag.

Redley, M., Hughes, J.C., and Holland, A. (2010). Voting without capacity: a cause for concern? *British Medical Journal*, **341**, 466–67.

Rhees, R. (ed.) (1981). *Ludwig Wittgenstein: Personal Recollections*. Oxford: Basil Blackwell.

Riley, K.P., Snowdon, D.A., and Markesbery, W.R. (2002). Alzheimer's neurofibrillary pathology and the spectrum of cognitive function: findings from the Nun Study. *Annals of Neurology*, **51**, 567–77.

Robertson, A. (1991). The politics of Alzheimer's disease: a case study in apocalyptic demography. In: *Critical Perspectives on Aging: The Political and Moral Economy of Growing Old* (eds. M. Minkler and C.L. Estes), pp. 135–50. Amityville, NY: Baywood.

Robinson, L., Hutchings, D., Dickinson, H.O., Corner, L., Beyer, F., Finch, T., et al. (2007). Effectiveness and acceptability of non-pharmacological interventions to reduce wandering in dementia: a systematic review. *International Journal of Geriatric Psychiatry*, **22**, 9–22.

Robinson, L., Brittain, K., Lindsay, S., Jackson, D., and Olivier, P. (2009). Keeping In Touch Everyday (KITE) project: developing assistive technologies with people with dementia and their carers to promote independence. *International Psychogeriatrics*, **21**, 494–502.

Rorty, A.O. (1990). Persons and *Personae*. In: *The Person and the Human Mind: Issues in Ancient and Modern Philosophy* (ed. C. Gill), pp. 21–38. Oxford: Clarendon Press.

Russell, J. (1954). Gerald Finzi–an English composer. *Tempo*, **33** (Autumn), 9–15.

Sabat, S.R. (1991). Turn-taking, turn-giving, and Alzheimer's disease: a case study of conversation. *The Georgetown Journal of Language & Linguistics*, **2**, 161–75.

Sabat, S.R. (2001). *The Experience of Alzheimer's Disease: Life Through a Tangled Veil*. Oxford: Blackwell.

Sabat, S.R. (2002). Selfhood and Alzheimer's disease. In: *The Person with Alzheimer's Disease: Pathways to Understanding the Experience* (ed. P.B. Harris), pp. 88–111. Baltimore and London: The Johns Hopkins University Press.

Sabat, S.R. (2006a). Mind, meaning, and personhood in dementia: the effects of positioning. In: *Dementia: Mind, Meaning, and the Person* (eds. J.C. Hughes, S.J. Louw, and S.R. Sabat), pp. 287–302. Oxford: Oxford University Press.

Sabat, S.R. (2006b). Mild cognitive impairment: what's in a name? *Philosophy, Psychiatry, & Psychology*, **13**, 13–20.

Sabat, S.R. and Harré, R. (1992). The construction and deconstruction of self in Alzheimer's disease. *Ageing and Society*, **12**, 443–61.

Sabat, S.R. and Harré, R. (1994). The Alzheimer's disease sufferer as a semiotic subject. *Philosophy, Psychiatry, & Psychology*, **1**, 145–60.

Sadler, J.Z. (2004). *Values and Psychiatric Diagnosis*. Oxford: Oxford University Press.

Sadler, J.Z. and Agich, G.J. (1995). Diseases, functions, values, and psychiatric classification. *Philosophy, Psychiatry, & Psychology*, **2**, 219–31.

Sampson, E.L., Blanchard, M.R., Jones, L., Tookman, A., and King, M. (2009). Dementia in the acute hospital: prospective cohort study of prevalence and mortality. *British Journal of Psychiatry*, **195**, 61–6.

Schulte, J. (1993). *Experience and Expression: Wittgenstein's Philosophy of Psychology*. Oxford: Oxford University Press.

Scruton, R. (2004). Understanding music. In: *Aesthetics and the Philosophy of Art: The Analytic Tradition* (eds. P. Lamarque and S.H. Olsen), pp. 448–62. Oxford: Blackwell. [First published in: Scruton, R. (1983). *The Aesthetic Understanding*, pp. 77–100, London: Metheun.]

Searle, J.R. (1995). *The Construction of Social Reality*. London: Penguin Books.

Sellars, W. (1997). *Empiricism and the Philosophy of Mind*. Cambridge, Mass.: Harvard University Press.

Seshadri, S., Fitzpatrick, A.L., Ikram, A., DeStefano, A.L., Gudnason, V., Boada, M., et al for the CHARGE, GERAD1, and EADI1 Consortia (2010). Genome-wide analysis of genetic loci associated with Alzheimer disease. *Journal of the American Medical Association*, **303**, 1832–40.

Shakespeare, T. (2006). *Disability Rights and Wrongs*. Abingdon and New York: Routledge.

Shear, J. (ed.) (1997). *Explaining Consciousness – The 'Hard Problem'*. Cambridge, Mass: MIT Press.

Siemers, E.R., Quinn, J.F., Kaye, J., Farlow, M.R., Parsteinsson, A., Tariot, P., et al. (2006). Effects of a gamma-secretase inhibitor in a randomized study of patients with Alzheimer disease. *Neurology*, **66**, 602–4.

Slors, M. (1998). Two conceptions of psychological continuity. *Philosophical Explorations*, **1**, 61–80.

Small, H. (2007). *The Long Life*. Oxford: Oxford University Press.

Small, N., Downs, M., and Froggatt, K. (2006). Improving end-of-life care for people with dementia – the benefits of combining UK approaches to palliative care and dementia care. In: *Care-Giving in Dementia – Research and Applications, Volume 4* (eds. B.M.L. Miesen and G.M.M. Jones), pp. 365–92. London: Routledge.

Small, N., Froggatt, K. and Downs, M. (2008). *Living and Dying with Dementia: Dialogues about Palliative Care*. Oxford: Oxford University Press.

Smith, A.D. and Jobst, K.A. (1996). Use of structural imaging to study the progression of Alzheimer's disease. *British Medical Bulletin*, **52**, 575–86.

Smith, P. (1990). Human persons. In: *The Person and the Human Mind: Issues in Ancient and Modern Philosophy* (ed. C. Gill), pp. 61–81. Oxford: Clarendon Press.

Smythies, J.R. (1992). Neurophilosophy. *Psychological Medicine*, **22**, 547–9.

Snowdon, D.A. (2003). Healthy aging and dementia: findings from the Nun Study. *Annals of Internal Medicine*, **139**, 450–4.

Snyder, L. (2006). Personhood and interpersonal communication in dementia. In: *Dementia: Mind, Meaning, and the Person* (eds. J.C. Hughes, S.J. Louw, and S.R. Sabat), pp. 259–76. Oxford: Oxford University Press.

Stansell, J. (2002). Volunteerism: Contributions by Persons with Alzheimer's Disease. In: *The Person with Alzheimer's Disease: Pathways to Understanding the Experience* (ed. P.B. Harris), pp. 211–27. Baltimore: The Johns Hopkins University Press.

Stephan, B.C.M., Matthews, F.E., McKeith, I.G., Bond, J., Brayne, C., and the Medical Research Council Cognitive Function and Aging Study. (2007). Early cognitive change in the general population: how do different definitions work? *Journal of the American Geriatric Society*, **55**, 1534–40.

Stern, D.G. (1995). *Wittgenstein on Mind and Language*. Oxford: Oxford University Press.

Stokes, G. (2008). *And Still the Music Plays: Stories of People with Dementia*. London: Hawker Publications.

Stokes, G. (2010). From psychological interventions to a psychology of dementia. In: *Supportive Care for the Person with Dementia* (eds. J.C. Hughes, M. Lloyd-Williams, and G.A. Sachs), pp. 159–69. Oxford: Oxford University Press.

Strawson, P.F. (1959). *Individuals. An Essay in Descriptive Metaphysics*. London: Methuen.

Stroud, B. (1996). Mind, meaning, and practice. In: *The Cambridge Companion to Wittgenstein* (eds. H. Sluga and D.G. Stern), pp. 296–319. Cambridge: Cambridge University Press.

Summerfield, D.M. (1990). On taking the rabbit of rule-following out of the hat of representation: a response to Pettit's 'The reality of rule-following'. *Mind*, **99**, 425–31.

Szasz, T.S. (1960). The myth of mental illness. *American Psychologist*, **15**, 113–18.

Taylor, C. (1985). *Human Agency and Language. Philosophical Papers I*. Cambridge: Cambridge University Press.

Taylor, C. (1989). *Sources of the Self: The Making of the Modern Identity*. Cambridge: Cambridge University Press.

Taylor, C. (1995). *Philosophical Arguments*. Cambridge, Mass: Harvard University Press.

ter Meulen, R.H.J., Nielsen, L., and Landeweerd, L. (2008). Ethical issues of enhancement technologies. In: *Principles of Health Care Ethics* (2nd edition) (eds. R.E. Ashcroft, A. Dawson, H. Draper, and J.R. McMillan), pp. 803–9. Chichester: John Wiley & Sons.

Thomas, A. (2008a). Clinical aspects of dementia: the syndrome of dementia. In: *Oxford Textbook of Old Age Psychiatry* (eds. R. Jacoby, C. Oppenheimer, T. Dening, and A. Thomas), pp. 423–4. Oxford: Oxford University Press.

Thomas, A. (2008b). Clinical aspects of dementia: Alzheimer's disease. In: *Oxford Textbook of Old Age Psychiatry* (eds. R. Jacoby, C. Oppenheimer, T. Dening, and A. Thomas), pp. 425–41. Oxford: Oxford University Press.

Thomas, E. (1981). *Selected Poems and Prose* (ed. D. Wright). Harmondsworth: Penguin Books.

Thornton, T. (1997a). Intention, rule following and the strategic role of Wright's order of determination test. *Philosophical Investigations*, **20**, 136–47.

Thornton, T. (1997b). Reasons and causes in philosophy and psychopathology. *Philosophy, Psychiatry, & Psychology*, **4**, 307–17.

Thornton, T. (1998). *Wittgenstein on Language and Thought: The Philosophy of Content*. Edinburgh: Edinburgh University Press.

Thornton, T. (2006). The ambiguities of mild cognitive impairment. *Philosophy, Psychiatry, & Psychology*, **13**, 21–7.

Thornton, T. (2007). *Essential Philosophy of Psychiatry*. Oxford: Oxford University Press.

Thornton, T. (2008). Should comprehensive diagnosis include idiographic understanding? *Medicine, Health Care and Philosophy*, **11**, 293–302.

Tomlinson, B.E., Blessed, G., and Roth, M. (1970). Observations on the brains of demented old people. *Journal of Neurological Science*, **11**, 205–42.

Toulmin, S. (1969). Ludwig Wittgenstein. *Encounter*, **32**, 58–71.

Toulmin, S. (1980). Agent and patient in psychiatry. *International Journal of Law and Psychiatry*, **3**, 267–78.

Trachtenberg, D.I. and Trojanowski, J.Q. (2008). Dementia: a word to be forgotten. *Archives of Neurology*, **65**, 593–5.

Tulving, E. (1972). Episodic and semantic memory. In: *Organization of Memory* (eds. E. Tulving and W. Donaldson), pp. 381–403. New York: Academic Press.

Tyrer. P. and Steinberg, D. (1993). *Models for Mental Disorder: Conceptual Models in Psychiatry*. Chichester: John Wiley.

van der Steen, J.T., Ooms, M.E., van der Wal, G., and Ribbe, M.W. (2002). Pneumonia: the demented patient's best friend? Discomfort after starting or withholding antibiotic treatment. *Journal of the American Geriatric Society*, **50**, 1681–8.

van der Steen, J.T., Kruse, R.L., Ooms, M.E., Ribbe, M.W., van der Wal, G., Heintz, L.L., et al. (2004). Treatment of nursing home residents with dementia and lower respiratory tract infection in the United States and the Netherlands: an ocean apart. *Journal of the American Geriatric Society*, **52**, 691–9.

van der Steen, J.T., Pasman, H.R., Ribbe, M.W., van der Wal, G., and Onwuteaka-Philipsen, B.D. (2009). Discomfort in dementia patients dying from pneumonia and its relief by antibiotics. *Scandinavian Journal of Infectious Diseases*, **41**, 143–51.

van Duijn, C.M., Clayton, D., Chandra, V., Fratiglioni, L., Graves, A.B., Heyman, A., et. al. (1991). Familial aggregation of Alzheimer's disease and related disorders: a collaborative re-analysis of case-control studies. EURODEM Risk Factors Research Group. *International Journal of Epidemiology*, **20**, S13–20.

Vaughan Williams, R. (1934). *National Music*. Oxford: Oxford University Press.

Vink, A.C., Birks, J., Bruinsma, M.S., and Scholten, R.J.P.M. (2004). Music therapy for people with dementia. *Cochrane Database of Systematic Reviews*, Issue 3. Art. No.: CD003477. DOI: 10.1002/14651858.CD003477.pub2 [accessed 17 July 2010].

Volicer, L. and Hurley, A. (1998). *Hospice Care for Patients with Advanced Progressive Dementia*. New York: Springer Publishing Company.

Vygotsky, L. (1934). *Thought and Language* (trans. E. Hanfmann and G. Vakar, (1962)). Cambridge, Mass.: MIT Press.

Wallace, D. (2010). The view of the person with dementia. In: *Supportive Care for the Person with Dementia* (eds. J.C. Hughes, M. Lloyd-Williams, and G.A. Sachs), pp. 21–6. Oxford: Oxford University Press.

Wakefield, J.C. (1992). The concept of mental disorder: on the boundary between biological facts and social values. *American Psychologist*, **47**, 373–88.

Wakefield, J.C. (1995). Dysfunction as a value-free concept: a reply to Sadler and Agich. *Philosophy, Psychiatry, & Psychology*, **2**, 233–46.

Weiner, M.F. and Lipton, A.M. (eds.) (2009). *The American Psychiatric Publishing Textbook of Alzheimer Disease and Other Dementias*. Washington DC: American Psychiatric Publishing.

Whitehouse, P.J. (2006). Demystifying the mystery of Alzheimer's as late, no longer mild cognitive impairment. *Philosophy, Psychiatry, & Psychology*, **13**, 87–8.

Whitehouse, P.J. and George, D. (2008). *The Myth of Alzheimer's: What You Aren't Being Told About Today's Most Dreaded Diagnosis*. New York: St. Martin's Press.

Whitehouse, P.J., Price, D.L., Clark, A.W., Coyle, J.T., and DeLong, M.R. (1981). Alzheimer disease: evidence for selective loss of cholinergic neurons in the nucleus basalis. *Annals of Neurology*, **10**, 122–6.

Whitman, W. (1995). *The Complete Poems of Walt Whitman*. Ware, UK: Wordsworth Editions.

Widdershoven, G.A.M. and Berghmans, R.L.P. (2006). Meaning-making in dementia: a hermeneutic perspective. In: *Dementia: Mind, Meaning, and the Person* (eds. J.C. Hughes, S.J. Louw, and S.R. Sabat), pp. 179–91. Oxford: Oxford University Press.

Widdershoven, G.A.M. and Widdershoven-Heerding, I. (2003). Understanding dementia: a hermeneutic perspective. In: *Nature and Narrative: An Introduction to the New Philosophy of Psychiatry* (eds. K.W.M. Fulford, K. Morris, J.Z. Sadler, and G. Stanghellini), pp. 103–11. Oxford: Oxford University Press.

Widdershoven, G., McMillan, J., Hope, T., and van der Scheer, L. (2008). *Empirical Ethics in Psychiatry*. Oxford: Oxford University Press.

Wiggins, D. (1987). The person as object of science, as subject of experience, and as locus of value. In: *Persons and Personality. A Contemporary Inquiry* (eds. A. Peacocke and G. Gillett), pp. 56–74. Oxford: Blackwell.

Wilcock, G. (2008). Clinical aspects of dementia: specific pharmacological treatments for Alzheimer's disease. In: *Oxford Textbook of Old Age Psychiatry* (eds. R. Jacoby, C. Oppenheimer, T. Dening, and A. Thomas), pp. 483–91. Oxford: Oxford University Press.

Wilkes, K.V. (1988). *Real People. Personal Identity without Thought Experiments*. Oxford: Clarendon Press.

Williams, M. (1999). *Wittgenstein, Mind and Meaning: Towards a Social Conception of Mind*. London: Routledge.

Winch, P. (1958). *The Idea of a Social Science and its Relation to Philosophy*. London: Routledge.

Wittgenstein, L. (1958). *The Blue and Brown Books*. Oxford: Blackwell.

Wittgenstein, L. (1968). *Philosophical Investigations* (eds. G.E.M. Anscombe and R. Rhees, trans. G.E.M. Anscombe). Blackwell, Oxford. (First edition 1953; second edition 1958; third edition 1967.)

Wittgenstein, L. (1974). *Tractatus Logico-Philosophicus* (trans. D.F. Pears and B.F. McGuiness). London and New York: Routledge. (This translation first published 1961; first published in German 1921; first English translation 1922.)

Wittgenstein, L. (1969). *On Certainty* (eds. G.E.M. Anscombe and G.H. von Wright, trans. D. Paul and G.E.M. Anscombe). Oxford: Blackwell.

Wittgenstein, L. (1974). *Philosophical Grammar* (ed. R. Rhees, trans. A. Kenny). Oxford: Blackwell.

Wittgenstein, L. (1978). *Remarks on the Foundations of Mathematics* (eds. G.H. von Wright, R. Rhees and G.E.M. Anscombe, revised edition). Oxford: Blackwell.

Wittgenstein, L. (1980). *Remarks on the Philosophy of Psychology Vol. I* (eds. G.E.M. Anscombe and G.H. von Wright, trans. G.E.M. Anscombe). Oxford: Blackwell.

Wittgenstein, L. (1981). *Zettel* (eds. G.E.M. Anscombe and G.H. von Wright, trans. G.E.M. Anscombe). Oxford: Blackwell.

Wittgenstein, L. (1992). *Last Writings on the Philosophy of Psychology. Vol II. The Inner and the Outer, 1949–1951*. (eds. G.H. von Wright and H. Nyman, trans. C.G. Luckhardt and M.A.E. Aue). Oxford: Blackwell.

Wittgenstein, L. (1980). *Culture and Value* (eds.; G.H. von Wright, H. Nyman, and P. Winch, trans.). Oxford: Basil Blackwell.

World Health Organization (WHO). (1992). The ICD-10 Classification of Mental and Behavioural Disorders. Clinical Descriptions and Diagnostic Guidelines. Geneva: WHO.

Wren, T.E. (1987). The psycho-heresy of Rom Harré. New Ideas in Psychology, **5**, 25–31.

Wright, C. (1981). *Wittgenstein on the Foundations of Mathematics*. London: Duckworth.

Wright, C. (1986). Rule following, meaning and constructivism. In: *Meaning and Interpretation*, (ed. C. Travis), pp. 271–97. Oxford: Blackwell.

Wright, C. (1989). Critical Notice: Colin McGinn, Wittgenstein on Meaning. *Mind*, **98**, 289–305.

Yale, R. and Snyder, L. (2002). The experience of support groups for persons with early-stage Alzheimer's disease and their families. In: *The Person with Alzheimer's Disease: Pathways to Understanding the Experience* (ed. P.B. Harris), pp. 228–45. Baltimore: The Johns Hopkins University Press.

Zeisel, J. (2009). *I'm Still Here: A New Philosophy of Alzheimer's Care*. New York: Avery (Penguin).

Index